Behavioral
Science
in Medicine

Behavioral Science in Medicine

BARBARA FADEM, *Ph.D.*

Professor of Psychiatry
Department of Psychiatry
University of Medicine and Dentistry of New Jersey
New Jersey Medical School
Newark, New Jersey

LIPPINCOTT WILLIAMS & WILKINS
A **Wolters Kluwer** Company

Philadelphia • Baltimore • New York • London
Buenos Aires • Hong Kong • Sydney • Tokyo

Acquisitions Editor: Betty Sun
Developmental Editor: Kathleen Scogna
Marketing Manager: Joseph Schott
Senior Project Editor: Paula C. Williams
Designer: Doug Smock
Compositor: International Typesetting and Composition
Printer: R.R. Donnelley & Sons—Crawfordsville

351 West Camden Street
Baltimore, Maryland 21201-2436 USA

530 Walnut Street
Philadelphia, Pennsylvania 19106-3621 USA

Printed in the United States of America

Library of Congress Cataloging-in-Publication Data
Fadem, Barbara.
   Behavioral science in Medicine / Barbara Fadem.
      p. ; cm.
   Includes bibliographical references and index.
   ISBN-13: 978-0-7817-3669-5
   ISBN-10: 0-7817-3669-2 (alk. paper)
  1. Social psychiatry. 2. Cultural psychiatry. 3. Mental illness. 4. Psychology, Pathological.
[DNLM: 1. Mental Disorders—diagnosis. 2. Mental Disorders—therapy. 3. Behavioral
Medicine—methods. WM 141 F144b 2003]
   RC455.F24 2003
   362.2'042—dc22

                                                                2003061202

The publishers have made every effort to trace the copyright holders for borrowed material. If they have inadvertently overlooked any, they will be pleased to make the necessary arrangements at the first opportunity.

To purchase additional copies of this book call our customer service department at **(800) 638-3030** or fax orders to **(301) 824-7390**. International customers should call **(301) 714-2324.**

Visit Lippincott Williams & Wilkins on the Internet: http://www.lww.com. Lippincott Williams & Wilkins customer service representatives are available from 8:30 am to 6:00 pm, EST, Monday through Friday, for telephone access.

                                                                     07
                                                   3 4 5 6 7 8 9 10

To Steve Simring, colleague, mentor, and friend.

TABLE OF CONTENTS

PART I.   THE LIFE CYCLE

PART II.   THE BIOLOGICAL BASES OF BEHAVIOR

PART III.   THE PSYCHOLOGICAL BASES OF
BEHAVIOR

PART IV.   PSYCHOPATHOLOGY

PART V.   SOCIAL BEHAVIOR

PART VI. THE DOCTOR–PATIENT RELATIONSHIP

PART VII. HEALTH CARE DELIVERY

In recent years, the intimate relationship between the mind and the physical health of individuals has become more apparent. ***Behavioral Science in Medicine*** addresses this relationship in a comprehensive but not encyclopedic primary text designed for medical students in the preclinical and clinical years. The book is also aimed at other medical professionals such as nurses, physical and occupational therapists, social workers, and psychologists, as well as at physicians already in practice.

The book contains 7 major sections and a total of 27 chapters covering essential subject material. The **Appendix** of the book contains clinically relevant information on epidemiology and biostatistics. Each chapter contains representative **clinical cases** that illustrate clinical scenarios that students are likely to encounter and **questions** with **annotated answers** illustrating important aspects of the material. These cases and questions not only provide a bridge between theory and practice but also focus on topics and concepts tested on standardized examinations such as the **United States Medical Licensing Examination (USMLE).** Also, much of the information in the book has been organized and summarized into tables, which facilitate learning and retention of the material and make studying more efficient.

The first section of the book, **the life cycle** includes material about stages of development from infancy to old age and information on death and normal vs. abnormal bereavement. In the second section, **the biological bases of behavior,** the genetics, anatomy, and biochemistry of normal and abnormal behavior and biological evaluation of patients with psychiatric symptoms and sleep and its disorders are discussed. In the third section, **the psychological bases of behavior,** psychoanalytic theory, learning theory, and psychological (clinical) assessment and treatment are described.

The fourth section of the book focuses on **psychopathology.** Using the most recent clinical criteria as described in the *Diagnostic and Statistical Manual of Mental Disorders,* Fourth Edition, Text Revision (DSM-IV-TR), psychotic, mood, anxiety, somatoform, factitious, eating, cognitive, dissociative, and related disorders and the use of biological therapies in their management are addressed.

In the fifth section of the book, **social behavior** in health is discussed with respect to cultural issues, sexuality, aggression and abuse, and substance abuse. Section six addresses aspects of **the doctor–patient relationship** including communication, personality styles and disorders, the role of stress in illness, and ethical and legal issues in medicine.

The seventh and final section, **health care delivery,** addresses the demographics of health care in the United States and includes information on costs, health insurance, and government involvement in paying for health care expenses.

Physical and emotional illnesses are among the most challenging of all life stressors. The goal of this book is to provide a framework of information for medical students, and other health care professionals that will assist them in helping their patients face and ultimately prevail over these challenges.

■ ACKNOWLEDGMENTS

I acknowledge with great appreciation the Chairman of the Department of Psychiatry, Dr. Charles Kellner, for his interest in and support for this effort and faculty members (in alphabetical order) at the New Jersey Medical School and elsewhere who generously and graciously gave their time to review (specific chapters in parentheses) the manuscript:

Shirley Berger, M.A. (1,2)
William Burke, M.A. (8,9,10,11)
Charles Cartright, M.D. (1,2)
Donald Ciccone, Ph.D. (16)
Amit Desai, M.D. (19)
James Fix, M.D. (5)
James Hill, Ph.D. (5)
Bart Holland, Ph.D. (Appendix)
Cheryl Kennedy, M.D. (23)
Patricia Murphy, Ph.D. (4, 24)
Moshe Rose, M.D. (5)
Debbie Salas Lopez, M.D. (20)
Steven Schleifer, M.D. (15,25)
Allan Siegel, Ph.D. (5,6)
Cynthia Stolman, Ph.D. (26)

Thanks are also due to the medical students, residents, faculty and staff who provided important, insightful comments on aspects of Chapters 19 and 20 including (but not limited to):

Chapter 19
Daniel Bleman, M.D.
Charles Kellner, M.D.
Reena Mathew, M.D.
Roberta Schwartzman, M.D.

Chapter 20
Deborah Brown
Rita Cominolli, M.D.
Rosa Godwin
Pooja Marria
Rita Mehta, M.D.
Annette Ortega
Ali Pashapour
Yissell Santana, M.D.
Margo Sabir
Lily Zhou-Gutterman, M.D.

Additionally, I am indebted to Kathleen Scogna, Paula Williams, and the staff at Lippincott Williams and Wilkins for the editorial expertise and assistance which has made my work easier and Matthew Chansky for his wonderful illustrations. All of these individuals have made the final result incalculably better. Finally, and as always, I thank with great affection and respect the medical students with whom I have had the honor of working and from whom I have had the fortune of learning.

The Beginning of Life: Pregnancy Through Preschool

1

An essential concept of human development is that people confront and master physical and social milestones not only during childhood, but also throughout adult life. The milestones of childhood are achieved at a rapid speed. Milestones achieved later are mastered more slowly but can be just as profound. A child is transformed in only one year from a self-involved newborn who can barely lift her head, into an interactive, mobile human being with specific desires and strong preferences. An impatient and insecure adolescent, anxious about what he will do and where he belongs in the world, becomes a confident adult, comfortable with who he is and what he is accomplishing in life.

Another important concept of development is that "normal" behavior at one age may be "abnormal" at another. A 3-year-old who puts the cat in the clothes dryer is considered "naughty" but not abnormal. A 10-year-old who does the same thing is likely to be given the diagnosis of **conduct disorder** (see Chapter 2). A 2-year-old who refuses to stay with a baby sitter is showing normal **separation anxiety.** A 9-year-old who will not go to school because he fears leaving his mother shows signs of **separation anxiety disorder** (see Chapter 2).

At all stages of development, a person has tasks to accomplish. The ability to carry out these tasks indicates that development is proceeding normally. Difficulty with these responsibilities suggests a developmental delay or even psychopathology. For example, a teen should be able to function academically and socially in a high-school setting. The possibility of depression or drug abuse arises if he is failing his classes or has no friends. Similarly, while a normal elderly person can live successfully on her own with little help from others, an illness that causes significant cognitive impairment will leave her unable to function safely and independently.

Physicians need to be aware of the physical, social, and cognitive changes that occur during all phases of normal development. Only then can they identify problems and provide treatment and direction to patients when things go wrong.

■ PRENATAL LIFE, BIRTH, AND THE POSTPARTUM PERIOD

In some cultural groups, the prenatal period is included in the calculation of an individual's age. Biological and environmental factors present during the prenatal period, birth, and just after birth significantly influence physical and mental development.

Prenatal life

Physical influences during pregnancy, like exposure to infectious agents and to drugs of use and abuse (see Chapter 23), can have a profound, pervasive, and persistent impact on fetal development. In the last few decades, research has shown that psychological influences can also have long-term effects on the fetus. For example, male offspring of female rats emotionally stressed during pregnancy show decreased masculine and increased feminine sexual behavior as adults. The mechanism of this effect is believed to involve a stress-related increase in maternal corticosteroid production, resulting in reduced fetal androgen secretion (Ward and Reed, 1985).

Sonographic observations indicate that human fetuses show a variety of behavior patterns that presage those they will show after birth. Facial grimacing, thumb sucking, responsiveness to taste and smell when substances are infused into the amniotic sac, and reactions to sound and light are seen prenatally. In addition to their diagnostic uses, fetal sonography and related technology have allowed parents to see their unborn child's face (Fig. 1–1), facilitating parent/infant bonding even before birth.

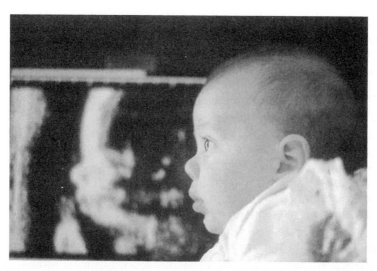

FIGURE 1-1. Photograph of a 6-month-old child along with the ultrasound sonography record taken 4 months into the infant's prenatal development.

((c) Jacques Pavlosky/SYGMA. Reprinted with permission from Santrock, J. W. (1999). Life span development. Boston: McGraw-Hill, 1999.)

Birth

The normal delivery of a healthy, full-term infant is usually a joyful event. Recent advances in childbirth analgesia and educational preparation have made vaginal birth more comfortable. The presence of the father in the delivery room, now commonplace, provides both support for the mother and the opportunity for the father to bond quickly with the new infant.

Although most deliveries are uneventful, problems related to the mother or fetus lead to **cesarean section** in about 23% of all births. This percentage decreased from 1989 to 1996, partly in response to increasing evidence that women often undergo unnecessary surgical procedures. In the last few years, however, the rate has increased and is now as high as it was in 1989. This recent increase reflects not only a rise in the primary cesarean rate, but also a fall in the number of women having a vaginal birth after cesarean delivery.

Premature birth and infant mortality

Unfortunately, not all infants are born full term and healthy; in 2000, approximately 12% were born prematurely (less than 37 completed weeks of gestation) and approximately 2% were born very prematurely (less than 32 completed weeks). Premature birth puts a child at risk for a variety of health problems, including physical disability and mental retardation, as well as emotional, behavioral, and learning problems.

In part because of its high rate of premature births, the United States has a high infant mortality rate compared with rates in other developed countries. In countries like England, Canada, France, and Germany, prenatal care without cost is available to most women. Because the U.S. health care system does not provide free prenatal care for all women (see Chapter 27), low income in the United States is associated with premature birth and high infant mortality. Mean annual income is lower in African Americans than in white Americans (see Chapter 20), and almost twice as many non-Hispanic African American infants than non-Hispanic white infants are born prematurely (17.4% vs 10.4%, respectively) and die in the first year of life (Table 1–1). Other causes for the high rate of premature births include the trend toward delayed childbearing and increased maternal age in the United States. Older mothers are more likely to require fertility treatments that often result in multiple births, in which infants tend to be born earlier and smaller.

Postpartum reactions

Women usually recover quickly from childbirth and have immediate and positive responses to their newborn infants. However, for a significant number of women who have had an uncomplicated delivery of a normal child, the postpartum period is characterized by an emotional state referred to as the **postpartum blues** or **baby blues.** This state of exaggerated emotionality and tearfulness usually lasts for a few days after birth. Although the cause of the baby blues is not always obvious, in some women it is related to physical events, like changes in hormone levels and fatigue. In other women, the baby blues are more closely related to social and psychological factors, such as a perceived lack of social support, the emotional stress of childbirth, and realistic feelings of additional responsibility. Psychological support and practical suggestions for child care from the physician are very helpful for women with postpartum blues, and most cases resolve on their own during the week or two after delivery.

A small percentage of women experience a more serious emotional reaction after childbirth. Mood disorders like **major depression,** character-

TABLE 1-1	Ethnicity and Infant Mortality in the United States (1998–2000)
ETHNIC GROUP	**INFANT DEATHS PER 1000 LIVE BIRTHS**
All ethnic groups	7.0
Asian or Pacific Islander	5.1
Hispanic/Latino	5.7
White	5.8
Native American	9.0
African American	13.9

From Matthews, T. J, Menacker, F., & MacDorman, M. Infant mortality statistics from the 2000 period: Linked birth/infant death set. *National Vital Statistics Report, 50,* 12. Hyattsville, MD: National Center for Health Statistics.

ized by feelings of hopelessness, helplessness, and even suicidal thoughts (see Chapter 13) occur in 5 to 10% of new mothers within a month after childbirth. Depressed mothers typically show a general lack of pleasure and interest in their child and in their usual activities, as well as poor self-care. If left untreated, a major depressive episode can persist for 1 year or more and can interfere with the development of the maternal-child bond. Infants of depressed mothers often themselves become depressed and fail to gain weight and reach developmental milestones at the expected ages— a condition known as **failure to thrive.**

Mood disorders such as depression can include psychotic features like hallucinations (i.e., false perceptions such as hearing voices) and delusions (i.e., false beliefs such as being spied upon) (see Chapter 12). Postpartum women who have **mood disorder with psychotic features** may experience a particular type of hallucination, **command hallucinations,** where voices instruct the mother to harm or actually kill her infant. Tragically, in some cases, the affected mother carries out these commands before the danger of her condition is recognized and treated.

A less common but also serious reaction to childbirth is **postpartum psychosis,** which occurs in 0.1 to 0.2% of postpartum mothers. Described in the **Diagnostic and Statistical Manual of Mental Disorders, 4th Edition, Text Revision (DSM-IV-TR)** (see Chapter 10) as **brief psychotic disorder with postpartum onset** (see Chapter 12), this condition is characterized by hallucinations, delusions, or other psychotic symptoms that are not better accounted for by mood disorder with psychotic features. Postpartum psychosis also begins in the postpartum month and lasts for up to 1 month.

CASE 1–1

THE PATIENT The day after giving birth to a healthy, 7 lb. 6 oz male infant, a 28-year-old woman reports that she feels "low" and has been crying intermittently throughout the day. She expresses distress at her reaction to this much-desired child and is surprised by her sad feelings. She denies thoughts of harming herself or the infant. Her pregnancy was uncomplicated and her medical history is unremarkable. Her social history reveals that she is married, and there is no record of marital problems or previous psychiatric illness. At discharge the next day, the patient reports that she is feeling better but still has episodes of crying during the daytime.

COMMENT This patient is showing the baby blues. In this state, the woman is emotional and tearful for a few days after the birth. Baby blues are believed to be related to factors like hormonal changes and the stress of childbirth.

TREATMENT There is no specific treatment for the baby blues. Most cases resolve on their own by the end of the first week after the birth. The patient should be monitored carefully over the next few weeks by phone calls and regular visits to the physician to be sure that she is free of early signs of the more serious and potentially dangerous reactions of postpartum depression and postpartum psychosis.

■ OVERVIEW OF DEVELOPMENT

Spheres of development

Development of children proceeds in many different areas and in a pre-dictable pattern. These areas can be divided for convenience into motor, social, and verbal/cognitive spheres. Motor development occurs in a cephalad to caudad and central to peripheral fashion. For example, the child gains control of his head before he can control his legs, and he can control his arms before he can control his fingers. Social development pro-ceeds from self to others, from total self-involvement to interactions with people in the outside world. Cognitive/verbal development progresses from understanding to expressing. A young child typically can under-stand more words than he can speak.

Most children achieve developmental milestones within a range of time at a similar pace in all spheres, although some show delays in one or more areas. For example, a 4-year-old child may be intellectually ad-vanced but socially immature. Sometimes, social stress can delay the ac-quisition of new skills or cause temporary regression in already acquired skills. For example, after the family moves to a new home, a toilet-trained child may begin to wet his bed again. It is important to identify develop-mental delays and address them as soon as possible because their persist-ence can become a source of social and school impairment.

Theories of development

Theorists who have studied the biological and sociological forces that af-fect the development of children have derived several impressions and schemes. Although an exhaustive discussion of these theories is beyond the scope of this book, knowledge of the most important concepts helps one understand how children acquire their behavior and skills.

It was once believed that all newborn children were **blank slates,** ready to be written on and shaped by life events. The important longitu-dinal work of Thomas and Chess showed instead that infants possess at birth endogenous differences in **temperament,** innate traits shown in re-sponse to the environment, and that these characteristics remained quite stable for at least the first 25 years of life. These traits include activity level, reactivity to stimuli, cyclic behavior patterns like sleeping, reac-tions to people, mood, distractibility, and attention span. Thomas and Chess further showed that children tend to fall into one of three tempera-ment categories:

- **Easy children** are adaptable to change, show regular eating and sleep-ing patterns, and usually have a positive mood. Fortunately, most chil-dren fall into this category.
- **Difficult children** are not adaptable to change, show irregular eating and sleeping patterns, and tend to have a negative mood.
- **Slow-to-warm-up children** show the traits of difficult children at first,

but adapt and improve over time as their experience with social contact increases.

As their studies progressed and their subjects approached adolescence, Thomas and Chess observed that, with respect to psychological problems, easy children were at low risk; slow-to- warm-up children were at some increased risk; and difficult children were at high risk.

Erik Erikson described development in terms of critical periods for the achievement of social goals. One implication of his theories is that if a specific goal is not achieved at a specific age, the individual will have difficulty achieving the goal in the future. For example, in Erikson's stage of **basic trust versus mistrust,** either the child learns to trust others during the first year of her life or she will have feelings of vulnerability in future social interactions.

Jean Piaget described development in terms of cognitive or learning capabilities of the child at each age. His research suggested that these capabilities were more closely related to neurological maturity than to a child's innate potential to learn.

Margaret Mahler described early development as a sequential process of separation of the child from the mother or primary caregiver. Her findings indicated that the ease with which a child negotiated this process of **separation-individuation** influenced his or her ability to enjoy trusting and emotionally fulfilling relationships in adult life.

Sigmund Freud described child development in terms of the parts of the body from which the most pleasure is derived at each stage. For example, the first year of life is the **oral stage,** a period when pleasure is derived primarily from sucking at the breast or bottle. Freud's theories, scrutinized more closely and discounted by some in recent years, are described in more detail in Chapter 8.

■ INFANCY: BIRTH TO 18 MONTHS

Like all social animals, humans need and seek the presence of others. From early life through old age, people who have strong social support report happier and more fulfilling lives than those who are isolated. This need is especially strong during infancy.

Attachment of the infant to the parent

One of the first tasks facing an infant is to form the most important social relationship of its life—an attachment to the person who has primary responsibility for its care. Although the father or other relative may assume this role, the **primary caregiver** usually is the mother. Attachment of the infant to its mother is a gradual process that takes place over the first few months of life.

In the first postnatal month, children are in what Margaret Mahler called the **normal autistic phase.** This term describes a state of self-involvement and lack of interest in others that, in older children, signifies psychopathology (see "autistic disorder" later in the chapter). At some time between the first and second months of life, children normally begin to respond to other people. Although a reflexive smile is present at birth, the **social smile** occurs in reaction to the sight of a human face and thus is one of the first markers of this responsiveness. Between the ages of 4 and 6 months, a child begins to show special responsiveness to his mother. Unfamiliar people get a polite if detached smile from the infant, but the sight of his mother provokes a bright-eyed, body-wriggling reaction, including smiles, laughs, and cooing vocalizations.

After a child has formed a strong attachment to his mother, he typically begins to show a reaction known as **stranger anxiety.** Whereas the child at 5 months was tolerant of being picked up by a stranger, the same child at 9 months will not tolerate this familiarity. Instead, he protests loudly and attempts to withdraw from the stranger. A well-meaning but unfamiliar relative may understandably be disturbed by this negative and vocal reaction, but its presence indicates that the infant has formed the desired attachment to his mother and that he can distinguish her from a stranger. Not surprisingly, children who have spent most of the time alone with their mothers are more likely to show stranger anxiety than those who have been exposed to multiple caretakers.

During the first months of life, objects and people that leave the child's line of sight essentially cease to exist for him. Toward the end of the first year, the child begins to understand that such objects and people continue to exist, even if out of view. Piaget described this understanding as **object permanence** (Fig. 1–2). The acquisition of object permanence may in part explain why, late in the first year, a child begins to show **separation anxiety** when unable to see his mother. That is, the child now realizes that his absent mother exists elsewhere and he anxiously and vocally tries to get to her.

The importance of attachment

Preserving the attachment that has formed between the infant and his mother is not only desirable for his development but may be essential for his survival. The normal 1-year-old protests loudly when first separated from his mother, but if the separation persists and no appropriate attachment figure is substituted, the infant ultimately becomes depressed, withdrawn, and unresponsive. He may also show poor physical growth and poor health or **failure to thrive,** a potentially life-threatening condition.

Studies of attachment in infant humans and other primates have shown that the effects of maternal-infant separation are long-lasting and extend to social behavior in adulthood. Harry Harlow demonstrated that infant monkeys reared in relative isolation by mechanical, surrogate, artificial mothers do not develop normal mating, maternal, and social behaviors as adults. Interestingly, males seemed to be more vulnerable to this isolation and showed more negative effects than females. The length of

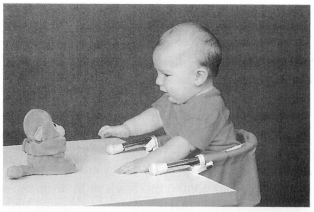

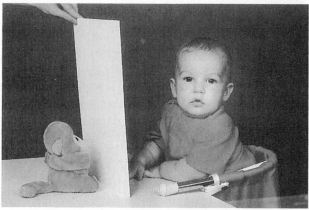

FIGURE 1-2. Object permanence—out of sight, out of mind. When a cardboard barrier is placed between this infant and the toy monkey, this child, about age 6 months, does not search for it. If this experiment is done later on in the child's first year, the child will attempt to find the missing toy.

(Reprinted with permission from Rathus, S. A. (1996). Psychology in the new millennium. Fort Worth, TX: Harcourt Brace College Publishers.)

time that an infant monkey was separated from its mother seemed to be crucial. Young monkeys raised in isolation for less than 6 months could be rehabilitated by playing with normal young monkeys. In those separated for more than 6 months, rehabilitation was not possible.

In the late 1940s, studies by researcher René Spitz of children in American orphanages suggested that humans also suffer serious long-term effects with prolonged separation from their primary attachment figure, a constellation of characteristics that Spitz called **hospitalism.** In particular, children in orphanages demonstrated severe developmental retardation (such as failure to sit or walk at the expected ages) and poor physical health. For example, deaths from rubeola (measles), relatively rare in the general population, were common among infected orphanage children. It is surprising and counterintuitive that institutions in which children were restricted to their cribs in order to maintain hygienic conditions had the highest death rates. Although not recognized at the time, current knowledge about psychoimmunology (see Chapter 25) suggests that this restrictive isolation and the social stress it caused had negative effects on immune system function, making isolated children particularly vulnerable to infection. Thus, preventing children from having social interaction ultimately proved to be as or even more dangerous than exposing them to a pathogen.

In the United States, these and related findings permanently changed the care of children whose relationships with their caregivers are temporarily interrupted due to a child's illness or family situation. For example, during the 1940s and 1950s, family visits to hospitalized children were restricted because of fear that the adults would infect the child. Now, visiting hours are commonly unrestricted, and family members are encouraged to spend as much time as possible with a hospitalized child.

For children whose families are temporarily unable to care for them, and for children who are awaiting approval for or are otherwise not yet available for adoption, **foster families** and **foster homes,** which are approved and funded by the state of residence, provide extended living situations. Ideally, a child in a foster home can form an attachment to her new caretaker and avoid the most serious dangers of institutionalization. Despite its shortcomings, foster care has proven to be a better choice for young children than institutional care.

It is important to note that depression and failure to thrive also may occur in a child living with his biological family, if they are physically abusive or physically and emotionally distant and insensitive to the child's needs. Although these conditions are more common in children in single-parent families and in severely financially and socially stressed families, they also occur in two-parent, middle- and high-income families.

Although protracted separation from the primary attachment figure can be devastating, there is no compelling evidence that daily separation from working parents in a high-quality day care setting has significant negative short- or long-term consequences for the physical or emotional development of young children.

Reactive attachment disorder of infancy or early childhood

The DSM-IV-TR term for the constellation of disturbances in social relatedness seen in otherwise normal infants and young children exposed to grossly pathological care is **reactive attachment disorder of infancy or early childhood,** inhibited type and disinhibited type.

In both subtypes of reactive attachment disorder, social circumstances such as institutionalization or an unstable home environment have prevented the child from forming a normal reciprocal attachment to a caregiver, resulting in abnormal behavior. In the **inhibited type** of reactive attachment disorder, the child is withdrawn and unresponsive, like Spitz's orphanage children. In the **disinhibited type,** the child approaches and cuddles up indiscriminately to strangers and to familiar people. Whichever the type, treatment is aimed at facilitating development of an ongoing, stable, one-on-one attachment to a primary caregiver. For children without families, this can be done through foster care or adoption. For children living in families, intervention is aimed at improving the existing family situation through counseling, practical help, and education for family members in child care.

Characteristics of the infant

A newborn infant is born with reflexes and instincts necessary for survival. He will move his head in the direction of the nipple or anything else that touches his cheek (the **rooting reflex**) in order to suck and obtain nourishment (the **sucking reflex**), and he will grip any object put into his palm (the **palmar grasp reflex).** Although these reflexes have obvious survival benefits, the benefits of other reflexes, such as the **Moro reflex,** where the limbs extend when the child is startled, and the **Babinski reflex,** which involves dorsiflexion of the toes when the sole of the foot is stroked, are obscure. Whatever their function now or in the ancestry of humans, most of these reflexes disappear during the first few postnatal months; Babinski's reflex disappears at about a year. Their persistence past infancy can indicate that the child has a neurological dysfunction. Motor, social, and verbal/cognitive characteristics of infants are summarized in Table 1–2.

■ THE TODDLER YEARS: 18 MONTHS TO 3 YEARS

Attachment and separation

The major task of the first year of life is to form an attachment to the mother or primary caregiver. During the second year of life, the child begins the process of separation from that person to become an autonomous individual. The child does this tentatively at first. At about age 18 months, she moves away from but then quickly returns to her mother for comfort and reassurance (Mahler's stage of **rapprochement**). At about age 2 years, while not yet independent, she asserts herself by being negative, and "no" becomes her favorite word. Because of the difficulty that parents typically have adjusting to the change from their compliant infant to this assertive 2-year-old, this age has been referred to as **"the terrible twos."** "Do you want to go upstairs?" or "Do you want to eat now?" are answered with an emphatic, foot-stamping "no." When the question "Do you want ice cream?" is answered with an affirmative headshake, it is clear that the child understands far more language than she is able to use.

Social interaction

Toddlers like to be in the company of other children but do not yet play with others in a cooperative fashion. Rather, play at this age takes the form of **parallel play,** that is, playing next to but not reciprocally with other chil-

TABLE 1-2	Motor, Social, Verbal, and Cognitive Characteristics of the Infant		
AGE (MONTHS)	**MOTOR CHARACTERISTICS**	**SOCIAL CHARACTERISTICS**	**VERBAL/COGNITIVE CHARACTERISTICS**
0–2	■ Follows objects with the eyes ■ Lifts head when lying prone	■ Is comforted by hearing a voice or being picked up	■ Shows different cries for hunger and discomfort
2–3	■ Lifts shoulders when lying prone	■ Smiles in response to a human face (the "social smile")	■ Vocalizes ("coos") in response to human attention
4–6	■ Rolls over ■ Holds a sitting position unassisted (6 months) ■ Reaches for objects ■ Uses a no-thumb "raking" grasp	■ Recognizes familiar people ■ Forms attachment to the primary caregiver	■ Repeats single sounds over and over ("babbles")
7–11	■ Crawls on hands and knees ■ Pulls self up to stand (10 months) ■ Uses a thumb and forefinger "pincer" grasp ■ Transfers objects from hand to hand	■ Shows discomfort and withdraws from unfamiliar people ("stranger anxiety") ■ Uses gestures (e.g., waves "bye-bye")	■ Responds to own name ■ Responds to simple instructions
12–15	■ Walks unassisted	■ Maintains the mental image of an object without seeing it ("object permanence") ■ Is fearful when separated from primary figure of attachment ("separation anxiety")	■ Says first words

dren. **Cooperative play,** such as waiting for your turn in games and sharing toys willingly, begins at about age 4 years. Motor, social, verbal, and cognitive characteristics of the toddler are summarized in Table 1–3.

TABLE 1-3 Motor, Social, Verbal, and Cognitive Characteristics of the Child 1½ to 3 years of Age

AGE (YEARS)	MOTOR CHARACTERISTICS	SOCIAL CHARACTERISTICS	VERBAL/COGNITIVE CHARACTERISTICS
1½	■ Stacks 3 blocks ■ Throws a ball ■ Climbs stairs one foot at a time	■ Moves away from and then toward the mother ("rapprochement")	■ Uses about 10 words ■ Says own name ■ Scribbles on paper
2	■ Stacks 6 blocks ■ Kicks a ball ■ Undresses herself ■ Uses a spoon or fork	■ Plays alongside other children ("parallel play") ■ Shows negativity; favorite word is "no"	■ Uses about 250 words and 2-word sentences ■ Names body parts ■ Uses pronouns
3	■ Stacks 9 blocks ■ Rides a tricycle ■ Uses scissors ■ Partially dresses herself ■ Climbs stairs using alternate feet	■ Has sense of self as male or female ("gender identity") ■ Achieves toilet training ■ Comfortably spends part of the day away from mother	■ Speaks in complete sentences ■ Identifies some colors ■ Copies a circle

Milestones at 3 years

The 3-year-old child shows important progress in her development. By this age, she can spend a few hours away from her mother in the care of other adults (e.g., in day care), a characteristic Erikson called **autonomy.** A child of this age who does not show evidence of autonomy may be demonstrating early signs of separation anxiety disorder. In school-age children, this disorder can manifest itself as **school refusal** (see Chapter 2).

For most children, bowel and bladder control training, which began at about age 2 years, is complete by age 3 years. Because some children take longer to toilet train, the disorders **encopresis** (soiling) and **enuresis** (wetting) cannot be diagnosed until the child is 4 and 5 years old, respectively.

Three-year-old children also now have a sense of **gender identity**— the understanding that they are either male or female. Although social factors may play some role, recent evidence suggests that gender identity is biologically determined (see Chapter 21). Children older than 3 years who believe they are really of the opposite gender or are unhappy with their physiological sex may ultimately be diagnosed with **gender identity disorder**.

■ THE PRESCHOOL CHILD: 3 TO 6 YEARS

Attachment and separation

Although the 3-year-child has gained some independence from his mother or primary caregiver, he still is strongly attached to that person. The birth of a sibling, often occurring when a child is about age 3 years in the United States, threatens that important primary relationship and may thus lead to jealousy or **sibling rivalry.** This emotion, competing with the child's natural feelings of affection for the infant, may lead him to hug the baby too tightly or kiss it too forcefully. Because of this and because preschoolers do not yet have an internalized sense of right and wrong, parents need to be present when the preschooler and the baby are together.

Another consequence of sibling rivalry, or in fact any other life stressor such as changing residence, may result in **regression,** a defense mechanism (see Chapter 8) in which the child behaves in a "babyish" way. For example, the child may demand to have his bottle back or, as noted earlier, begin to wet the bed again. This reaction is usually temporary and, with the parent-promoted realization that being a big brother or big sister has advantages such as staying up later than the baby, the child's behavior shortly improves to its presibling level.

Social interaction

Between the ages of 2 and 4 years, the child's vocabulary increases rapidly. Some of this newly acquired vocabulary may not please the parents. For example, preschool children commonly find humor in repeating bathroom words (e.g., "pee pee" or "poo poo") at particularly inappropriate times, like when grandparents come to visit.

Preschool children have an active fantasy life. Some, particularly first or only children, may even have **imaginary friends** with whom they converse and play when they feel lonely. However, although the line between fantasy and reality may not be drawn sharply, children can distinguish between them at this age and know that imaginary friends are not real people. The ability to play cooperatively with other real-life children, like waiting for a turn in board games, usually starts at around age 4.

Preschool children typically have a strong fear of bodily injury. Because of this, elective surgery should be postponed if possible until at least school age (6 to 7 years). Many children act out these fears of injury and curiosity about bodies and bodily functions by undressing each other in the guise of **playing doctor.** Although some play of this type is expected in preschoolers, excessive or exclusive use of such play or evidence of detailed knowledge about adult sexual practices suggests that the child has been inappropriately exposed to adult sexuality or even to sexual abuse (see Chapter 18). Other motor, social, and verbal/cognitive characteristics of preschool children are listed in Table 1–4.

TABLE 1-4	Motor, Social, Verbal, and Cognitive Characteristics of the Child 4 to 6 Years of Age		
AGE (YEARS)	MOTOR CHARACTERISTICS	SOCIAL CHARACTERISTICS	VERBAL/COGNITIVE CHARACTERISTICS
4	■ Creates simple drawing of a person ■ Fastens garments with buttons and zippers ■ Combs hair, brushes teeth ■ Hops on one foot	■ Shows overconcern about illness and injury ■ Shows curiosity about sex, where babies come from, and bodily functions ■ Has nightmares and phobias ■ Has imaginary companions	■ Shows good verbal self-expression ■ Copies a cross
5	■ Draws a person in detail ■ Skips using alternate feet	■ Plays cooperatively with other children ■ Seeks the affection of the opposite-sex parent	■ Copies a square
6	■ Ties shoelaces ■ Rides a bicycle Motor skills	■ Begins to develop moral values ■ Begins to understand the finality of death	■ Begins to read ■ Copies a triangle ■ Prints letters

Milestones at 6 years

Many important milestones characterize the age of 6 years. Although the 3- and 4-year-old does not yet have an inner sense of right and wrong, at about 6 years of age, development of the child's **conscience** (the superego of Freud) and sense of **morality** are underway. For example, the 3-year-old is gentle with his baby brother in order to please his mother, but the 6-year-old is gentle because he understands that hurting the baby is wrong. At this age, the child learns that lying is also wrong and that one should tell the truth. Morality and empathy increase further during the school-age years (see Chapter 2).

At about age 6, the child also begins to understand the finality of death. He now realizes that dead people do not wake up and that his dead pet will not come back to life. This realization can be accompanied by fears that his parents will die and thus abandon him. Parents should be counseled to be

THE PATIENT A mother brings her 3-year-old daughter to the family physician for a well-child checkup. The child is in the 50th percentile for weight and height and, except for recurrent upper respiratory infections, physical examination is normal. The mother reports that the child can go up and down stairs using alternate feet and has begun to pedal her tricycle. She can say about 20 words, interacts well with her mother, and seems bright and alert. Her preschool teacher has told the mother that, although the child plays next to and is interested in socializing with other children, she does not play cooperatively with them.

COMMENT This 3-year-old appears to be normal with respect to motor skills. Three years is the age at which most children can climb stairs using alternate feet and ride a tricycle. She also seems to be developing normally with respect to social skills; 3-year-old children play next to (in parallel) but not cooperatively with other children. Although the child is apparently normal in these areas, her verbal skills are delayed. Children 3 years of age should speak in complete sentences and have a vocabulary of about 900 words. This delay in verbal skills requires further evaluation.

TREATMENT One of the most common causes of delayed speech is hearing loss caused by persistent ear infections. Therefore, the first step in the management of this case is to schedule a hearing test and a speech and language assessment. If problems are found, otolaryngology (ear, nose, and throat) referral is necessary to identify the cause of the hearing loss. Although pervasive developmental disorders like autism, mental retardation, or a learning disability are also characterized by delayed language acquisition, this child's normal social and motor development suggests that these diagnoses are less likely.

honest with the worried child about death. For example, they should not tell the child that a dead person is sleeping or on a long trip. Rather, the parents should try to follow the child's lead as to how much to tell him, and be open to talking with the child about his fears of loneliness and loss.

■ PERVASIVE DEVELOPMENTAL DISORDERS

Some children do not acquire verbal and social skills at the expected age. Among the reasons for this delay are mental retardation (discussed in Chapter 2) and the **pervasive developmental disorders (PDDs).**

The PDDS are characterized by failure to acquire, or the early loss of, reciprocal social interactions and communication skills such as language (despite normal hearing). Children with PDDs also show a restricted range of interests and repetitive behaviors as well as problems in motor coordination, such as clumsiness. The PDDs, including autistic disorder, Asperger's disorder, Rett's disorder, and childhood disintegrative disorder are more common than previous estimates indicated, occurring in about 63 children per 10,000.

The PDDs are not reversible. Their associated deficits result in lifelong problems in social and occupational functioning. Although there is no cure, treatment, which involves behavioral therapy and educational programs to increase social, communicative, and self-care skills, can increase the child's level of functioning and decrease behavior problems like self-injury. Medication can also be used to control associated symptoms such as agitation and hyperactivity. Because caring for children with PDDs involves significant physical and psychological stress, intervention also should include providing supportive therapy and counseling to caregivers.

Autistic disorder

The prototype of the PDDs is **autistic disorder.** Characteristics of autistic disorder are seen before age 3 years and include deficits in socialization and severe problems with language and communication. Autistic children have significant problems forming social relationships, even with their parents. They do not play or use toys normally, and they typically show active resistance to alterations in their environment. Just changing the child from pajamas into clothing can be a daily battle for caretakers. Many also engage in repetitive behavior such as spinning and self-injurious behavior such as head banging, often with little evidence of pain. Some autistic children have unusual abilities such as memory or calculation skills, which are referred to as **savant skills.** Most autistic children do not have special abilities and, although their social and language deficits make measurement difficult, between 26% and 75% can be classified as mentally retarded.

Autistic disorder occurs in about 17 children per 10,000 with no ethnic differences. Autism is 4 to 5 times more common in boys; however, when girls are affected, their symptoms are often more severe. No psychological or social causes of autistic disorder have been identified. Rather, its etiology is believed to be biological.

Neuroanatomical and neurochemical differences may exist between autistic children and normal children. Research studies suggest that, in autistic children, the amygdala and hippocampus are smaller, the cerebellum has fewer Purkinje cells, and the blood contains less oxytocin, a hormone involved in the regulation of social behavior in animals (Stokstad, 2001).

There appears also to be a strong genetic component in autistic disorder. The concordance rate in monozygotic twins is at least three times higher than in dizygotic twins, and the disorder is more prevalent in siblings of autistic children than in the general population. Many genes have been implicated in autism (Stokstad, 2001). The strongest susceptibility locus appears to be on chromosome 7q, but others include 2q and 16p. Genes on chromosome 15 also have been implicated. Other factors that have been associated with autism include immunological incompatibility between mother and fetus and perinatal complications leading to cerebral dysfunction.

Approximately 25% of autistic children develop seizures. Because common immunizations of childhood—the DTP (diphtheria, tetanus, and pertussis) and MMR (measles, mumps, and rubella) vaccines—also may cause seizures, it has been suggested that childhood immunizations increase the risk of autistic disorder. Fortunately, the results of a recent study of 639,000 children (Barlow et al., 2001) and other studies (Hilts, 2001) do not support such a link.

Other pervasive developmental disorders

Asperger's disorder has been described as a mild form of autism. As in autism, the child with this disorder has significant problems forming social relationships and engages in repetitive behavior. Children with Asperger's disorder also have intense, obsessional interests in obscure topics that can be learned by memorization, such as brands of lawn mowers or names of World War II battles. In contrast to autistic disorder, the child with Asperger's disorder has normal cognitive development and little or no developmental language delay, although conversational language skills are often significantly impaired.

Rett's disorder involves diminished social, verbal, and cognitive development after up to 4 years of normal functioning. Stereotyped, hand-wringing movements (Fig. 1–3); breathing problems; mental retardation; and psychomotor abnormalities like ataxia are common. As the child with

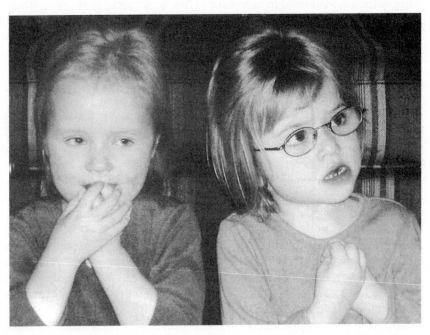

FIGURE 1-3. Rett syndrome. These two girls with Rett syndrome show the abnormal hand gestures seen in this pervasive development disorder.

(Reprinted with permission from Society for Women's Health Research. Rett syndrome. Sexx Matters, Winter 2003, p. 4.)

Rett's disorder gets older, motor skills decline but social skills tend to improve. In most cases, the gene responsible for Rett's disorder is X-linked and the locus maps to Xq28 (Shastry, 2001; Willemsen-Swinkels & Buitelaar, 2002). Because most male fetuses with the abnormal gene die before or shortly after birth, Rett's disorder is seen almost exclusively in girls. **Childhood disintegrative disorder** is a rare condition characterized by diminished social, verbal, cognitive, and motor development after 2 to 10 years of normal functioning. The disorder may be more common in boys.

REVIEW QUESTIONS

1. A 5-year-old child is the only survivor of a car accident in which both her parents died. She is uninjured. Although she has been told that her mother has died, she repeatedly asks for her mother. The best explanation for this child's behavior is

   (A) an acute reaction to severe stress

   (B) a normal reaction for her age

   (C) delusional disorder

   (D) brief psychotic disorder

   (E) an undiagnosed head injury

2. After the family moves to a new apartment, a 4-year-old girl comes into her parent's bed at about 2:00 AM every night. She says that a "monster" is in her room. She continues to do well in nursery school and enjoys playing with friends. The best explanation of this girl's behavior is

   (A) separation anxiety disorder

   (B) normal behavior with regression

   (C) pervasive developmental disorder

   (D) lack of basic trust

   (E) lack of separation-individuation

3. A normal 8-month-old child is brought to the pediatrician for his monthly well-baby examination. The child is the family's first and he is cared for at home by his mother. When the doctor approaches the child in his mother's arms, the child's behavior is most likely to be characterized by

   (A) clinging to the mother

   (B) smiling at the doctor

   (C) indifference to the doctor

   (D) holding his arms out to the doctor to be picked up (i.e., an anticipatory posture)

   (E) withdrawal from both the doctor and the mother

4. The mother of a 2-year-old child tells the physician that although she instructs the child to sit still at the dinner table, the child cannot seem to do so for more than 10 minutes at a time. The child squirms in her seat and gets out of her chair. The child's motor and verbal skills are appropriate for her age. Which of the following best fits this picture?

(A) normal behavior

(B) attention-deficit hyperactivity disorder (ADHD)

(C) Autistic disorder

(D) Rett's disorder

(E) Conduct disorder

5. A 4-year-old child who has never spoken voluntarily shows no interest in or connection to his parents, other adults, or other children. His hearing is normal. His mother tells the doctor that he persistently spins around in place and that he screams and struggles fiercely when she tries to take him outside of the house. The best explanation for this child's behavior is

(A) separation anxiety disorder

(B) normal behavior with regression

(C) pervasive developmental disorder

(D) lack of basic trust

(E) failure of separation-individuation

ANSWERS AND EXPLANATIONS

1-B. This 5-year-old child is showing a normal reaction for her age. Children under the age of 6 years do not understand the finality of death and fully expect dead people to come back to life. That is why she asks for her mother even though she has been told that her mother has died. This child has been severely stressed by the loss of her mother, but she is not out of touch with reality. Therefore, the diagnoses of delusional disorder or brief psychotic disorder (see Chapter 12) are not appropriate. There is no evidence of an undiagnosed head injury.

2-B. The best description of this girl's behavior is normal with regression, a defense mechanism in which a person acts like that they did when they were younger. Because she continues to play well when away from her mother, this child is not showing evidence of separation anxiety disorder. There is also no evidence of a pervasive developmental disorder, lack of basic trust, or problems with separation-individuation.

3-A. Stranger anxiety (the tendency to cry and cling to the mother in the presence of an unfamiliar person) develops in infants who have established a normal relationship with a primary caregiver at 7 to 9 months of age. This child's behavior indicates that he can now distinguish familiar from unfamiliar people. Stranger anxiety is more common in children who are cared for by only one person and less common in those exposed to many different caregivers.

4-A. It is normal for a 2-year-old child to have difficulty sitting still for any length of time. By school age, children should be able to sit still and pay attention for longer periods. This child does not exhibit signs or symptoms of attention-deficit hyperactivity disorder (ADHD) or conduct disorder. The child's motor and verbal skills are appropriate for her age and thus do not fit the picture of autistic disorder or Rett's disorder.

5-C. A child who has never spoken voluntarily and who shows no interest in or connection to his parents, other adults, or other children but has normal hearing, is showing evidence of autistic disorder, a pervasive developmental disorder. He spins because, as with many autistic children, repetitive motion calms him. Any change in his environment, such as going out of the house, leads to intense discomfort, struggling, and screaming. Children with separation anxiety disorder, lack of basic trust, normal behavior with regression, and problems with separation-individuation are able to form relationships with others. This child's failure to form such relationships precludes these diagnoses.

REFERENCES

Baker, J. E., Sedney, M. A., & Gross, E. (1992). Psychological tasks for bereaved children. *Am J Orthopsychiatry, 62,* 105.

Barlow, W. E., Davis, R., Glasser, J. W., Rhodes, P. H., Thompson, R. S., Mullooly, J. P., et al. (2001). The risk of seizures after receipt of whole-cell pertussis or measles, mumps, and rubella vaccine. *N Engl J Med, 345,* 656–661.

Bowlby, J. (1969). *Attachment and loss.* New York: Basic Books.

Chess, S., & Thomas, A. (1986). *Temperament in clinical practice.* New York: Guilford Press.

Erikson, E. H. (1963). *Childhood and society* (2nd ed.). New York: Norton.

Ghaziuddin, M., & Butler, E. (1998). Clumsiness in autism and Asperger syndrome: a further report. *J Intellect Disabil Res, 42,* 43–48.

Harlow, H. F. (1961). The development of affectional patterns in infant monkeys. In B.M. Foss (Ed.), *Determinants of infant behavior* (Vol. 1). New York: Wiley.

Hilts, P. J. (2001, August 30). Study clears two vaccines of any long-lasting harm. *The New York Times,* A18 (co. 5).

Kaplan, H. I., & Sadock, B. J. (1998). *Synopsis of psychiatry* (8th ed.). Baltimore: Williams & Wilkins.

Lerner, J. V., & Abrams, L.A. (1994). Developmental correlates of maternal employment influences on children. In C. B. Fisher & R. M.

Lerner (Eds.), *Applied developmental psychology.* New York: McGraw-Hill.

Mahler, M. (1968). *On human symbiosis and the vicissitudes of individuation.* New York: International Universities Press.

Martin, J. A., Hamilton, B. E., Ventura, S. J., Menacker, F., & Park, M. M. (2002). Births: Final data for 2000. *National Vital Statistics Reports, 50* (5), 4–5, 14–15.

Piaget, J., & Inhelder, B. 1969. *The psychology of the child.* New York: Basic Books.

Rofe, Y., Blittner, M., & Lewin, I. (1993). Emotional experiences during the three trimesters of pregnancy. *J Clin Psychol, 49,* 3.

Shastry, B. S. (2001). Molecular genetics of Rett syndrome. *Neurochem Int, 38,* 503–508.

Silverstein, L. B. (1991). Transforming the debate about child care and maternal employment. *Am Psychol, 46,* 1025–1032.

Spitz, R. A. (1945). Hospitalism: An inquiry into the genesis of psychiatric conditions in early childhood. *Psychoanal Study Child, 1,* 53–74.

Stokstad, E. (2001). New hints into the biological basis of autism. *Science, 294,* 34–37.

Thomas, A. Chess, S., & Birch, H. G. (1970). The origins of personality. *Sci Am, 223,* 102–109.

Ward, I. L., & Reed, J. (1985). Prenatal stress and prepubertal social rearing conditions interact to determine sexual behavior in male rats. *Behav Neurosci, 99,* 301–309.

Willemsen-Swinkels, S. H. N., & Buitelaar, J. K. (2002). The autistic spectrum: subgroups, boundaries and treatment. *Psychiatr Clin N Am, 25,* 811–836.

School Age and Adolescence **2**

In certain cultural and religious groups, the age of 7 years is a significant developmental milestone. The Catholic Church considers children of this age to have attained the ability to reason and thus designates it the age for the First Holy Communion. Formal schooling, the development of conscience and morality, and the ability to function in the world independent from the family, all start at about this age.

The age of 20 years is another significant development milestone. Childhood is over, adolescence is coming to an end, and the individual must now be physically and socially prepared to face the challenges and enjoy the privileges of adult life.

■ SCHOOL AGE: 7–11 YEARS

Compared with earlier and later ages, the school-age years of 7 to 11 are a relatively carefree time for children. Many difficult physical and psychological tasks have been mastered, and psychosexual issues are dormant. The child can now refine her motor, social, and intellectual skills and, as an independent person, experience the outside world of peers and new experiences. Erikson, describing this stage as **industry versus inferiority,** said that development of these skills with hard work (i.e., industry) can lead to a lifelong sense of competence. In contrast, failure to achieve these goals can result in persistent feelings of low self-esteem.

School and learning

As in most modern societies, formal schooling in the United States begins at about the age of 7 years. At this age, children acquire the capacity for **logical thought.** Piaget noted that it was necessary to have this skill to be able to reason and learn mathematical concepts, and he called this developmental period the stage of **concrete operations.** For example, a child with concrete operational skills can understand that objects can have more than one property—a toy can be both red and metal—and that the quantity of any substance remains the same regardless of the size of the container it is in. The latter concept Piaget called the concept of **conservation.** For example, the 7-year-old child, but not the 4-year-old child, can understand that two containers contain the same amount of water even though one is a tall, thin tube and one is a short, wide bowl (Fig. 2–1). Because of the speed at which these abilities must be gained, previously unidentified learning problems often become obvious at the start of formal schooling.

Conservation of substance (6–7 years)

A

The experimenter presents two identical plasticene balls. The subject admits that the balls have equal amounts of plasticene.

B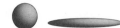

One of the balls is deformed. The subject is asked whether the balls still contain equal amounts.

Conservation of liquids (6–7 years)

A

Two beakers are filled to the same level with water. The subject sees that they are equal.

B

The liquid of one container is poured into a tall tube (or flat dish). The subject is asked whether each contains the same amount.

Conservation of area (9–10 years)

A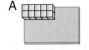

The subject and the experimenter each have identical sheets of cardboard. Wooden blocks are placed on the sheets in identical positions. The subject is asked whether each sheet has the same amount of space remaining.

B

The experimenter scatters the blocks on one of the sheets. The subject is asked the same question.

FIGURE 2-1. Tests evaluating the concept of conservation.

(From OF CHILDREN 1st edition. (c) 1973. Reprinted with permission of Wadsworth, a division of Thomson Learning: www.thomsonrights.com. FAX 800 730-2215.)

Play and peer relationships

The social life of school-age children revolves around school, as well as sports and other extramural activities. It is through these pursuits that children gain a sense of mastery and self-esteem and begin to form social relationships with adults who are not their caregivers. Teachers, sports coaches, and scout leaders become supplemental role models, and their approval and support grow in importance to the child. Children also develop a sense of competence through the pursuit of hobbies. Here they can use their newly acquired organizational skills to catalogue and track collections of objects, such as stamps, coins, dolls, or trading cards.

Peer relationships, particularly with children of the same sex, also increase in importance during the school-age years. Children of this age typically have a small group of friends with whom they talk, often about their similarities in attitudes and beliefs and the dissimilarities of children outside of the group. Popular children typically have good interpersonal skills and follow the rules. Children who do not "fit in" and are rejected by the group commonly fall into one of two types: those that are depressed, anxious, and have low self-esteem, and those that are overly aggressive or "bossy." Exercises aimed at helping unpopular children learn and practice social skills can help them make new friendships. Also, because these children typically have poor attitudes toward school, such interventions have the added benefit of improving school performance.

Sexuality

With the sexual and romantic feelings of adolescence yet to come, the quiescent sexuality that characterizes the 7- to 11-year age group led Freud to describe this developmental period as **latency.** The latency-age child typically identifies himself or herself with the parent or caregiver of the same sex and wants to be just like that person when he or she grows up. Children of this age also have little social interest in those of the opposite sex. Boys prefer to play with boys and girls with girls. They may even describe children of the opposite sex as "silly" or "yucky." This attitude will change dramatically in just a few years.

The development of morality

In contrast to younger children, who are almost totally self-involved (see Chapter 1), 6- to 7-year-old children have begun to develop the ability to put themselves in another person's position and to internalize a sense of right and wrong. Development of these feelings of empathy and morality continue throughout the school years.

In the first stages of the transition from self-involvement to understanding others, and like a convert to a new religion, the child has more of an awareness of right and wrong and is more rule-conscious than an older child or adult. The 7-year-old insists that the Monopoly board game be played strictly by the rules; no player "gets out of jail" until he gives up three turns. Later, as the child begins to understand another person's point of view, he becomes more accepting and flexible in social interactions. The 12-year-old can bend the rules and allow players who are losing to leave jail and resume the game after only one missing turn.

Maturation of the nervous system permits the latency-age child to engage in complex motor tasks. This, coupled with the child's growing internal sense of morality, results in her interest in and ability to follow the often complex rules of team sports.

Illness

Compared with younger or older children, school-age children cope well with illness and hospitalization. Thus, when there is a choice, this is the best age to perform elective surgery. Although most cope well, some school-age children (and adolescents) who are ill or who have an ill sibling or parent may respond by misbehaving at school or home (i.e., using the defense mechanism of **acting out** [see Chapter 8]). Others may become anxious, depressed, or withdrawn.

Another important milestone of this age is comprehending the finality of death. As discussed in Chapter 1, the 6-year-old child begins to understand that death is final and fears that his parents will die and leave him. At about the age of 9 years, the child begins to understand that children also can die and he may begin to fear his own death. If a child is in fact seriously or even terminally ill, the question of whether, when, and how to tell him about the prognosis is a difficult one for parents and physicians (see Chapter 24).

■ ADOLESCENCE: 11–20 YEARS

For convenience, adolescence can be divided into **early** (ages 11–14 years), **middle** (ages 15–17 years), and **late** (ages 18–20 years) **phases.** All three phases are characterized by the further development of independence and autonomy as well as the new requirements of personal decision-making.

Early adolescence (11-14 years)

Puberty is the physical indicator of the start of adolescence. This milestone is marked by increased skeletal growth and the development of primary and secondary sex characteristics. Girls reach puberty earlier than boys. In the United States, the average age of the start of pubertal development is 10.5 years in girls (normal range 8.0–13.5 years) and 11.5 years in boys (normal range 9.5–13.5 years). First menstruation, or **menarche,** usually occurs between 11 and 14 years, and **first ejaculation,** a marker of puberty in boys, occurs between 12 and 15 years. The physical process of puberty is usually complete by an average age of 13.5 years in girls and 15.0 years in boys, with normal ranges of 10.5–17.0 and 13.5–17.0 in girls and boys, respectively. **Tanner staging** classifies puberty into five levels—

TABLE 2-1	Tanner Stages of Sexual Development		
TANNER STAGE	**CHARACTERISTICS**		
	FEMALE	**MALE**	**BOTH**
Stage 1	Preadolescent	Preadolescent	Preadolescent
Stage 2	■ Nipples (papillae) slightly elevated ■ Areola enlarges ■ Breast tissue slightly elevated	■ Testes enlarge ■ Penis enlarges ■ Scrotum enlarges and develops some texture	■ Scant, straight pubic hair
Stage 3	■ Breast and areola enlarge but no separation in contour	■ Penis increases further in length ■ Testes enlarge further	■ Pubic hair increases over the pubis and becomes curly
Stage 4	■ Areola rises above the rest of the breast	■ Penis increases in width ■ Glans develops ■ Scrotal skin darkens	■ Pubic hair resembles adult type but less in quantity
Stage 5	■ Breast and pubic hair like adult	■ Male sex organs and pubic hair like adult	■ Pubic hair also on medial surface of thighs

from immature, Stage 1 to mature, Stage 5 based on the development of secondary sex characteristics (Table 2–1).

The remarkable physical changes of adolescence, coupled with a teenager's increased concern about physical appearance, can render any alteration in the expected pattern of development (like acne, obesity, or late breast development) particularly stressful.

Although sensitive to the opinions of peers, early adolescents usually are obedient (unlike older teens) and are unlikely to seriously oppose parental authority.

Middle adolescence (15–17 years)

By about age 15 years, the adolescent has a great interest in body image and in popularity with same- and opposite-sex peers. To fit in with peers, the middle adolescent embraces current fashions in clothing and music and prefers to spend time with friends rather than family. This behavior is expected and normal, but it can lead to conflict with parents.

In part because of a readiness to challenge the rules and feelings of invulnerability, the middle adolescent is also more likely than younger or older adolescents to engage in risk-taking behavior. This behavior can take the form of failure to use birth control, smoking cigarettes, and taking drugs, and thus can have potentially serious medical consequences. Warning an adolescent of the long-term consequences of her risk-taking behavior has limited effectiveness. Education about obvious short-term benefits, particularly on physical appearance or popularity, is more likely to decrease a teenager's unwanted behavior. For example, pointing out that smoking will darken her teeth or cause bad breath is more likely to influence a teenager's smoking behavior than telling her that she is at increased, long-term risk for lung cancer.

Because they may lose, albeit temporarily, their valued, newly acquired autonomy and need for privacy, medically ill middle adolescents may be reluctant to comply with medical advice. This reaction can challenge the patience of parents and even the most dedicated doctor.

Late adolescence: Identity versus role confusion

Late adolescence is associated with an **identity crisis,** in which the teen must define and refine his place in the world. Resolution of this crisis usually results in the further development of morals, ethics, and self-control, as well as the ability to realistically appraise one's own abilities. In most countries, this age group (usually college students) becomes vocal about humanitarian issues and world problems and initiates protest movements for social change. Erikson said that adolescents who have difficulty forming their identities and finding their places in the world demonstrate **role confusion.** With role confusion, the teen may display behavioral abnormalities, such as criminality, drug abuse, or an interest in cults.

As for learning, some, but not all, late adolescents develop the ability for abstract, hypothetical, or formal reasoning like that required for calculus. Piaget called this stage of cognitive development **formal operations.**

Teenage sexuality and pregnancy

Adolescence is marked not only by cognitive maturation and personality formation, but also by the onset of sexual feelings. These feelings are expressed through physical activity and through **masturbation.** Daily masturbation throughout adolescence (and later) is a normal occurrence, and heterosexual or homosexual **crushes**—feelings of love for an unattainable person such as a rock star—are common. Homosexual experiences may occur during adolescence and may or may not be initial expressions of a homosexual sexual orientation. And, although parents may become alarmed, such practicing is part of normal development.

In the United States, the average age of first sexual intercourse is about 16 years. By 19 years of age, most men and women have had intercourse. Because the average age of first marriage is about 23 years, sex before marriage is the norm in this society.

Fewer than half of all sexually active teenagers regularly use contraceptives. The reasons for this are varied, but teenagers are often convinced that they are "special" and "different" and thus will not get pregnant or develop a sexually transmitted disease. This conviction is not based on fact. In 2000, the 15- to 19-year-old age group had the highest age-specific gonorrhea rate among women (716 cases per 100,000) and the third highest rate among men (328 cases per 100,000). In fact, chlamydia is more common in adolescent women (2,400 cases per 100,000) than in older women. Other reasons for failure of teens to use contraceptives include lack of access to them or not knowing which methods are effective.

Emotional and social factors that predispose teens to pregnancy include depression, poor school achievement, and divorced parents. Although the pregnancy rate in American teenagers is currently decreasing, in 2000 this age group gave birth to approximately 469,000 infants; at least 8,500 were born to mothers younger than 15 years. In contrast, the pregnancy rate among older women, particularly those over age 40 years, is increasing (Fig. 2–2). Pregnant teenagers can present a challenge to physicians because they are at higher risk for obstetric complications than

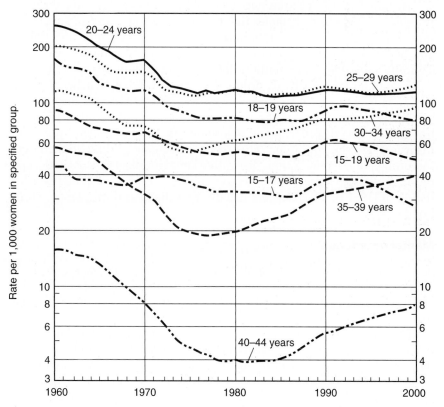

NOTE: Rates are plotted on a log scale.

FIGURE 2-2. Birth rates in the United States by age of mother: 1960–2000.

(Reprinted with permission from Martin, J. A., Hamilton, B. E., Ventura, S. J., Menacker, F, & Park, M. M. (2002). Births: Final data for 2000. Natl Vital Stat Rep, 50(5), 1–101.)

older patients. This is true in part because teens are less likely to seek prenatal care than older patients and also because they are physically immature.

Most medical care to minors (those under age 18 years) requires parental consent. However, it is usually both ethical and legal for physicians to provide minors with sexual counseling and contraceptives without parental knowledge or consent, as well as provide treatment for sexually transmitted diseases, problems associated with pregnancy, and drug and alcohol abuse (see Chapter 26).

The Supreme Court decision of **Roe versus Wade** in 1973 made first-trimester **abortion** legal in every state. Second trimester abortion is legal only in certain states. Teenagers have about half a million abortions annually; however, in at least half of the states, they must obtain parental consent for the procedure.

■ PROBLEMS AFFECTING DEVELOPMENT

Although most children negotiate latency and adolescence with few problems, others face obstacles that interfere with learning and socialization. For example, mental retardation can cause developmental delays, and behavioral problems can result from disruptive behavior disorders, Tourette's disorder and attention-deficit/hyperactivity disorder (ADHD).

Except for personality disorders (see Chapter 24), which, according to the DSM-IV-TR cannot be diagnosed in children, children can have the same psychiatric disorders as adults, including anxiety disorders like post-traumatic stress disorder, mood disorders like depression, and psychotic disorders like schizophrenia. This section discusses childhood disorders, including mental retardation, disruptive behavior disorders, ADHD, separation anxiety disorder, and selective mutism. Table 2–2 contains a full listing of DSM-IV-TR disorders usually first diagnosed in infancy, childhood or adolescence.

Mental retardation

Not all children reach their cognitive milestones at the expected age. If the child's intellectual functioning is significantly below that expected for her age (see Chapter 10) and affect her ability to function, she may be classified as mentally retarded.

Mental retardation has both biological and environmental causes. Among genetic causes, the most common are **Down's syndrome** and **Fragile X syndrome** (FXS). Approximately 95% of cases of Down's syndrome involve trisomy of chromosome 21 resulting from meiotic nondisjunction and, in about 4% of cases, translocation and fusion of chromosomes 21 and 13, 14, or 15. The remaining 1% of cases is due to mosaicism caused by mitotic nondisjunction. Individuals with this rare form of Down's syndrome have some normal and some abnormal cells and may show fewer characteristics of the disorder. The physical characteristics of Down's syn-

TABLE 2-2 DSM-IV-TR Classification of Disorders Usually First Diagnosed in Infancy, Childhood, or Adolescence

CLASSIFICATIONS	DISORDERS
Mental retardation	Mild, moderate, severe, profound, or severity unspecified
Learning disorders	Reading disorder, mathematics disorder, disorder of written expression, learning disorder NOS
Motor skills disorder	Developmental coordination disorder (not due to a general medical condition)
Communication disorders	Expressive and mixed receptive-expressive language disorders, phonological disorder (use of inappropriate speech sounds), stuttering, communication disorder NOS
Pervasive developmental disorders (PDD)	Autistic disorder, Rett's disorder, childhood disintegrative disorder, Asperger's disorder, PDD NOS
Feeding and eating disorders	Pica (eating non-food items), rumination disorder (regurgitating and rechewing food), feeding disorder of infancy or early childhood
Tic disorders	Tourette's disorder, chronic motor or vocal tic disorder, transient tic disorder, tic disorder NOS
Elimination disorders	Encopresis: with or without constipation and overflow incontinence Enuresis (not due to a general medical condition)
Other disorders of infancy, childhood, or adolescence	Separation anxiety disorder, selective mutism, reactive attachment disorder of infancy or early childhood, stereotypic movement disorder (nonfunctional motor behavior), disorder of infancy, childhood or adolescence NOS

NOS, not otherwise specified.

drome include a single palmar transverse crease, protruding tongue, flat facies, hypotonia, epicanthal folds, small ears, and a thick neck. Down's syndrome has also been linked to a higher risk of premature aging and Alzheimer's disease (see Chapter 18). Down's syndrome occurs about equally in both sexes.

In FXS, abnormalities are present in a single gene on the long arm of the X chromosome at the Xq27 site (the fragile site). This disorder also is present in both sexes but usually affects males more severely. Boys with

FXS typically show delayed cognitive function, behavior problems like hyperactivity, and stereotypic movements such as hand-flapping. Physical abnormalities include hyperextensible joints, large ears, an elongated face, and post-pubertal enlargement of the testes.

Other biological causes of mental retardation include metabolic factors affecting the mother or fetus; prenatal and postnatal infection such as **rubella** and **toxoplasmosis;** and maternal substance abuse. Many cases of mental retardation are of unknown etiology. Mental retardation may also occur in conjunction with developmental disorders such as autism, neurological dysfunctions, such as seizures, hearing problems, and visual problems.

Mildly (IQ of 50–69; see Chapter 8) and moderately (IQ of 35–49) mentally retarded children and adolescents face many social challenges. As they get older, they come to understand that they are different and often become frustrated by their efforts to fit in and be like others. The poor self-esteem that results may lead to increasing social withdrawal and even more difficulty communicating with peers. Avoidance of pregnancy can become an issue for retarded people after they experience puberty, particularly in residential social settings like school or summer camp. For these individuals, education and supervision as well as long-acting, reversible contraceptive methods (such as subcutaneous hormone implants) can be particularly useful.

Disruptive behavior disorders of childhood

The normal toddler is defiant and has little regard for the feelings of others. However, by about age 7 years, most children are compliant with parental rules and show empathic feelings toward others. Some school-age children, however, demonstrate persistent patterns of defiant, difficult behavior that are ultimately disruptive.

The disruptive behavior disorders, which include **conduct disorder** and **oppositional defiant disorder,** are characterized by inappropriate behavior that causes problems in social relationships and school performance. In conduct disorder, the child shows behavior that significantly violates social norms (e.g., mistreating or torturing animals or younger children; stealing; truancy; and setting fires). In contrast to the child with conduct disorder, the child with oppositional defiant disorder is defiant, argumentative, resentful, and noncompliant, but his behavior does not grossly violate social norms.

The disruptive behavior disorders are more common in boys and are not associated with frank mental retardation. They are seen in 2 to 16% of children under age 18 years (depending on the research study), but these disorders may be overdiagnosed. Like those coping with physical illness, depressed or anxious children and teenagers may **act out** (see Chapter 8) their personally unacceptable emotions by showing inappropriate, negative behavior.

Genetic factors are believed to be involved in the etiology of the disruptive disorders. Relatives show more of these disorders in childhood, and in adulthood are more likely to show antisocial personality disorders, substance abuse, and mood disorders. Marital discord and child abuse can also characterize the families of children with these disorders.

Most children with behavior-disruptive disorders show remission by adulthood. Some, particularly those with conduct disorder, continue to have symptoms. Conduct disorder that persists after age 18 years is re-named **antisocial personality disorder** and is associated with criminal be-havior, substance abuse, and mood disorders (see Chapter 18).

Tourette's disorder

Tourette's disorder is a relatively rare chronic disorder characterized by involuntary motor movements and vocalizations (tics). It begins before 18 years of age, is much more common in boys, and usually starts with a mo-tor tic, such as facial grimacing or blinking, that first occurs between ages 7 and 8 years. Vocal tics like grunting, barking, or the involuntary use of profanity follow. Children who have Tourette's may be misdiagnosed with behavior problems because their tics are likely to be disruptive in class and at home.

Tourette's disorder is associated with dysfunctional regulation of dopamine in the caudate nucleus (see Chapter 5) and is treated with an-tipsychotic agents like haloperidol (Haldol) and pimozide, as well as atyp-ical agents like risperidone (Risperdal) (see Chapter 19). Although all other characteristics are similar to those of Tourette's disorder, **motor and vocal tic disorders** are characterized by involuntary motor tics or vocal tics, but not both.

Attention-deficit/hyperactivity disorder (ADHD)

Like children with behavior-disruptive disorders and Tourette's disorder, children with ADHD have difficulty controlling their behavior. However, in ADHD, the reasons for the lack of self-control are closely related to the excessive activity and inattention characteristic of this condition. Al-though ADHD may not be diagnosed until the symptoms interfere with learning and social interactions in school, the DSM-IV-TR diagnosis re-quires evidence of the disorder before age 7 years and persistence of the symptoms for at least 6 months. It must also occur in at least two settings, such as at school and at home. The DSM-IV-TR lists three types of ADHD: **combined type, predominately inattentive type,** and **predominantly hy-peractive type** (Table 2–3).

The etiology of ADHD is largely unknown. Minor brain dysfunction may be present, but there is no compelling evidence of serious structural neurological problems or frank mental retardation. Anecdotal information exists, but scientific studies have not revealed an association between ADHD and improper diet, excessive sugar intake, or allergy to food addi-tives, such as artificial colors or flavors. Although the etiology of ADHD is

TABLE 2-3	DSM-IV-TR Symptoms of Attention-Deficit/Hyperactivity Disorder Subtypes

SYMPTOMS OF HYPERACTIVITY-IMPULSIVITY (H-I)	SYMPTOMS OF INATTENTION
■ Shows restlessness and fidgeting, squirms in seat ■ Shows inappropriate or excessive running and climbing ■ Shows excessive talking ■ Cannot remain seated ■ Cannot play quietly ■ Acts as if motor-driven ■ Answers before questions are completed ■ Cannot await turn ■ Interrupts or intrudes on conversations of others	■ Makes careless mistakes due to inattention ■ Has limited attention span ■ Does not listen to direct speech ■ Does not finish work or chores ■ Cannot organize tasks and activities ■ Avoids sustained mental effort ■ Loses necessary objects like books or pencils ■ Is easily distracted ■ Is forgetful
ATTENTION-DEFICIT/HYPERACTIVITY DISORDER, COMBINED TYPE	
At least 6 symptoms of H-I	At least 6 symptoms of inattention
ATTENTION-DEFICIT/HYPERACTIVITY DISORDER, PREDOMINATELY INATTENTIVE TYPE	
Fewer than 6 symptoms of H-I	At least 6 symptoms of inattention
ATTENTION-DEFICIT/HYPERACTIVITY DISORDER, PREDOMINATELY HYPERACTIVE TYPE	
At least 6 symptoms of H-I	Fewer than 6 symptoms of inattention

not related to parenting style like excessive punishment or leniency, children with ADHD are more likely to be physically abused by their parents because of their problematic behavior. They are also more likely to show behavior-disruptive disorders.

Treatment of ADHD involves psychosocial and educational interventions, as well as pharmacologic treatments. The latter are primarily central nervous system (CNS) stimulants like **methylphenidate (Ritalin)** and **dextroamphetamine sulfate (Dexedrine)** (see Table 19–6). Although the mechanism of their action on ADHD is not completely clear, CNS stimulants apparently help reduce activity level and increase attention span, thereby improving the child's ability to concentrate. Because stimulant drugs also decrease appetite (see Chapter 9), children taking them may show inhibited growth and failure to gain weight. However, both growth and weight usually return to normal once the child stops taking the medication. These negative effects can be reduced by using the agents only when needed, such as on school days. Other medications are used to treat associated features of ADHD, like anxiety and depression.

Many children with ADHD show some improvement in symptoms in adolescence, particularly decreased activity level. Most adolescents with ADHD show further improvement in all symptoms by adulthood.

The diagnosis and treatment of ADHD are controversial. Some argue that certain children diagnosed with ADHD may in fact simply be more active than their parents or teachers can tolerate, leading to unnecessary pharmacotherapy and its associated side effects, as well as to increased risk for drug abuse later in life. More accurate diagnostic criteria for ADHD and increased use of social and psychological interventions for very active children and their parents can reduce the potential problems associated with misdiagnosis. Even if the child does need medication, recent evidence suggests that children who take stimulants for ADHD are not at increased risk for drug abuse in adulthood (Wilens et al., 2003).

Separation anxiety disorder

Often called **school phobia** or **school refusal** because refusal to go to school is the major manifestation, **separation anxiety disorder** is characterized by an overwhelming fear of loss of a major attachment figure, particularly the mother. Because of this fear, the child avoids going to school and leaving the mother by complaining of physical symptoms like stomach pain or headache.

CASE   2-1

THE PATIENT   Over the past 2 years, a 9-year-old boy has been caught stealing money from other children in school. His mother reports that she recently found his goldfish dead on the floor with a pencil through it. The child denies that he killed the fish and says that he steals from the other children because it is "just fun." His parents are divorced and he lives with his mother. The father, who has a history of alcohol abuse, visits the child about twice yearly.

COMMENT   This child shows evidence of conduct disorder. Children with conduct disorder have a poorly developed conscience and sense of morality, and their behavior markedly violates social norms. Torturing animals is a common manifestation of this disorder, and the brutal way that the child killed the fish illustrates this characteristic. One of the differential diagnoses of conduct disorder is oppositional defiant disorder. The latter condition also involves problems dealing with authority figures like parents and teachers; however, unlike conduct disorder, it is associated with relatively unimpaired relationships with friends and family pets.

TREATMENT   Treatment of conduct disorder is multimodal and includes counseling to help parents provide structure and reasonable discipline for the child. Treatment also includes family therapy to normalize what is likely to be a dysfunctional and unbalanced family system (see Chapter 11).

Separation anxiety disorder affects as many as 4% of school-age children. Although the most common age of onset is 7 to 8 years, the disorder may start later. The late-onset type of separation anxiety disorder has a poorer prognosis. Both social and familial factors are involved in the etiology of separation anxiety disorder. For example, the disorder may be precipitated by a stressful life event, such as moving or the death of a family member or pet. Parents of children with this disorder are more likely themselves to have anxiety disorders and often appear to be overly concerned about the child's well-being. The children themselves are at increased risk for anxiety disorders in adulthood, particularly agoraphobia. Gradual reintroduction to school, coupled with family therapy, is the most effective treatment for children with this disorder. Medications such as antidepressants are also useful for the associated symptoms.

Selective mutism

Selective mutism is a rare disorder in which children (more commonly girls) speak in some social situations (e.g., at home) but not in others (e.g., at school). Sometimes the child whispers or communicates with hand gestures. Aside from the problem with speech, the child's behavior with others is appropriately interactive. Thus, selective mutism is not simply normal shyness. The age of onset of selective mutism is commonly about 6 years, and it can last from months to years. The disorder has a poorer prognosis when it persists after age 10 years. As in separation anxiety disorder, selective mutism often follows a stressful life event, and the most effective treatments are family and behavioral therapy.

REVIEW QUESTIONS

1. A 15-year-old girl tells her physician that she has been smoking cigarettes for the past year. She relates that her best friends and both of her parents smoke. The most likely reason that this teenager does not stop smoking is because

   (A) she is depressed

   (B) her parents smoke

   (C) her peers smoke

   (D) she does not know that smoking is harmful

   (E) smoking is addictive

2. After her 6-year-old brother is diagnosed with juvenile rheumatoid arthritis, a formerly outgoing 9-year-old girl begins to spend most of her free time in her room watching television. A previously good student, she also begins to do poorly in school. The parents are very stressed by caring for the younger child but do not ask the older child

for help. The most appropriate suggestion for the doctor to make with respect to the 9-year-old is to tell the parents to

(A) insist that the girl take more responsibility for caring for her brother

(B) ignore her behavior

(C) remove the television from her room

(D) pay more attention to her

(E) tell her not to worry

Questions 3–5

A 10-year-old boy with normal intelligence has few friends. He does poorly in school because he frequently interrupts his teacher and leaves his seat to walk around the classroom. Twice each week the child is taken out of class to work alone with a private tutor. The tutor reports that the child works well and productively with her.

3. The best explanation for this child's behavior is

(A) attention-deficit/hyperactivity disorder (ADHD)

(B) separation anxiety disorder

(C) oppositional defiant disorder

(D) conduct disorder

(E) autistic disorder

4. The etiology of this child's difficulty is most closely associated with

(A) food allergy

(B) neurological dysfunction

(C) improper diet

(D) excessive punishment

(E) excessive leniency

5. Of the following, the most effective single treatment for this child is

(A) an opioid

(B) an antidepressant

(C) a central nervous system (CNS) sedative

(D) individual psychotherapy

(E) a CNS stimulant

ANSWERS AND EXPLANATIONS

1-C. Peer pressure has a major influence on the behavior of adolescents, who tend to do what other adolescents are doing. Depression, the smoking behavior of her parents, and the addictive quality of cigarettes have less of an influence. Most teenagers have been educated with respect to the dangers of smoking.

2-D. The doctor should remind the parents to pay more attention to the older child. The child is likely to be frightened by her younger sibling's illness and the attitudes of her parents toward him. School-age children like this one may become withdrawn or "act out" by showing bad behavior when fearful or depressed. Although she can be included in the care of her brother, it is not appropriate to insist that she take more responsibility for him. Ignoring her behavior or punishing her can increase her fear and withdrawal. Simply telling her not to worry will not be effective.

3-A, 4-B, 5-E. This 10-year-old boy who gets into trouble at school because he disturbs the teacher and the other students and cannot seem to sit still is showing symptoms of attention-deficit/hyperactivity disorder (ADHD). Children with ADHD can often learn well when there are few distractions (e.g., when he is alone with a private tutor). ADHD is believed to result from neurological dysfunction. Associations between the disorder and improper diet or food allergy have not been demonstrated scientifically. The disorder is also not a result of excessive punishment or leniency. The most effective pharmacological treatment for children with ADHD is use of central nervous system stimulants, including methylphenidate (Ritalin) and dextroamphetamine sulfate (Dexedrine). Although family therapy and educational strategies are helpful in ADHD, individual psychotherapy (see Chapter 11) is not particularly useful for children with this condition.

REFERENCES

Brown, W. T. (1989). The fragile X syndrome. *Neurol Clin, 7,* 107.

Centers for Disease Control (CDC). (2000). *STDs in adolescents and young adults.* National STD Surveillance Report.

Clawson, J. A. (1996). A child with chronic illness and the process of family adaptation. *J Pediatr Nursing, 11,* 52–61.

Dunn, J., & McGuire, S. (1992). Sibling and peer relationships in childhood. *J Child Psychol Psychiatr, 33,* 67–105.

Faust, M. S. (1977). Somatic development of adolescent girls. *Monogr Soc Res Child Dev, 42,* 75–82.

Piaget, J., & Inhelder, B. (1969). *The psychology of the child.* New York: Basic Books.

Sadler, T. W. (2000). *Langman's medical embryology* (8th ed.). Baltimore: Lippincott Williams & Wilkins.

Shapiro, T., & Hertzig, M. (1988). Normal child and adolescent development. In J. A. Talbott, R. E. Hales, & S. C. Yudofsky (Eds.), *American psychiatric press textbook of psychiatry.* Washington, DC: American Psychiatric Press.

Shapiro, T., & Perry, R. (1976). Latency revisited: The age 7 plus or minus 1. *Psychoanal Study Child, 31,* 79–105.

Tanner, J. M. (1970). Physical growth. In P. H. Mussen (Ed.), *Carmichael's manual of child development* (3rd ed., pp. 77–155). New York: Wiley.

Wilens, T. E., Faraone, S. V., Biederman, J., & Gunawardene, S. (2003). Does stimulant therapy of attention-deficit/hyperactivity disorder beget later substance abuse? A meta-analytic review of the literature. *Pediatrics, 111,* 179–185.

The Challenges of Early and Middle Adulthood

3

L ike childhood and adolescence, adulthood is characterized by transitional periods. In adults, these periods commonly involve the reappraisal of one's desires, goals, and values, and can therefore provide important opportunities for growth and development. If an individual does not negotiate these transitions successfully and instead becomes emotionally "stuck" at some developmental point, long-term consequences can result. The heterosexual 45-year-old man who has lived with a succession of different women over the years but has been unable to make a commitment to any of them may face isolation and loneliness in the future.

Some people not only stop developing during transitional periods, but may actually retreat or regress to an earlier stage of development. The young adult who, after being diagnosed with a chronic illness, begins to show the volatility and acting-out characteristics of adolescence, must accept and adapt to a new image of herself if she is to progress in her life.

People may be particularly vulnerable to physical and emotional illness during periods of life change. An alert physician can identify such patients and help them successfully negotiate these milestones. Such intervention may also help reduce the likelihood of future medical as well as social problems for the patient.

■ DEMOGRAPHICS AND CURRENT TRENDS

Marriage

An old joke poses the question, "Do married people live longer?" The comical punch line is, "Not really, it only *seems* longer." In fact, not only do married people, particularly men, live longer, but research shows that they also are mentally and physically healthier than non-married people. When matched for age, race, and sex, married people have less cancer, heart disease, and other disorders than divorced people. It is not clear whether these health benefits result from being married or whether physically and emotionally well people are more likely to be married. In either case, in the United States, the average age of first marriage is about 25 years for women and 27 years for men. By age 30, most Americans are married.

Families

With marriage, the birth of a child, or the adoption of a child, a new family is formed. Although there are many types of families in the United States, the most common type of family includes mother, father, and dependent children (i.e., under age 18 years) living together in one household—a configuration known as the **nuclear family.**

Approximately 60% of American children live with their married biological parents (Harden, 2001). Other types of American families include cohabiting heterosexual and gay parent families and single-parent families. The extended family includes other family members such as grandparents who, in this country, usually live outside of the nuclear household.

In most two-parent American families, both parents work. In 2001, both parents worked outside of the home in more than half of all married couples with at least one child of preschool age, and almost 70% of couples with school-age children. Only about 25% of children live in a **traditional family** configuration, in which the father works outside of the home and the mother is a full-time homemaker. No matter what the family configuration, parenting children is expensive; the cost of raising a child to age 17 years in the United States is more than $100,000. And, as medical students and their families know too well, post-secondary education can effectively double this figure.

Divorce

Currently, close to half of all marriages in the United States end in divorce. Unhappily, when at least one spouse is a physician, the divorce rate is up to 20% higher than when neither spouse is a physician. A study of graduates of The Johns Hopkins University School of Medicine from 1948 through 1964 showed that, among married physicians, gender, specialty choice, and time of marriage were related to rates of divorce. Female physicians, physicians choosing psychiatry, and medical students married before medical school graduation had the highest divorce rates (Rollman et al, 1997).

In the general American population, factors that have been associated with the high rate of divorce include short length of the courtship period, marriage during teenage years, and premarital pregnancy. Other factors relate to the couple's family of origin and include absence of family support for the couple, prior divorce in the family, and differences in religion or socioeconomic background between the couple. Although it might be expected that life stress draws couples together, the unfortunate reverse seems to be true. Couples that experience the serious illness or death of a child are more likely than other couples to divorce.

Single-parent families

Approximately 25% of all American children live in single-parent families, a percentage that varies by ethnic group (Table 3–1). Most single-parent families are headed by women and, although many unmarried mothers belong to low socioeconomic groups, the fastest growing population of single mothers is actually made up of educated, professional women who choose to bear or adopt children on their own.

For reasons not yet clear, in recent years the percentage of children living in single-parent families has been declining while the number of two-parent families has been increasing. The fact that two-parent families have higher incomes contributes to the positive finding that, in 2000, fewer children than in past years were living below the poverty line.

Single-parent families face unique challenges. Studies have consistently demonstrated that all members of single-parent families are at increased risk for physical and mental illness. Although the issue is complex, it is believed that the lower incomes and less social support that characterize single-parent families are related to this increased risk. Another sobering finding of this research is that children whose parents divorce are at particularly high risk for failure in school, depression, drug abuse, suicide, criminal activity, and for divorce themselves in the future.

TABLE 3-1	Distribution by Ethnic Group of Percentage of Children Living in Different Family Types in the United States			
ETHNIC GROUP	MARRIED PARENTS	SINGLE MOTHER	COHABITING PARENT OR SINGLE FATHER	NO PARENT
African American	39%	43%	8%	9%
Hispanic American	66%	21%	7%	5%
White American	78%	12%	7%	3%

Reprinted with permission from Harden, B. (2001, August 12). 2-parent families rise after change in welfare laws. *The New York Times*, p. 1A.

Child custody

When the parental unit is broken, it must be decided which of the involved adults will have **custody,** or primary responsibility for the children, and with whom the children will live. Until the last few decades, the most common type of custody arrangement after divorce was **sole custody.** In this scheme, the parent with whom the child lived, usually the mother, had legal responsibility for the child and made decisions about his care. The other parent, usually the father, contributed to the child's financial support and had the right to visit the child on a regular schedule. In recent years, **joint residential custody** has become more popular than sole custody. In this arrangement, the child spends part of the time living with each parent; the parents share legal responsibility and jointly make decisions about the child's care. If the parents live close to each other, the child may spend part of the week with each parent. A now familiar sight for grade-school teachers is a child—toting a bulging backpack filled with clothing, toys, and schoolwork—arriving at school from his father's home and leaving school bound for his mother's home. If parents with joint custody live some distance from each other, the child may spend the school year with one and summers and vacations with the other.

An alternative custody choice is **split custody.** In this option, usually reserved for teenagers, each parent has custody of at least one child in the family. That child may be asked to choose which parent to live with, or his living situation may be decided for him by parents or ordered by the court. In contrast to past years, fathers are increasingly asking for and being granted the custodial care of their children. No matter what the custody type determined after divorce, children who continue to have regular contact with the noncustodial parent have fewer emotional and behavioral problems than those who have no contact with that parent.

Assisted reproduction and adoption

Although most couples bear children within a few years of marriage, more Americans now than in the past are choosing to postpone having children. Because fertility tends to decrease with age, this choice increases the likelihood of infertility. Thus, more frequently than in the past, couples must enhance their chances for conception using new reproductive technologies like *in vitro* **fertilization** with its resultant risks (see Chapter 1).

Another option for couples and single people who want children but are unable or unwilling to bear a child is **adoption.** Although the outcome of most adoptions is positive—the couple or single person has a child to love and care for and the child gains a family—adoptive parents can also face special challenges. In addition to dealing with the expected problems associated with the developmental stages of childhood (see Chapters 1 and 2), some adopted children, particularly those adopted after infancy, are at increased risk for behavioral problems in childhood and adolescence. Another unique issue faced by adoptive parents is when and how much to tell their child about the adoption. It is generally accepted that children should be told that they are adopted at the earliest age possible and that they should be told all that is known about their biological parents. This strategy has many benefits, including decreasing the chance that a person other than a parent will tell the child these facts and details before the parent is able to do so.

■ EARLY ADULTHOOD: 20–40 YEARS

Daniel Levinson, who studied early adulthood, noted that at age 30, one's role in society is defined, physical development has peaked, and the individual is independent. Not uncommonly, a critical period of reappraisal of one's life, which has been called the **age 30 transition** or **crisis,** also occurs at about this time.

Love and work

Most people emerge from the turmoil of adolescence with a sense of who they are and where they belong in the world. This sense makes it possible for a person to establish intimacy with another individual without feeling a loss of his or her own sense of identity. When Erikson described early adulthood as the stage of **intimacy versus isolation,** he implied that an individual who does not develop a loving, emotional, and sexual relationship with another person at this time may be unable to do so in later years. Most individuals develop this intimate relationship through marriage or other type of committed relationship.

Sigmund Freud said that, in addition to love, gratifying work is an essential component of emotional health in adulthood. Such work can take place both inside and outside of the home. In the United States, most men work outside of the home and develop their careers throughout early adulthood. Women who initially choose one career path, like full-time homemaker or career person, often change paths in their middle thirties, either by returning to work or school after their children reach school age, or by becoming full or part-time homemakers after developing a professional career.

■ MIDDLE ADULTHOOD: 40–65 YEARS

Although young adults tend to look at middle adulthood with dread, age does have its advantages. The middle-aged person usually possesses good health and has more money, power, and authority than at any other life stage. Despite its financial benefits, middle age nowadays is associated with unique social responsibilities. With their aging parents living longer but not necessarily in better health, and their adult children remaining financially dependent on them for longer, people now in middle age, who have responsibilities to both older and younger relatives, have been called the **"sandwich generation."**

Generativity versus stagnation

Most middle-aged individuals are active and productive and have a sense of contributing to the world. However, if a person has not achieved his goals by middle age, the realization that there is more of life behind him than in front of him can result instead in a sense of emptiness—Erikson's stage of **generativity versus stagnation.** In response to this sense, some people develop what has been called a **midlife crisis.** This phenomenon, which occurs primarily in men in their middle forties or early fifties, may be precipitated by severe or unexpected lifestyle changes, such as the death of parents or spouse, loss of a job, or serious medical illness. It can lead to a change in profession, infidelity, divorce, or increased use of alcohol or drugs. Physicians need to be aware that their middle-aged patients, who are sandwiched between needy relatives in older and younger generations or who experience significant changes in lifestyle, may be at increased risk for health problems.

The climacterium

The physiological changes that occur in men and women during mid-life have been called the climacterium. In men, although hormone levels do not change significantly in middle age, a decrease in muscle strength, endurance, and sexual performance (see Chapter 18) occurs. In women, these changes are identified by **menopause,** a time when the ovaries stop functioning and menstruation ceases. Absence of menstruation for 1 year is one definition of the end of menopause. Although some women experience emotional distress during menopause, most women have few significant

CASE 3-1

THE PATIENT A successful, 54-year-old attorney tells his physician that he has decided to leave his wife of 20 years and start dating again. He explains, "I love my wife but I feel like life is passing me by." The patient has a history of hypertension and recently was diagnosed with coronary artery disease. When interviewing him, the doctor discovers that both of the attorney's elderly parents died in the past year.

COMMENT This attorney is showing signs of a midlife crisis. This transitional period, occurring primarily in middle-aged men, often leads to a change in profession or marital status—in this case, divorce. A midlife crisis can be precipitated by a medical illness (the patient's diagnosis of coronary artery disease here) or important lifestyle changes, such as the death of a close relative (the patient's parents in this case).

TREATMENT People who change lifestyles in middle age may be at particular risk for physical and psychological problems. In fact, suicide is more common in middle-aged and elderly divorced men than in any other group (see Chapter 14). Because of this and because of this patient's medical history, the physician should follow him closely with regularly scheduled visits. Because the midlife crisis may be associated with risk-taking behavior, the physician should remember to question the patient about his alcohol and drug use and provide counseling and treatment where appropriate.

physical or psychological problems. Many women feel instead that menopause has given them new freedom from menstrual problems and fears of unwanted pregnancy.

Vasomotor instability, called **hot flashes** or **flushes,** is a common physical problem associated with menopause in women in all countries and cultural groups. The flushes are characterized by a sudden onset of an intense feeling of heat accompanied by profuse sweating that lasts up to a few minutes. These experiences, which can interrupt sleep and lead to chronic tiredness, may continue for years but can be relieved by **estrogen replacement therapy (ERT).** Although ERT can also prevent or slow the progression of menopausal symptoms like vaginal dryness and bone changes leading to osteoporosis, other claims for ERT, such as reduction in risk of psychiatric symptoms or cardiovascular disease, have little scientific support (see Chapter 21). On the negative side, long-term use of ERT has been associated with an increased risk of cancer of the uterus and, when used in combination with progesterone, of the breast as well. Alternatives to ERT include specific medications, such as alendronate sodium (Fosamax), to prevent or reverse bone loss. Claims of efficacy for the relief of menopausal symptoms or for the safety of phyto (plant-derived) estrogens, like those found in soy products, have not been substantiated scientifically (Baber et al, 1999).

REVIEW QUESTIONS

1. A 52-year-old woman in the United States has a 52-year-old female friend in Australia. Both are in good general health and neither has menstruated for about 1 year. Which of the following symptoms are *both* women most likely to experience at this time?

   (A) Severe depression

   (B) Severe anxiety

   (C) Hot flashes

   (D) Fatigue

   (E) Lethargy

2. A 59-year-old woman tells her physician that she has been taking estrogen and progesterone replacement therapy since she stopped menstruating, 5 years ago. Compared with women of her age who have not taken hormone replacement therapy, this patient is likely to be at decreased risk for

   (A) breast cancer

   (B) uterine cancer

   (C) cardiovascular disease

   (D) osteoporosis

   (E) depression

3. A 29-year-old man and a 25-year-old woman get married after a 1-year engagement. She is pregnant. They are both Methodists and are from middle-class families. Both sets of parents are married. Which of the following factors puts this couple at highest risk for divorce?

(A) Her pregnancy

(B) Their parents' marital histories

(C) Their socioeconomic backgrounds

(D) Their religious backgrounds

(E) The length of their engagement

4. A couple who has just adopted a male infant asks the pediatrician whether they should tell the child he is adopted and, if so, when they should tell him. The best recommendation that the physician can make is to suggest that the parents

(A) tell him he is adopted but wait until he is at least 3 years old

(B) tell him he is adopted as soon as he can understand language

(C) tell him he is adopted but wait until he enters school

(D) do not tell him he is adopted until he asks

(E) do not tell him he is adopted until there is a medical reason to do so

5. The superintendent of schools in a large, ethnically diverse school district is trying to estimate how many of the school's students live in single-parent families. If the school's population is representative of the United States population, her best guess is approximately

(A) 5%

(B) 10%

(C) 25%

(D) 45%

(E) 65%

ANSWERS AND EXPLANATIONS

1-C. These 52-year-old women in good general health are going through menopause. The most common symptom of menopause occurring cross-culturally is hot flashes, a purely physiological phenomenon. In most women, menopause is not characterized by psychopathology, such as severe depression or anxiety, or physical symptoms like fatigue and lethargy.

2-D. In menopausal women, estrogen replacement therapy (ERT) is most closely associated with decreased risk for osteoporosis. ERT has also been associated with increased risk of breast cancer (when administered in combination with progesterone) and uterine cancer (when administered without progesterone), but not with prevention of cardiovascular disease or psychiatric illness.

3-A. Of these factors, the one that puts this couple at highest risk for divorce is pregnancy at the time of marriage. The socioeconomic and religious backgrounds, parents' marital states, and length of engagement of this couple do not put them at higher risk for divorce.

4-B. The best recommendation that the physician can make is to tell the child he is adopted as soon as he can understand language. Waiting until he is of a certain age or until he asks or enters school or until there is a medical reason to do so increases the risk that someone other than the parent will tell him first.

5-C. If the school's population is representative of the United States population, the principal's best guess is that 25% of the students live in single-parent families.

REFERENCES

Baber, R. J., Templeman, C., Morton, T., Kelly, E. G., & West, L. (1999). Randomized placebo-controlled trial of an isoflavone supplement and menopausal symptoms in women. *Climacteric, 2,* 79–84.

Erikson, E. H. (1987). *A way of looking at things: Selected papers from 1930 to 1980.* New York: Norton.

Freud, S. (1935). *A general introduction to psychoanalysis* (Rev. ed.) (J. Riviere, Trans.). New York: Liverright.

Gould, R. L. (1972). The phases of adult life: A study in developmental psychology. *Am J Psychiatry 129,* 521–531.

Harden, B. (2001, August 12). 2-parent families rise after change in welfare laws. *The New York Times,* p. 1A.

Institute of Medicine. (2000). *Exploring the biological contributions to human health: Does sex matter?* Washington, DC: National Academy Press.

Levinson, D. J., Darrow, C. M., Klein, E. B., et al. (1978). *The seasons of a man's life.* New York: Alfred A. Knopf.

Lewin, T. (2001, July 19). Child well-being improves, U.S. says. *The New York Times,* p. A14.

Lynch, J. J. (1977). *The broken heart: The medical consequences of loneliness.* New York: Basic Books.

Rollman, B. L., Mead, L. A., Wang, N.-Y., & Klag, M. J. (1997). Medical specialty and the incidence of divorce. *N Engl J Med 1997, 336,* 800–803.

Sloutsky, V. M. (1997). Institutional care and developmental outcomes of 6- and 7-year old children: A contextualist perspective. *Intl J Behavior Dev, 20,* 131–151.

Sotile, W. M., & Sotile, M. O. (1995). *The medical marriage: A couple's survival guide.* Washington, DC: American Medical Association Press.

U.S. Bureau of the Census. (1994). *Statistical abstracts of the United States, 1994* (114th ed.). Washington DC: U.S. Government Printing Office.

Vaillant, G. (1977). *Adaptation to life.* Boston: Little, Brown & Co..

Wallerstein, J. S., & Blackslee, S. (1989). *Second chance: Men, women and children a decade after divorce.* New York: Ticknor and Fields.

Aging, Death, and Bereavement

4

It is predicted that, by the year 2020, more than 15% of the population will be over 65 years of age. In fact, the fastest-growing segment of the population is what has been referred to as the **"old-old,"** people over age 85. In Britain, the medical care of the elderly is commonly referred to as "old age medicine." In the United States, such a descriptor for this group of citizens is avoided. Rather, the care of aging patients is called **geriatrics;** the study of aging is termed **gerontology;** and the patients themselves are most commonly referred to as **senior** or **mature citizens.** Whatever the terminology, the care of the steadily growing elderly population has become an important branch of medicine.

Although death is an unfortunate reality at any age, most deaths occur in the elderly population. Because of this, a discussion of death and grief, or **bereavement,** is included in this chapter.

■ OLD AGE: 65 YEARS AND OLDER

How can one identify the point at which a middle-aged person becomes a senior citizen? The Federal Government defines this milestone as age 65. At this age, individuals become eligible to collect Federal pension **(Social Security)** and health insurance **(Medicare)** (see Chapter 27) benefits, which are funded by monies accrued throughout one's working life by a combination of employee, employer, and government contributions. The benefits continue until death of the contributor and may, for his spouse and dependents, even continue beyond his death. Because it is the recognized age of retirement from work, 65 years is considered by many to be the transition point where middle age ends and old age begins.

The losses of aging

Americans tend to place a high value on work and independence and on youth and physical beauty (see Chapter 20). Therefore, retired, aging people may be perceived as less valuable. Unfortunately, the loss of social status associated with this perception is only one of the losses the elderly face. They must also deal with loss by death of spouses, family members, and friends, and they must confront the inevitable declines in their own health and strength.

Although the losses and changes associated with aging can contribute to the development of **depression** (see below and Chapter 13) in some people, most elderly people adjust well to these changes and continue to learn, to contribute to, and enjoy life. On the positive side, freedom from the responsibilities of work and childrearing allow older people to pursue interests and education that they did not have time for when they were younger.

Erikson described old age as the stage of **ego integrity versus despair;** a time when a person either has satisfaction and pride in her past accomplishments or feels that she has wasted her life. It is reassuring for younger people to learn that most elderly people achieve ego integrity in the last years of life.

Independence versus care by others

Many people believe that, invariably, the elderly will ultimately have to be cared for by others. In fact, this is not true. Although in certain cultural groups aging people are typically cared for by relatives (see Chapter 20). Less than one fourth of the American elderly are cared for by younger family members, and fewer than that spend their last years in long-term care facilities like nursing homes (see Chapter 27). In fact, most elderly Americans live independently and care for themselves. Newer options, such as **assisted living,** in which people live in complexes consisting of private rooms or apartments and receive help with meals, shopping, and housework, allow elderly Americans to remain relatively independent for longer periods of time.

Nursing homes provide inpatient, long-term care for about 5% of the elderly population. This care, often costing more than $1,000 per week, is not covered by Medicare. Therefore, a serious illness or injury that requires long-term inpatient care can effectively pauperize an elderly patient. Congress is currently addressing ways of helping the elderly pay for long-term nursing home care and assisted living services through government-funded programs.

Cognitive function in the elderly

The idea that elderly people usually have significant cognitive impairment is another pervasive but unsupported stereotype. Although slight memory and learning problems occur in normal aging, they generally do not interfere with the person's ability to function independently. **Dementia,** which has been referred to by the now outmoded term "senility," is a relatively uncommon disorder, occurring in less than 10% of the total elderly population (see Chapter 18).

The prevalence of dementia does, however, increase with age, and some degree of cognitive impairment is present in up to half of the over-age-85 population. Innovative pharmacologic treatments such as the acetylcholinesterase inhibitors (see Chapter 19) for the most common type of dementia, Alzheimer's disease, promise that, in the future, these cognitive changes can be prevented or treated effectively.

Longevity

In the United States, the average life expectancy at birth is currently 76–77 years, a figure that varies greatly by gender and ethnicity (Fig. 4–1). Although demographic differences in life expectancy have been decreasing over the past few years, they still extend to more than 20 years between the longest- (Chinese-American women) and the shortest- (African-American men) lived groups. While women tend to live longer than men, this

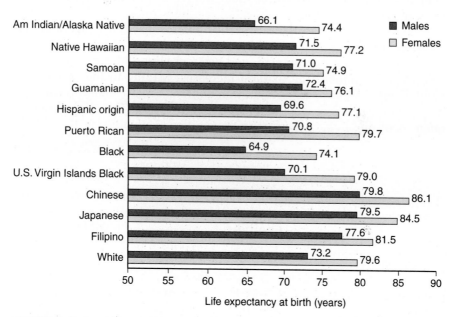

FIGURE 4-1. Life expectancy (in years) at birth in the United States by sex and ethnic group.

(Reprinted with permission from National Center for Health Statistics (1996) and National Institutes of Health, Office of Research on Women's Health (1998). Institute of Medicine (2001). Exploring the biological contributions to human health: Does sex matter? Washington, DC: National Academy Press.)

advantage comes with a burden. Elderly women are more likely than elderly men to have disabling health problems.

Research in gerontology suggests that longevity is associated primarily with a family history of longevity. It is also associated with continued physical and occupational activity, work satisfaction, advanced education, and, as discussed in Chapter 3, the presence of social support systems such as marriage.

Physical and neurological changes in aging

It has been said that aging is not for cowards. Physical strength and health gradually decline, and cardiovascular, renal, pulmonary, gastrointestinal, musculoskeletal, and immune functions are ultimately compromised. It is ironic that about the only thing that increases with aging is the ratio of body fat to muscle mass.

Neurological changes that occur in normal aging include decreased cerebral blood flow and decreased brain weight. Senile plaques and neurofibrillary tangles may also appear, albeit to a lesser extent in normally aging brains than in brains of patients with Alzheimer's disease (see Chapter 18). Despite these brain changes, which can be accompanied by mild reductions in memory and learning speed, intelligence (in the absence of dementia or other brain disease;) (See Chapter 10) remains approximately the same throughout life.

Neurotransmitter availability in the brain decreases with age. This decrease occurs via several mechanisms. First, secretion of norepinephrine, dopamine, γ-aminobutyric acid, and acetylcholine diminish. Also, concentration of monoamine oxidase increases, leading to the accelerated breakdown of some of these neurotransmitters. Finally, neurotransmitter receptors may be less responsive in the aging brain. The clinical consequences of these changes in neurotransmitter availability in the elderly

TABLE 4-1	Neurochemical Changes in the Aging Brain	
NEUROCHEMICAL	CHANGE WITH AGING	POSSIBLE PSYCHIATRIC RESULT
Norepinephrine	Decrease	Depression
Dopamine	Decrease	Depression
γ-aminobutyric acid	Decrease	Anxiety
Acetylcholine	Decrease	Dementia
Monoamine oxidase	Increase	Psychiatric symptoms

can include increased likelihood of psychiatric symptoms (Table 4–1) and of negative side effects associated with psychopharmacological treatment.

Psychosocial changes in aging

The common physical health problems associated with aging are uncomfortable, and they can have serious emotional and social consequences. For example, the embarrassing problem of reduced bladder control seen in some aging patients can impair one's ability to leave home. Age-associated losses in muscle strength and in sensory functions like vision and hearing can further decrease social opportunities and increase social isolation, well-known contributors to the occurrence of depressive symptoms in people of any age.

Another, often undetected, serious social problem associated with aging is the **abuse** of cognitively or physically impaired elderly people by their caretakers (see Chapter 22).

Psychopathology in the elderly

Depression in the elderly is commonly characterized by memory loss and cognitive problems. These symptoms can mimic and be misdiagnosed as dementia. This misdiagnosed disorder, known as **pseudodementia** (see Chapter 14), must be identified because depression can increase suicide risk. Also, in contrast to dementia, pseudodementia is highly responsive to treatment.

Suicide resulting from social loss, physical illness, or depression is more common in the elderly than in the general population. **Anxiety** and fearfulness also are more common in the elderly, who must deal with the realistic possibility of developing a serious illness or of falling and breaking a bone. In addition, daytime confusion due to unidentified **alcohol- or benzodiazepine-related disorders** (see Chapter 23) as well as **sleep disorders** (see Chapter 10) can exacerbate anxiety and depression in the elderly. Sometimes, depression or medical illness leading to delirium (see Chapter 18) in the elderly can be accompanied by delusions, often of the persecutory type. These delusions include the belief that a spouse is unfaithful or that a caregiver is stealing money or household objects.

Although common, depression and anxiety are not inevitable, nor are they normal in the elderly. With medical and pharmacological interventions and practical suggestions for self-care, the primary care physician can aggressively and successfully treat these disorders. Unfortunately, because Medicare currently does not completely cover outpatient prescription drugs (see Chapter 27), elderly patients without sufficient resources may be unable to use some of the newer and often more expensive pharmacologic agents (see Chapter 19). Supportive psychotherapy (e.g., cognitive therapy; see Chapter 11) and electroconvulsive therapy (see Chapter 19) can also help relieve depression in the elderly. The latter is particularly useful for seriously depressed elderly patients who are intolerant of or who do not respond to other treatments.

■ DYING, DEATH, AND BEREAVEMENT

The losses of youth usually revolve around jobs and relationships. In contrast, the most significant loss facing the elderly is loss of life itself. Confronting the end of life requires that a person separate from friends, family, and possessions. This painful task requires that one pass through a variety of psychological stages. Ideally, the last of these stages includes resolution and acceptance.

Stages of dying

Many researchers have studied the psychology of dying. While there is no one typical way of dying, the physician Elizabeth Kübler-Ross, described the process of dying and loss as a sequence of five stages: **denial, anger, bargaining, depression,** and **acceptance.** She noted that some people who anticipate their own or a loved one's death go through only two or three of the stages, whereas others go through the stages simultaneously or in a different order. Most commonly, however, people experience the stages in the following sequence:

- In the first stage, **denial**, the patient unconsciously cannot accept the diagnosis and refuses to believe that she is dying. She may make statements like "the laboratory made an error" or "that must be someone else's diagnosis." This stage generally resolves within a few hours or, at most, days.
- The stage that follows is characterized by **anger,** often directed at the physician and hospital staff. Verbal confrontations initiated by the patient such as "you should have done more tests," are common. Physicians must learn not to take such comments personally; instead, they should try to understand the fear and anxiety in the patients that provoke the outbursts.
- After the anger stage is resolved, the patient frequently tries to strike a bargain with God or some higher being. This stage of **bargaining** is characterized by statements like "I will give half of my money to charity if I can get rid of this disease" in an unconscious effort to "undo" (a defense mechanism, see Chapter 8) a negative life event.
- The stage of **depression,** including preoccupation with death and emotional detachment, follows. In this stage, the patient feels distant from others and seems sad and hopeless. In a normal grief reaction, depression is short-lasting and is quickly followed by acceptance.
- In the **acceptance** phase, the patient deals calmly with her fate and is able to use and even enjoy her remaining time with friends and family.

Interestingly, the stages of dying can also occur with other life losses, such as the loss of a body part through amputation or mastectomy or, for younger people, a natural or induced abortion.

Bereavement (normal grief) versus depression (abnormal grief)

It is normal to feel great sadness after the loss of a loved one or in anticipation of one's own death. This normal reaction, also called **bereavement,** can, like the stages of dying, occur with life losses other than death. Although most grief reactions after a severe life loss are considered normal, others are extreme enough to be considered pathological. For example, both normal grief and pathological grief are characterized initially by shock and even denial that the event has actually occurred. However, whereas denial tends to last up to a few hours in normal grief, the denial of pathological grief may persist over days or weeks. Both normal grief and pathological grief include sadness, crying, and other expressions of sorrow, particularly in the early stages. In normal grief, these expressions gradually subside over a 1- to 2-year period. However, they commonly and normally recur on holidays or special occasions, a phenomenon called the **anniversary reaction.** In contrast, in pathological grief, the characteristics of bereavement persist and may even intensify over time.

Cultural differences are notable in normal grief reactions. In some cultures, the bereaved are expected to outwardly express their distress with verbalizations and actions. In others, such displays are discouraged (see Chapter 20). No matter what the culture, the characteristics of normal grief can sometimes mimic those of mental illness. For example, **illusions** (e.g., misperceptions that the deceased person is physically present) are seen in normal grief reactions. In contrast, the presence of frank **delusions,** such as a belief that the dead person is controlling one's

---

CASE 4-1

THE PATIENT A 72-year-old diabetic patient whose wife died 8 months ago appears unkempt and unshaven. He reports that he cries frequently during the day when he thinks about his wife and has recurrent nightmares about the circumstances of her death. Although previously gregarious, he states that he now prefers to be alone and has no interest in interacting with friends and family. There is no evidence of a thought disorder or suicidal ideation. Physical examination, although essentially normal, reveals that the patient's blood sugar, formerly well controlled, is elevated and he has lost 12 pounds since his checkup the previous year. He explains that he has forgotten to give himself his daily insulin injection a few times in the last few weeks and has little appetite for food.

COMMENT This patient demonstrates an abnormal grief reaction. He is showing signs of depression (e.g., poor grooming, significant weight loss, social withdrawal, and lack of self-care; see Chapter 12). Although forgetting to take his insulin could indicate the development of dementia, it is better explained as another symptom of depression (pseudodementia).

TREATMENT For this patient, the best first recommendation of the physician is antidepressant medication. This recommendation should be coupled with frequent, scheduled visits and regular phone conversations with the doctor. If the patient does not respond to or has significant side effects from the medication, another option for this elderly man is electroconvulsive therapy (ECT) (see Chapter 15). The patient's difficulties with appetite, sleep, and self-care will improve as his mood improves.

thoughts, or **hallucinations,** such as hearing the dead person talking, suggests an abnormal grief reaction. See Table 12–3 for further clarification of these terms. Comparisons between normal and abnormal grief reactions are shown in Table 4–2.

The role of physicians in dying and death

Physicians play an important role for the dying patient and bereaved family. First, it is up to the physician to make the dying patient (and, with the patient's permission, the family) completely aware of the diagnosis and prognosis (see Chapter 24). Next, the doctor can provide reassurance to the patient and family that their intense responses to the news are normal

TABLE 4-2	Comparison between Normal Grief Reactions and Abnormal Grief Reactions	
NORMAL GRIEF REACTION (BEREAVEMENT)	**ABNORMAL GRIEF REACTION (DEPRESSION)**
Minor weight loss (<5 pounds)	Significant weight loss (>5% of body weight)
Minor sleep disturbances (e.g. some difficulty falling asleep)	Significant sleep disturbances (e.g. repeated nighttime awakenings and early morning awakenings)
Some guilty feelings	Intense feelings of guilt and worthlessness
Illusions	Hallucinations and delusions
Attempts to return to work and to socialize	Resumes few, if any, work or social activities
Cries and expresses sadness	Considers or attempts suicide
Severe symptoms resolve in <2 months	Severe symptoms persist for >2 months
Moderate symptoms subside in <1 year	Moderate symptoms persist for >1 year
Treatment includes increased contact with the physician, supportive psychotherapy, support groups, and short-acting benzodiazepines for problems with sleep	Treatment includes antidepressants, antipsychotics, or electroconvulsive therapy and professional psychotherapy

Adapted from Fadem, B. (2001). *Behavioral science* (3rd ed.). Baltimore: Lippincott, Williams & Wilkins.

and to be expected. The doctor also can be an important support person for the dying patient and for the family before and after the death.

Physicians have the training to make the distinction between normal and pathological grief reactions. They also have the training and tools to support the patient or family member experiencing the former, and to aggressively treat the person showing the latter. On a practical note, doctors need to medically follow bereaved family members because the risk of morbidity and mortality is increased for close relatives (especially widowed men) in the first year of bereavement (see Chapter 25).

Physicians often feel a sense of failure when they cannot prevent the death of their patients. Doctors who recognize this reaction can resist the emotional detachment it can lead to, ultimately making them even more effective in guiding the patient and family through this most important of all of life's transitions.

REVIEW QUESTIONS

1. A 69-year-old patient whose husband of 50 years died 6 months ago reports that she sometimes cannot fall asleep at night and often cries when she thinks about her husband. She also tells the doctor that on one occasion she followed a man down the street who resembled her late husband but felt foolish about it later. The patient also relates that she enjoys visits from her grandchildren and has resumed her daily walks with a friend. For this patient, the best recommendation of the physician is to suggest

   (A) antidepressant medication

   (B) regular phone calls and visits to "check in" with the doctor

   (C) regular sessions with a psychotherapist

   (D) a neuropsychological evaluation for Alzheimer's disease

   (E) a hypnotic benzodiazepine daily for sleep

2. A terminally ill 55-year-old patient who says to his doctor, "I would not be dying if you had taken better care of me" is most likely to be in the stage of dying that Kübler-Ross described as

   (A) denial

   (B) anger

   (C) bargaining

   (D) depression

   (E) acceptance

3. A physician has just diagnosed terminal liver cancer in a 70-year-old man. Which of the following is the most appropriate behavior for the physician?

(A) Prior to telling the patient, she should inform his adult children of the diagnosis and prognosis.

(B) She should limit her contact with the family until after the patient dies.

(C) She should provide a barbiturate for the patient until the initial shock of his diagnosis abates.

(D) She should address the patient's concerns directly with him.

(E) She should see the patient less frequently as his death approaches.

Questions 4 and 5

An 82-year-old patient tells his doctor that he is concerned because he sometimes forgets the phone numbers of new acquaintances and the fact that his bowling score is not as high as it once was. He reports that he is comfortable living alone and taking care of his own needs and that he has a number of friends with whom he eats out regularly. Physical examination is unremarkable.

4. Which of the following is most likely to be true about this patient?

(A) He should be advised to live in an assisted care facility

(B) He has early signs of Alzheimer's disease

(C) He is showing signs of depression

(D) He is likely to develop an anxiety disorder in the near future

(E) He is showing signs of normal aging

5. Which of the following is most likely to be found on psychological and physical examination of this patient?

(A) Inability to remember his address

(B) Increased muscle mass

(C) Decreased size of brain ventricles

(D) Decreased bladder control

(E) Increased immune responses

ANSWERS AND EXPLANATIONS

1-B. This patient whose husband died 6 months ago is showing a normal grief reaction. Although she sometimes has difficulty falling asleep and cries when she thinks about her husband, she is showing efforts to return to her social life with family and friends. The illusion of believing she sees a man who resembles her late husband is seen in a normal grief reaction. For a normal grief reaction, recommending regular phone calls and visits to "check in" with the doctor are the appropriate interventions. There are no indications that sleep medication, antidepressants, psychotherapy, or neuropsychological evaluation are necessary for this patient.

2-B. During the anger stage of dying, the patient is likely to blame the physician.

3-D. Ideally, the physician should speak to the patient directly and not through his adult children. With the patient's permission, they can be told the diagnosis and prognosis later. While a physician may become emotionally detached from the patient in order to deal with his impending death, she should see the patient more, not less frequently as his death approaches. Heavy sedation is rarely indicated for a dying patient.

4-E. This active, independent 82-year-old man is showing normal aging. He can function well living alone and enjoys social activities. There is no evidence that this patient has Alzheimer's disease, depression, or an anxiety disorder.

5-D. Decreased bladder control is a common finding in normal aging. In normal aging, immune responses and muscle mass decrease and brain ventricles increase in size because of brain shrinkage. Although mild memory problems may occur, severe memory problems such as forgetting one's address do not occur in normal aging.

REFERENCES

Erikson, E. H. (1987). *A way of looking at things: Selected papers from 1930 to 1980.* New York: Norton.

Erikson, K., & Vallas, S. P. (Eds.). (1990). *The nature of work.* New Haven: Yale University Press.

Freud, S. (1935). *A general introduction to psychoanalysis* (Rev. ed.) (J. Riviere, Trans.). New York: Liverright.

Institute of Medicine. (2001). *Exploring the biological contributions to human health: Does sex matter?* Washington, DC: National Academy Press.

Kastenbaum, R. (1998). *Death, society and human experience* (6th ed.). Boston: Allyn and Bacon.

Levinson, D. J., & Goodeneh, W. E. (1985). The life cycle. In: H. I. Kaplan & B. J. Sadock (Eds.), *Comprehensive textbook of psychiatry.* Baltimore: Williams & Wilkins.

Stroebe, M., Hansson, R., Stroebe, W., & Schut, H. (2001). *Handbook of bereavement research.* Washington, DC: American Psychological Association.

Vaillant, G. (1977). *Adaptation to life.* Boston: Little, Brown.

Genetics, Anatomy, and Biochemistry of Behavior   **5**

L ike physical health, emotional health is a result of complex interactions among biological, social, and environmental influences. Disorders of either type of health result from aberrations or distortions in one or more of these influences at any time in a person's life.

Theoretical difficulties exist when trying to separate biological from social and environmental factors in the etiology of psychiatric illness. Therefore, the term **organic mental disorder,** used in past years to describe behavioral symptoms with causes outside of the emotional range, is rarely used. Furthermore, the development over the past few decades of advanced techniques in neuroimaging and neurophysiology have shown that psychiatric function is influenced significantly by neuroanatomical and neurochemical factors. This chapter focuses on the contributions of these and other biological components to the expression of normal behavior and its disorders.

■ GENETICS

The role of genetic influences on the development of physical conditions like heart disease, diabetes, and cancer has been well-documented. Genetic influences are also important in the display of behavior and its disorders. Because behavioral disorders are expressed in and thus are confounded by the social setting, it is more difficult in behavioral than in physical disorders to isolate genetic from social and environmental etiologies. Research tools that can help separate and identify these factors include family, twin, and adoption studies.

Research studies

Family risk studies are used to distinguish between genetic and other risk factors in the etiology of disorders. For a behavioral disorder or trait, the frequency of its occurrence in the relatives of an affected individual, or **proband,** is compared with its frequency in the general population. If a genetic component is involved in its etiology, a disorder would be expected to have a higher **concordance rate** (i.e., if concordant, the disorder occurs in both relatives) in close relatives of people with the disorder than in more distant relatives or in the general population.

Twin studies also are employed to identify genetic factors in disorders. These studies work on the assumption that, because monozygotic twins have the same genetic makeup, the likelihood of both twins having a disorder will be higher than that of dizygotic twins, who are only as similar genetically as siblings. Furthermore, this assumption should hold true whether the twins are raised in the same home or in separate adoptive homes. For many psychiatric and behavioral traits and disorders, anecdotal and documented findings in twin and **adoption studies** strongly support this hypothesis.

Psychiatric disorders

Research studies provide evidence that genetic factors are involved in the etiology of major psychiatric disorders like schizophrenia and bipolar disorder (see Chapters 12 and 13). Although each of these disorders occurs in about 1% of the general population, persons with a close genetic relationship to patients with schizophrenia or bipolar disorder are more likely than those with more distant relationships to develop these disorders (Table 5–1). Recent studies suggest also that the volume of brain areas known to be involved in the symptoms of schizophrenia (e.g., gray matter in frontal lobes and language areas) is more similar in monozygotic than in dizygotic twin pairs (Thompson et al., 2001).

Although it has been difficult to link specific chromosomal markers with psychiatric illnesses, in some studies, schizophrenia has been associated with markers on the long arms of chromosomes 5, 11, 18, and 22; the short arm of chromosome 19; and, recently with chromosomes 6, a genetic variation in the dysbindin gene (Staub et al., 2002), 8, a genetic variate of the neureregulin 1 gene (Stefansson et al., 2003), and 13, a gene associated with disturbed transmission of glutamate (Chumakov et al., 2002). Also, although the significant association previously found between bipolar disorder and genetic markers on chromosome 11 was not

TABLE 5-1	Risk of Developing Schizophrenia and Bipolar Disorder in Relatives of Patients	
RELATIONSHIP TO PATIENT	APPROXIMATE RISK FOR SCHIZOPHRENIA (%)	APPROXIMATE RISK FOR BIPOLAR DISORDER (%)
No relationship (general population)	1	1
First-degree relative (sibling, dizygotic twin, or parent) of a patient with the disorder	10	20
Child of two parents with the disorder	40	60
Monozygotic twin of a patient with the disorder	50	75

CASE 5-1

THE PATIENT A physician confirms that a 26-year-old woman is in her first trimester of pregnancy. During the discussion after the examination, the woman tells the doctor that her identical twin sister recently entered a psychiatric hospital. The patient explains that over the past few months her sister reported hearing the voice of God telling her that she was chosen for a special "mission." The patient does not know her sister's diagnosis but expresses concern that her own unborn child will develop the same illness.

COMMENT Although more information must be gained to make a definitive diagnosis of the sister's illness, the presence of auditory hallucinations (hearing voices) lasting over several months suggests schizophrenia (see Chapter 12). Alternatively, the patient's sister may be showing the manic phase of bipolar disorder characterized by delusions of grandeur (being chosen for a special mission) (see Chapter 13). Although other factors are involved in their etiology, there is a significant genetic component to the development of both of these disorders. Because the patient has the same genetic makeup as her monozygotic twin sister, the risk to her own child is the same as it would be for her sister's child or for any first-degree relative.

TREATMENT The patient should be advised that there are other nongenetic factors involved in the etiology of major psychiatric illness; however, if her sister has schizophrenia, her own child's genetic risk for developing the illness is about 10%. Bipolar disorder has a higher concordance rate and her child's genetic risk is about 20%. Counseling should be provided to help the patient understand the two disorders and their treatments.

retained when the subject pool was extended, recent evidence suggests that loci for increased risk for bipolar disorder may be present on chromosomes 12 (Ewald et al., 1998), 16 (Ewald and Kruse, 1997), and 18 (Ewald et al., 1997).

Genetic factors also play a role in the etiology of personality characteristics. For example, personality features such as responsiveness to stimulation, fearfulness, activity level, and distractibility have a higher concordance rate in monozygotic twins than in dizygotic twins. Such factors also play a role in the etiology of **personality disorders (PDS),** a diagnosis that is made when an individual has significant difficulties in social or occupational functioning because of his or her personality characteristics (see Chapter 24).

The personality disorders are organized in three groups or "clusters" by similarities in their presentations (Table 24-2). When compared with the general population, relatives of patients in each of the clusters tend to have specific psychiatric problems. For example, patients with cluster A disorders (schizoid, schizotypal, paranoid) are more likely to have relatives with psychotic disorders like schizophrenia, whereas cluster B (histrionic, narcissistic, antisocial, borderline) disorder patients are more likely to have relatives with major depressive and substance abuse disorders. Cluster C (avoidant, obsessive-compulsive, dependent) disorders have been associated with anxiety disorders in relatives (Bouchard et al., 1990).

Neuropsychiatric disorders

There is strong support for genetic influences in the etiology of neuropsychiatric disorders like Alzheimer's disease (see Chapter 18). Family risk studies show that, although this disease is present in only 10% of nonrelatives, 25 to 50% of close relatives of Alzheimer's patients eventually develop the disease. There is also a higher concordance rate for Alzheimer's in monozygotic than in dizygotic twins.

Several chromosomes have been linked to the development of Alzheimer's. Most well-known is the association of Alzheimer's with chromosome 21—individuals with Down's syndrome (trisomy 21) who live beyond age 40 ultimately develop behavioral and neuroanatomical evidence of Alzheimer's. Chromosomes 1 and 14 have also been linked to Alzheimer's, particularly in the **early onset type** that is evident before age 60. Also, the presence on chromosome 19 of the **apolipoprotein E$_2$ (Apo E$_2$) allele** appears to decrease and the **E$_4$ allele (Apo E$_4$)** to increase the likelihood of developing Alzheimer's disease, particularly in women (Bartrez-Faz, D. et al., 2002).

Other neuropsychiatric disorders with strong genetic components include Huntington's disease and Tourette's disorder (see Chapter 2). Offspring of one affected parent with Huntingon's disease, a fatal autosomal-dominant disorder associated with an abnormal gene on the short end of chromosome 4, have a 50% chance of developing the disorder. A high percentage of patients with Tourette's disorder have a family member who is also affected by the illness, and its concordance rate is higher in monozygotic than in dizygotic twins.

Substance abuse disorders

Many people believe that substance abuse disorders are caused by an individual's weak self-control or poor choice of social peers. Although such social difficulties clearly exist among abusers, much recent evidence suggests that substance abuse disorders such as alcoholism also have a genetic component. Evidence of genetic associations in alcoholism includes findings that:

- The concordance rate for alcoholism is about twice as high for monozygotic twins as it is for dizygotic twins
- Adopted children tend in adulthood to show the drinking patterns characteristic of their biological rather than their adoptive parents
- Alcoholism is about four times more prevalent in the biological children of alcoholics than of nonalcoholics

Furthermore, the genetic component of alcoholism is related to both sex and age of onset; sons of alcoholics are at greater risk than daughters, particularly if the sons begin to abuse alcohol before age 20.

Cocaine abuse is also associated with genetic factors. Recently (McHugh et al., 2002), a polymorphism in the promoter region of the prodynorphin gene was shown to be associated with protection against cocaine abuse.

■ BEHAVIORAL NEUROANATOMY

The human nervous system consists of the **central nervous system (CNS)** and the **peripheral nervous system (PNS).** The CNS contains the brain (cerebral hemispheres, basal ganglia, and thalamus); brainstem (pons, medulla, and midbrain); and the spinal cord. The PNS consists of somatosensory (afferent) neurons, motor (efferent) neurons, and autonomic neurons. Although anatomically separate, the CNS and PNS function interactively.

The cerebral cortex

The area of the brain most closely associated with behavior is the **cerebral cortex,** although subcortical areas are also involved. The activity of the cortex can be segregated functionally into **sensory, motor,** and **association areas** that act together to ultimately affect behavior.

The cortex also can be divided anatomically into **frontal, temporal, parietal,** and **occipital lobes,** as well as **limbic lobes** that contain the medial parts of the frontal, temporal, and parietal lobes. Behavioral alterations seen in people with brain lesions caused by accident, disease, or surgery illustrate the major neuropsychiatric functions of these areas and of other cortical regions (Table 5–2).

TABLE 5-2	Neuropsychiatric Anatomy: Function and Dysfunction	
REGION/DIVISION	MAJOR FUNCTIONS	EFFECTS OF LESION ON BEHAVIOR
Frontal lobes		
Dorsolateral convexity	■ Planning for future action (executive functions)	■ Decreased motivation, concentration and attention ■ Disorientation ■ Mood disturbances
Orbitofrontal cortex	■ Control over biological drives	■ Disinhibition and inappropriate behavior ■ Poor judgment ■ Lack of inhibition or remorse ("pseudo-psychopathic" behavior)
Medial cortex	■ Control of movement	■ Apathy ■ Decreased spontaneous movement (akinesia) ■ Gait disturbances ■ Incontinence
Temporal lobes	■ Memory ■ Learning ■ Emotion ■ Auditory processing	■ Impaired memory ■ Psychomotor seizures ■ Changes in aggressive behavior ■ Inability to understand language (i.e., Wernicke's aphasia [left-side lesions])
Limbic lobes		
Hippocampus	■ Memory storage	■ Poor new learning
Amygdala	■ Coordination of emotional states, particularly anger and aggression, with somatic responses	■ Klüver-Bucy syndrome (decreased aggression, increased sexuality, hyperorality) ■ Decreased conditioned fear response ■ Inability to recognize facial and vocal expressions of anger in others

TABLE 5-2 Neuropsychiatric Anatomy: Function and Dysfunction
(Continued)

REGION/DIVISION	MAJOR FUNCTIONS	EFFECTS OF LESION ON BEHAVIOR
Parietal lobes	■ Somatic sensation and body image	■ Impaired IQ ■ Impaired processing of visual-spatial information, (i.e., cannot copy a simple line drawing or a clock face correctly [right-sided lesions]) ■ Gerstmann's syndrome (i.e., cannot name fingers, write, tell left from right, or do simple math, and impaired processing of verbal information [left-sided lesions])
Occipital lobes	■ Vision	■ Visual hallucinations and illusions ■ Inability to identify camouflaged objects ■ Blindness

IQ = Intelligence quotent

Frontal lobes. The frontal lobes have four major subdivisions. The first two, the **motor strip** and the **supplemental motor area,** are involved in motor behavior; the third (**Broca's area**) in language. The fourth division is the **prefrontal cortex.**

Clinically occurring events, surgically imposed changes, and neuroimaging studies provide evidence for the behavioral functions of the prefrontal cortex. The famous case of Phineas Gage, a man who received a large prefrontal lobe lesion in an accident in the mid-nineteenth century, first demonstrated the personality functions of the frontal lobes (Harlow, 1868). Although he had remarkably few obvious neurological problems, Gage demonstrated a significant personality change after his brain lesion healed. A formerly nonaggressive person, Gage showed outbursts of anger after the accident. A respectful, energetic, persistent, and organized person before his accident, he began to show an inability to carry out plans and a lack of self-control and concern for others. In a similar way, some patients who have had bilateral **prefrontal lobotomy,** a surgical procedure used in the past to treat serious psychiatric illness, retain intellectual functioning but show uncharacteristic apathy and lack of "goal-directed" behavior after the surgery.

Perseveration, engaging in repeated unnecessary behavior and thought, disinhibition, and sudden outbursts of temper, as well as reinstatement of the infantile sucking and rooting reflexes (**frontal release signs**) are seen in patients with prefrontal lobe damage; this is now known as **prefrontal lobe syndrome.** Interestingly, schizophrenia and obsessive-compulsive disorder (OCD), both of which are characterized by personality and affective changes, are associated with decreased bilateral prefrontal cortical activity as measured by functional magnetic resonance imaging (fMRI) and positron emission tomography (PET) (Baxter, 1999) (see Chapter 6).

Although personality changes are associated with damage to the entire prefrontal cortex, clinical and other evidence indicates that the three major prefrontal subdivisions—the orbitofrontal region, the dorsolateral convexity, and the medial region—have specialized behavioral functions. The **dorsolateral convexity** influences behavior and personality and has "executive" responsibilities involving activities like formulating plans, maintaining attention and concentration, and changing problem-solving strategies when needed. The **orbitofrontal cortex** is a center for the biological control of inhibition, emotions, and drive states. It is also part of the dopamine-driven **"reward circuit"** of the brain and is activated in addicts exposed to drug-related cues (Goldstein and Volkow, 2002). The **medial region** has connections to the basal ganglia and accessory cortical motor areas and is involved primarily in motor activity. Damage to each of these subdivisions results in characteristic behavioral abnormalities (see Case 5–2 and Table 5–2).

The emotional-behavioral functions of the frontal lobes are lateralized. Lesions of the left prefrontal area, both cortical and subcortical, can result in depression, whereas lesions of the right are more likely to produce manifestations of elevated mood. Similarly, fMRI studies reveal that positive mood is associated with activation of the left prefrontal cortex and stress with activation of the right prefrontal cortex (Davidson and Irwin, 1999).

Limbic lobe. Because the neurons within the limbic lobe form circuits that play a major role in emotions, the limbic lobe has been called the **limbic system.** Its primary functions are to mediate between the hypothalamus and cerebral cortex and to modulate the activity of the autonomic nervous system (ANS). First described by Papez in 1937 and expanded later to include other areas, the limbic system or **Papez circuit** contains the **hippocampus, fornix, amygdala, septum,** part of the **thalamus,** the **cingulate gyrus,** and related structures (Fig. 5–1). The limbic system also acts on the hypothalamus, which in turn influences endocrine control of emotions via secretion of hormones. Damage to the limbic lobe, particularly the amygdala and hypothalamus, results in behavioral abnormalities (see Table 5–2). Recently, neuroimaging studies indicate that, like the prefrontal cortex, the volume of limbic structures like the amygdala and hippocampus are reduced in patients with schizophrenia.

THE PATIENT After a mild stroke, a hospitalized 64-year-old former firefighter begins to show uncharacteristic impulsivity and mood changes. The nurses report that when the patient was found walking down the hospital hallway naked, he explained that he was "just trying to cool off." The patient's wife believes that his strange behavior is due to post-traumatic stress disorder as a result of a life-threatening fire he witnessed the previous month. The physician believes instead that the patient's behavior fits the DSM-IV-TR diagnosis of "personality change due to a general medical condition" and is a direct result of the injury to his brain caused by the stroke. To further evaluate this patient, the doctor orders a computed tomography scan, a magnetic resonance imaging (MRI), and a series of neurological tests.

COMMENT It can be difficult to gauge whether a change in behavior after a neurological insult is due to damage to the brain. This case is problematic because of the temporal juxtaposition of an intense psychosocial stressor (the fire) with the physical insult to this patient's brain caused by a stroke. Tests used to distinguish neurological from emotional symptoms include the Mental Status Examination, the Folstein Mini-Mental State Examination, and neuropsychiatric tests like the Bender Visual Motor Gestalt Test (see Chapter 6).

TREATMENT The results of the MRI and neuropsychiatric tests suggest that the patient has sustained damage to the orbitofrontal cortex (see Table 5–2). The behavioral abnormalities he shows (e.g., personality changes and lack of characteristic modesty) give further evidence that this is the site of damage. No surgery is indicated at this time, and treatment involves providing supportive treatment and a structured environment as the lesion heals.

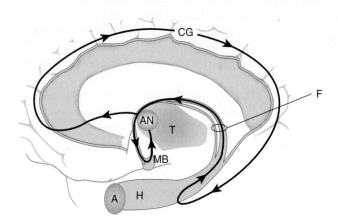

FIGURE 5-1. Papez circuit. A, amygdala; AN, anterior nucleus of the thalamus; CG, cingulate gyrus; H, hippocampus; MB, mamillary body; F, fornix; T, thalamus. The arrow represents the anatomy of the loop believed to be involved in the processing of emotions.

(Reprinted with permission from Filley, C. M. (1995). Neurobehavioral anatomy. Niwot, CO: University Press of Colorodo.)

The basal ganglia

The basal ganglia are a group of nuclei that receive information from the entire cerebral cortex and project it to the frontal lobes via the thalamus. There are four structural components of the basal ganglia:

- **Striatum** (containing the **caudate nucleus** and the **putamen**)
- **Pallidum** (also called the **globus pallidus**)
- **Substantia nigra**
- **Subthalamic nucleus**

The basal ganglia function to translate the desire to execute movement into actual movement. Conditions causing damage to its nuclei can result in neuropsychiatric illnesses with motor symptoms. For example, over-activity of the striatum or damage to the substantia nigra results in Parkinson's-like symptoms like the inability to initiate movement (bradykinesia). Underactivity of the striatum and shrinking of the caudate nucleus are associated with the symptoms of Huntington's disease. Damage to the caudate is associated also with Tourette's syndrome, whereas lesions of the pallidum and subthalamic nucleus result in conditions characterized by sudden, uncontrolled limb movements.

Hemispheric specialization

The left side of the brain controls the right side of the body. Because approximately 90% of the population preferentially uses the right hand, the left hemisphere of the brain is referred to as the **dominant hemisphere.** Communication between the cerebral hemispheres occurs via structures including the **corpus callosum, anterior commissure, hippocampal commissure,** and **habenular commissure.** Clinical studies using patients in whom these structures, particularly the corpus callosum, have been divided surgically to treat severe epilepsy, or who have sustained injury to only one side of the brain, demonstrate that the hemispheres are functionally lateralized.

Because the left hemisphere is associated with language function, damage to this hemisphere results in impairment of skills such as speech, writing, and reading in almost all right-handed people and in most left-handed people. The right, or **nondominant hemisphere,** is associated primarily with perception and also with spatial relations, body image, recognition of faces and music, puzzle-solving, map-reading, and musical and artistic ability. Damage to the right hemisphere has motor sequelae and indirect effects on behavior but does not usually affect intelligence or personality directly.

There are sex differences in functional organization of the brain. For example, women generally have a larger corpus callosum and anterior commissure and appear to have better interhemispheric communication than men. When doing a verbal task, women typically use both hemispheres, whereas men show activation of only one hemisphere (Fig. 5–2) (Shaywitz et al., 1995). The better-developed right hemispheres of men

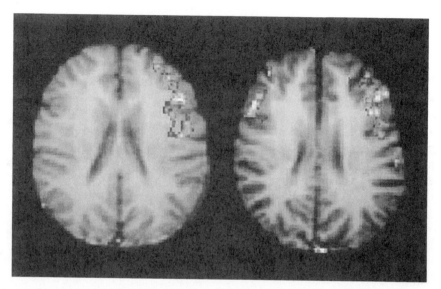

FIGURE 5-2. Composite functional magnetic resonance (fMRI) images of male and female brains. These composite fMRI images in males (left image) and females (right image) show the distribution of activation of a cognitive task—in this case, phonological processing involving identifying whether nonsense words (e.g., leet and jeet) rhymed or not. Males show unilateral activation in the left inferior frontal gyrus, whereas females show activity in both the left and right inferior frontal gyri.

(Reprinted with permission from Shaywitz, B.A., Shaywitz, S. E., Pugh, K. R., Constable, R. T., Skudlarski, P., Fulbright, R. K., et al. (1995). Sex differences in the functional organization of the brain for language. Nature, 373, 607–609.)

may in part explain the consistently documented male advantage in executing spatial tasks (Halpern, 2000). *— ♂ better in spatial tasks*

Consciousness, coma, and brain death

The **thalamus** and **reticular formation,** a network of neurons in the brainstem, are the brain regions most closely involved in arousal and consciousness. In contrast to cortical lesions (particularly left-sided lesions), which must be extensive to cause loss of consciousness, relatively small, localized lesions of either of these structures, particularly the reticular formation, can cause profound loss of consciousness or coma, nonsleep loss of consciousness that extends for a prolonged period (Kandel et al, 2000). Similarly, lesions that disrupt connections between the brainstem and thalamus can result in coma. Levels of consciousness can be scored on a scale of 3 to 15 using the **Glasgow Coma Scale** (see Chapter 6, Table 6–4).

A patient in a profound coma has no conscious cognitive function. If the eyes are open and there is a sleep-wake cycle, the person is said to be in a **persistent vegetative state.** Whether to maintain a person who is in this state on life support is an important ethical issue in medicine (see Chapter 26).

Peripheral nervous system

The PNS contains sensory, motor, and autonomic fibers outside of the CNS, including the spinal nerves, cranial nerves, and peripheral ganglia. The PNS carries sensory information to the CNS and motor information away from the CNS.

The autonomic nervous system. The **ANS** is the part of the PNS most closely involved in behavior. The **parasympathetic** division of the ANS acts mainly to maintain homeostasis and conserve resources while the **sympathetic** division is closely involved in response to stress. In tandem, these divisions innervate the internal organs and coordinate emotions with visceral responses, such as heart rate, blood pressure, and peptic acid secretion. Exacerbation of these visceral responses as a result of psychological stress is implicated in the development and progression of physical illnesses like hypertension, peptic ulcer disease, and rheumatoid arthritis (see Chapter 25).

The hypothalamus. The **hypothalamus** lies between the thalamus and the pituitary gland and has an important role in the biological control of emotion, particularly rage and aggression. The hypothalamus is important also in the maintenance of homeostasis, specifically in the regulation of body temperature and drinking and eating behavior. Damage to the **ventromedial nucleus (the satiety center)** of the hypothalamus results in increased appetite leading to obesity, whereas **lateral nucleus** damage results in decreased appetite and weight loss. The hypothalamus also is associated with coordinating the autonomic nervous system with pituitary gland function.

Mediated by the pituitary gland, which regulates gonadal hormone secretion, the hypothalamus is also involved in the regulation of sexual activity in adulthood. Animal studies demonstrate that differential exposure of males and females to gonadal hormones during perinatal life results in permanent sex differences in the volume of certain hypothalamic nuclei. Some controversial studies suggest that similar anatomic sex differences in these nuclei are associated with sexual orientation in men (LeVay, 1991).

■ NEUROTRANSMISSION

Neurotransmitters are chemical messengers that are closely involved in cellular function at all levels of the nervous system. Emotions and psychopathology are believed to result from interactions and imbalances among these messengers in the brain. The three major classes of neurotransmitters are the **biogenic amines (monoamines), amino acids,** and **peptides.** Biogenic amines and amino acids are synthesized in presynaptic terminals, whereas peptides are synthesized in neuronal cell bodies. Endocrine hormones and other substances can also function as neurotransmitters.

Presynaptic and postsynaptic receptors are proteins present in the membranes of neurons that can recognize specific neurotransmitters. When the presynaptic neuron is stimulated, the neurotransmitter is released, travels across the synaptic cleft (i.e., the space between the axon terminal of the presynaptic neuron and the dendrite of the postsynaptic neuron), and acts on receptors on the postsynaptic neuron. Neurotransmitters are excitatory if they increase the chance that a neuron will fire, and they are inhibitory if they decrease this chance.

Regulation of neurotransmitters

The concentration of neurotransmitters in the synaptic cleft is closely related to mood and behavior. Both passive and active mechanisms affect this concentration. After release by the presynaptic neuron, neurotransmitters are removed from the synaptic cleft passively by simple diffusion into local tissue. Active removal is accomplished by reuptake by the presynaptic neuron or by degradation by enzymes such as **monoamine oxidase** or acetylcholinesterase. Recent evidence indicates that not only lowered availability of neurotransmitters, but changes in the number, or affinity (sensitivity) of receptors for specific neurotransmitters (**neuronal plasticity**) and the efficiency with which a neurotransmitter signal is changed into a message, can regulate neuron responsiveness.

When stimulated by neurotransmitters, postsynaptic receptors also may alter the metabolism of neurons by the use of **second messengers** like cyclic adenosine and guanosine monophosphate, lipids like diacylglycerol, and Ca^{2+}. The eicosanoid metabolites and gases like nitric oxide also may act as second messengers as well as neurotransmitters.

Increased or decreased availability of specific neurotransmitters is associated with common psychiatric disorders and conditions (Table 5–3). Normalization of neurotransmitter availability by pharmacologic agents is associated with symptom relief for some of these disorders (see Chapter 19).

Biogenic amines

The **biogenic amines,** or **monoamines,** include catecholamines, indolamines, ethylamines, and quaternary amines. The monoamine theory of mood disorder hypothesizes that altered monoamine activity and related changes in monoamine receptors result in abnormalities of mood.

Dopamine. Dopamine, a catecholamine, is involved in the pathophysiology of Parkinson's disease, mood disorders, the conditioned fear response (see Chapter 9), and the "rewarding" nature of drugs of abuse (see Chapter 23). Dopamine has also been implicated in the pathophysiology of schizophrenia and other psychotic disorders (see Chapter 12).

At least five dopamine receptor subtypes have been identified and cloned (D_1, D_2, D_3, D_4, and D_5). Whereas the D_2 receptor subtype seems to be the major site of action for traditional antipsychotic agents, the D_1 and

TABLE 5-3	Neuropsychiatric Conditions, Associated Neurotransmitter Activity, and Implicated Brain Areas		
CONDITION	NEUROTRANSMITTER (MAJOR METABOLITE) ACTIVITY INCREASED ($\uparrow$) OR DECREASED ($\downarrow$)	PRIMARY BRAIN AREAS IMPLICATED IN SYMPTOM PRODUCTION	OTHER BRAIN AREAS IMPLICATED
Depression	Norepinephrine (MHPG) ($\downarrow$), serotonin (5-HIAA) ($\downarrow$), dopamine (HVA) ($\downarrow$)	Left prefrontal cortex	Limbic system
Mania	Dopamine (HVA) ($\uparrow$)	Right prefrontal cortex	Limbic system
Psychosis	Dopamine (HVA) ($\uparrow$), serotonin (5-HIAA) ($\uparrow$), glutamate ($\uparrow$)	Bilateral prefrontal cortex	Limbic system
Anxiety	γ-aminobutyric acid (GABA) ($\downarrow$), serotonin (5-HIAA) ($\downarrow$), norepinephrine (MHPG) ($\uparrow$)	Locus ceruleus	Right parahippocampal gyrus
Dementia	Acetylcholine (ACh) ($\downarrow$), glutamate ($\uparrow$)	Hippocampus	Nucleus basalis of Meynert (ACh production)

HVA, homovanillic acid; 5-HIAA, 5-hydroxyindoleacetic acid; MHPG, 3-methoxy-4-hydroxyphenyl-glycol.

D_4 subtypes are implicated in the action of the newer, "atypical" antipsychotics like clozapine (see Chapter 19). The three major dopaminergic tracts in the brain are the nigrostriatal tract, the tuberoinfundibular tract, and the mesolimbic-mesocortical tract (Fig. 5–3).

The **nigrostriatal tract** is involved in the regulation of muscle tone and movement and its degeneration is seen in Parkinson's disease. Treatment with traditional antipsychotic drugs, which block postsynaptic dopamine receptors receiving input from the nigrostriatal tract, can result in parkinsonism-like symptoms.

Dopamine acts on the **tuberoinfundibular tract** to inhibit the secretion of prolactin from the anterior pituitary. Blockade of dopamine receptors by antipsychotic drugs prevents this inhibition, ultimately leading to elevated prolactin levels and side effects like breast enlargement, galactorrhea, and sexual dysfunction.

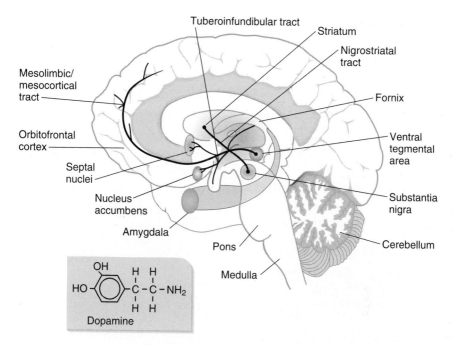

FIGURE 5-3. Distribution of dopaminergic axons in the central nervous system. Most dopamine-containing fibers arise from the substantia nigra (which projects to the striatum) and the ventral tegmental area.

The **mesolimbic/mesocortical tract** is associated with the manifestations of psychosis and may have a role in expression of emotions because it projects into the limbic system and prefrontal cortex. Hyperactivity of the mesolimbic tract is associated with the positive symptoms and hyperactivity of the mesocortical tract with the negative symptoms of schizophrenia (see Chapter 12) (Stahl, 2001).

Another important dopaminergic pathway in the brain runs from the ventral tegmental area to the nucleus accumbens (Fig. 5–3). This pathway becomes activated following use of some drugs of abuse, suggesting that it is involved in the rewarding and addictive nature of these agents (see Chapter 23).

Norepinephrine. Norepinephrine, a catecholamine, plays a role in mood, anxiety, arousal, learning, and memory. Like dopaminergic neurons, noradrenergic neurons synthesize dopamine. After synthesis, dopamine β-hydroxylase, present in noradrenergic neurons, converts this dopamine to norepinephrine. Most noradrenergic neurons (approximately 10,000 per hemisphere in the brain) are located in nuclei in the upper brainstem; the most important of these is the **locus ceruleus** (Fig. 5–4).

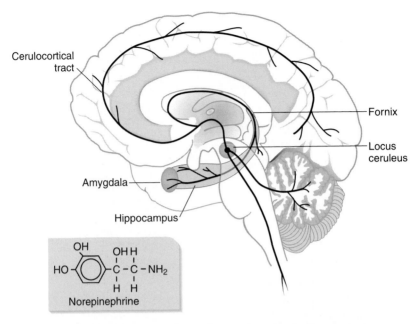

FIGURE 5-4. Distribution of noradrenergic axons in the central nervous system (CNS). Most noradrenaline-containing fibers arise from the locus ceruleus and are distributed throughout the CNS.

Serotonin. Serotonin, an indolamine, plays a role in mood, sleep, pain sensitivity, appetite, sexuality, and impulse control. In the synthesis of serotonin, the amino acid tryptophan is converted to serotonin (also known as 5-hydroxytryptamine) by the enzyme tryptophan hydroxylase as well as by an amino acid decarboxylase. Anatomically, most serotonergic cell bodies in the brain are located in the **dorsal raphe nucleus** in the upper pons and lower midbrain (Fig. 5–5).

Increased brain serotonin concentrations are associated with positive effects like improved mood and sleep, as well as negative effects like decreased sexual function (particularly delayed orgasm) and, in high concentrations, psychotic symptoms. Because of this, newer antipsychotic medications work on normalizing serotonergic as well as dopaminergic systems (see Chapter 19). Decreased serotonin availability is associated with depression of mood, poor impulse control, violent behavior, alcoholism, chronic pain syndromes, sleep disorders, and anxiety disorders like OCD. Through different mechanisms, all antidepressant medications currently in use increase the availability of serotonin and other biogenic amines in the synaptic cleft (see Chapter 19).

Acetylcholine and histamine. Acetylcholine (ACh), a quaternary amine, and **histamine**, an ethylamine, are neurotransmitters involved in behavior and in the troubling side effects of psychoactive medication.

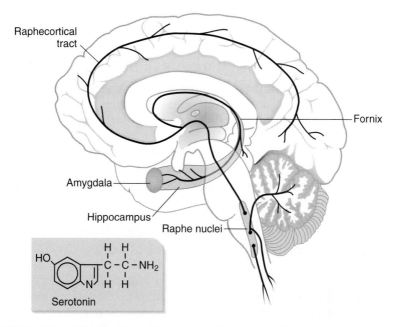

FIGURE 5-5. Distribution of serotonergic axons in the central nervous system (CNS). Most serotonin-containing fibers arise from the raphe nuclei and are distributed throughout the CNS.

Acetylcholine is used by nerve-skeleton-muscle junctions. Cholinergic neurons synthesize ACh from acetyl coenzyme A and choline using the enzyme choline acetyltransferase. The enzyme **acetylcholinesterase (AChE)** breaks ACh down into choline and acetate. Involved but probably not causal in mood disorders, cholinergic mechanisms are critical in cognitive functioning. Loss of cholinergic neurons or decreased availability of acetylcholine due to decreased production of the synthesizing enzyme **choline acetyltransferase** results in cognitive disorders like dementia of the Alzheimer type (Alzheimer's disease). Down's syndrome, movement disorders, and sleep disorders (see Chapter 7) also are related to decreased availability of ACh. Although no pharmacologic treatment has been able to reverse lost function in patients with Alzheimer's disease, blocking the action of AChE with drugs such as donepezil (Aricept), rivastigmine (Exelon), and galantamine (Reminyl) can delay progression of the disease (see Chapter 19).

Muscarinic ACh receptors play a greater role in behavior and in the side effects of psychoactive agents than **nicotinic** ACh receptors. Blockade of muscarinic receptors with drugs such as antipsychotics and tricyclic antidepressants results in the classic **anticholinergic side effects** seen with use of these drugs, including dry mouth, blurred vision, urinary hesitancy, and constipation.

The availability of histamine is also altered by psychoactive agents. Histamine-receptor blockade with drugs such as antipsychotics and tricyclic antidepressants is responsible in part for common side effects of these agents, such as sedation and increased appetite leading to weight gain.

Other neurotransmitters involved in behavior

Amino acid neurotransmitters like **g-aminobutyric acid (GABA), glycine,** and **glutamate** are involved in most synapses in the brain. These and neuropeptides, like the **endogenous opioids,** have a role in behavior.

Amino acids. γ-**Aminobutyric acid** is the principal inhibitory neurotransmitter in the CNS and is closely associated with the symptoms of anxiety. The effectiveness of the antianxiety agents, like the benzodiazepines (e.g., diazepam [Valium]) and barbiturates (e.g., secobarbital [Seconal]) (see Chapter 19), involves their ability to increase the affinity of GABA for its binding site, allowing chloride to enter the neuron. As a result, the neuron becomes hyperpolarized and inhibited, decreasing neuronal firing and ultimately decreasing anxiety.

Glycine is an inhibitory neurotransmitter found primarily in the spinal cord. It works on its own and as a regulator of the excitatory neurotransmitter glutamate. **Glutamate** itself has been associated with epilepsy, neurodegenerative illnesses, memory formation, mechanisms of cell death, and schizophrenia. Symptoms of schizophrenia have been linked specifically to alterations in the major glutamate receptor, N-methyl-D-aspartate (NMDA). Drugs that block NMDA induce psychotic symptoms in healthy volunteers (Tamminga & Frost, 2001), and genes linked to the development of schizophrenia are associated with disruption of the NMDA-receptor pathway (Chumakov et al., 2001).

Neuropeptides. Neuropeptides that act on behavior include the endogenous opioids, the **enkephalins** and **endorphins.** These neurotransmitters are produced by the brain itself, serve to decrease pain and anxiety, and have a role in addiction and mood.

Placebo effects (i.e., subjective responsiveness to inactive pharmacologic agents) may be mediated by the endogenous opioid and dopaminergic systems. Prior treatment with an opioid-receptor blocker like naloxone can inhibit placebo effects (Sher, 1997). Placebo-induced release of endogenous dopamine in the striatum of patients with Parkinson's disease has also been demonstrated (de la Fuente-Fernandez et al., 2001).

Other neuropeptides associated with psychiatric disorders include:

- **Cholecystokinin** (CCK) and **neurotensin** with schizophrenia
- **Somatostatin, substance P, vasopressin, oxytocin,** and **vasoactive intestinal peptide** (VIP) with mood disorders
- Somatostatin, and substance P with Huntington's disease
- Somatostatin and VIP with dementia of the Alzheimer's type
- Substance P and CCK with anxiety disorders
- Substance P with pain and aggression

REVIEW QUESTIONS

Questions 1–2

Blood plasma analysis of a 25-year-old female patient shows an increased concentration of homovanillic acid (HVA).

1. Of the following disorders, this finding is most closely associated with
   - (A) Parkinson's disease
   - (B) Untreated depression
   - (C) Treated schizophrenia
   - (D) Pheochromocytoma
   - (E) Untreated schizophrenia

2. If this diagnosis is appropriate, the size of cerebral ventricles, glucose utilization in the frontal lobes, and size of limbic structures in this patient are most likely to be respectively
   - (A) Increased, decreased, decreased
   - (B) Increased, decreased, increased
   - (C) Increased, increased, decreased
   - (D) Decreased, decreased, decreased
   - (E) Decreased, increased, decreased
   - (F) Decreased, increased, increased

Questions 3–4

A right-handed 61-year-old stroke patient tells the physician that since the stroke he feels "down" and no longer has interest in food or in any of the activities he formerly enjoyed.

3. This patient's mood symptoms suggest that the part of his brain most likely to have been affected by the stroke is the
   - (A) right temporal lobe
   - (B) left temporal lobe
   - (C) right parietal lobe
   - (D) left parietal lobe
   - (E) right frontal lobe
   - (F) left frontal lobe

4. Analysis of the body fluids of this depressed patient are most likely to show
   - (A) increased 3-methoxy-4-hydroxyphenylglycol (MHPG)
   - (B) increased acetylcholine

(C) increased 5-hydroxyindoleacetic acid (5-HIAA)

(D) decreased 5-HIAA

(E) increased homovanillic acid (HVA)

5. A 25-year-old male patient who is withdrawing from heroin shows intense anxiety, increased pulse, elevated blood pressure, and hand tremor. When he is given clonidine, his symptoms improve. The area of the brain most likely to be involved in the improvement in this patient's symptoms is (are) the

(A) right parietal lobe

(B) basal ganglia

(C) locus ceruleus

(D) raphe nuclei

(E) amygdala

(F) substantia nigra

6. A 33-year-old woman shows side effects such as sedation, increased appetite, and weight gain while being treated with antipsychotic medication. Of the following, the mechanism most closely associated with these effects is

(A) blockade of serotonin receptors

(B) blockade of dopamine receptors

(C) blockade of norepinephrine receptors

(D) blockade of histamine receptors

(E) decreased availability of serotonin

7. A 70-year-old former college professor cannot tell you the name of the current president and has difficulty identifying the man sitting next to her (her son). She began having memory problems 3 years ago. Her motor function is essentially normal. Of the following, the areas of the brain most likely to be affected in this patient are the

(A) right parietal lobe and basal ganglia

(B) basal ganglia and left parietal lobes

(C) hippocampus and nucleus basalis of Meynert

(D) reticular system and hippocampus

(E) amygdala and left temporal lobe

(F) right frontal lobe and nucleus basalis of Meynert

ANSWERS AND EXPLANATIONS

1-E, 2-A. Although not diagnostic, increased body fluid concentrations of homovanillic acid (HVA), a major metabolite of dopamine, are more likely to be seen in unmedicated schizophrenic patients. Decreased HVA is more likely to be seen in Parkinson's disease, depression, and in medicated schizophrenic patients. Increased vanillylmandelic acid (VMA), a metabolite of norepinephrine, is characteristic of pheochromocytoma. Decreased body fluid concentrations of 5-HIAA, a metabolite of serotonin, are more likely to be seen in depression. Although neuroimaging cannot be used to diagnose psychiatric illness, the brains of schizophrenics show increased size of cerebral ventricles; decreased size of the hippocampus and limbic structures such as the amygdala; and decreased glucose usage in the frontal lobes.

3-F, 4-D. Of the listed brain areas, depression is most likely to be associated with damage to the left frontal lobe. Decreased body fluid concentrations of 5-HIAA, a metabolite of serotonin, as well as decreased HVA and MHPG, metabolites of dopamine and norepinephrine, respectively, are seen in depression.

5-C. Clonidine is an alpha-2-adrenergic receptor agonist. Its effectiveness in treating withdrawal symptoms associated with use of opiates and sedatives is believed to be due to its action on noradrenergic neurons in the locus ceruleus.

6-D. Sedation, increased appetite, and weight gain are side effects of treatment with certain antipsychotic agents. The mechanism most closely associated with these side effects is blockade of histamine receptors. Blockade of dopamine receptors by these antipsychotic medications is associated also with side effects such as parkinsonism-like symptoms and elevated prolactin levels.

7-C. This patient probably has dementia of the Alzheimer type. Of the listed brain areas, the ones most closely implicated in this disorder are the hippocampus and nucleus basalis of Meynert.

REFERENCES

Bartrés-Faz, D., Junqué, C., Moral, P., López-Alomar, A., Sánchez-Aldeguer, J., & Clemente, I. C. (2002). Apolipoprotein E gender effects on cognitive performance in age-associated memory impairment. *J Neuropsych Clin Neurosci, 14,* 80–83.

Baxter, L.R. (1999). Functional imaging of brain systems mediating obsessive compulsive disorder. In D. S. Charney, E. J. Nestler, & B. S. Bunney (Eds.). *Neurobiology of mental illness* (pp. 534–547). New York: Oxford University Press.

Bouchard, T. J., Lykken, D. T., McGue, M., Segal, N. L., & Tellegen, A. (1990). Sources of human psychological differences: The Minnesota study of twins reared apart. *Science, 250,* 223.

Bouchard, T. J., & McGue, M. (1981). Familial studies of intelligence: A review. *Science, 212,* 1055–1059.

Carlsson, A. (2001). A paradigm shift in brain research. *Science, 294,* 1021–1024.

Chumakov, I., Blumenfeld, M., Guerassimenko, O., Cavarec, L., Palicio, M., Abderrahim, H., et al. (2002). Genetic and physiological data implicating the new human gene G72 and the gene for D-amino acid oxidase in schizophrenia. *Proc Natl Acad Sci, 99,* 13675–13680.

Davidson, R. J., & Irwin, W. (1999). The functional neuroanatomy of emotion and affective style. *Trends Cog Sci, 3,* 11–21.

de la Fuente-Fernandez, R., Ruth, T. J., Sossi, V., Schulzer, M., Calne, D. B., & Stoessl, A. J. (2001). Expectation and dopamine release: Mechanism of the placebo effect in Parkinson's disease. *Science, 293,* 1164–1166.

Ewald, H., Koed, K., Mors, O., Flint, T., & Kruse, T. A. (1997). Linkage analysis between manic-depressive illness and chromosome 18. A review and a study of Danish families. *Psych Gen, 7,* 1–12.

Ewald, H., & Kruse, T. A. (1997). Bipolar affective disorder, chromosome 16p13.3 and recessive disease genes. *Am J Med Genet, 72,* 549–550.

Ewald, H., Degn, B., Mors, O., & Kruse, T. A. (1998). Significant linkage between bipolar affective disorder and chromosome 12q. *Psychiatr Genet, 8,* 131–140.

Goldstein, R. Z., & Volkow, N. D. (2002). Drug addiction and its underlying neurobiological basis: Neuroimaging evidence for the involvement of the frontal cortex. *Am J Psychiatry, 159,* 1642–1652

Goy, R. W., & McEwen, B. S. (1980). *Sexual differentiation of the brain.* Cambridge: MIT Press.

Halpern, D. F. (2000). *Sex differences in cognitive abilities* (3rd ed.). Mahwah, NJ: Lawrence Ehrlbaum Associates.

Harlow, J. M. (1868). Recovery after severe injury to the head. *Publ Mass Med Soc, 2,* 327–346.

Heninger, G. R. (1995). Indoleamines: The role of serotonin in clinical disorders. In F. E. Bloom & D. J. Kupfer (Eds.), *Psychopharmacology: The fourth generation of progress.* New York: Raven Press.

Joffe, R. (2000). Thyroid hormones. In B. J. Sadock & V. A Sadock (Eds.), *Comprehensive textbook of psychiatry* (7th ed., Vol. II). Philadelphia: Lippincott, Williams & Wilkins.

Kandel, E. R., Schwartz, J. H., & Jessell, T. M. (2000). *Principles of neural science* (4th ed.). New York: Appleton and Lange.

Kingsley, R. E. (2000). *Concise text of neuroscience.* Philadelphia: Lippincott, Williams & Wilkins.

LeVay, S. (1991). A difference in hypothalamic structure between heterosexual and homosexual men. *Science, 253,* 1034–1037.

Loehlin, J. C., & Nicholas, R. C. (1976). *Heredity, environment and personality.* Austin: University of Texas Press.

McHugh, P. F., Kellogg, S., Bell, K., Schluger, R. P., Leal, S. M., & Kreek, M. J. (2002). Potentially functional polymorphism in the promoter region of prodynorphin gene may be associated with protection against cocaine dependence or abuse. *Am J Med Genet,* 114(4), 4.

Nestler, E. J., Hyman, S. E., & Malenka, R. C. (2001). *Molecular neuropharmacology.* New York: McGraw Hill.

Shaywitz, B. A., Shaywitz, S. E., Pugh, K., Constable, R. T., Skudlarski, P., Fulbright, R. K., et al. (1995). Sex differences in the functional organization of the brain for language. *Nature, 373,* 607–609.

Sher, L. (1997). The placebo effect on mood and behavior: the role of the endogenous opioid system. *Med Hypotheses, 48,* 347–349.

Stahl, S. M. (2001). 670 "hit-and-run" actions at dopamine receptors, part 1: Mechanism of action of atypical antipsychotics. *J Clin Psychiatry, 62,* 923.

Stefansson, H., Sarginson, J., Kong, A., Yates, P., Steinthorsdottir, V., Gudfinnsson, E., et al. (2002). Association of neuregulin 1 with schizophrenia confirmed in a Scottish population. *Am J Hum Genet, 72,* 83–87.

Straub, R. E., Jiang, Y., MacLean, C.J., Ma, Y., Webb, B. T., Myakishev, M. V., et al. (2002). Genetic variation in the 6p22.3 gene DTNBP1, the human ortholog of the mouse dysbindin gene, is associated with schizophrenia. *Am J Hum Genet, 71,* 337–478.

Tamminga, C. A., & Frost, D. O. (2001). Changing concepts in the neurochemistry of schizophrenia. *Am J Psychiatry, 158,* 1365–1366.

Teasdale, G., & Jennett, B. (1974). The Glasgow coma scale. *Lancet, 2,* 81–83.

Thompson, P. M., Cannon, T. D., Narr, K. L., van Erp, T., Poutaned, V., Huttunen, M., et al. (2001). Genetic influences on brain structure. *Nat Neurosci, 4,* 1253–1258.

Biological   **6**
Assessment
of Patients
With Psychiatric
Symptoms

B iological abnormalities, unidentified medical illnesses and substance abuse can cause psychiatric symptoms in otherwise mentally healthy individuals and can exacerbate such symptoms in persons already diagnosed with psychiatric illnesses. For example, hypo- or hyperglycemia can present with symptoms of anxiety, while depression may be an early sign of pancreatic carcinoma. To identify and treat the underlying medical problem, physical examination and specific biological tests and procedures are used in the clinical evaluation of patients who exhibit behavioral symptoms.

▓ PHYSICAL EXAMINATION

A complete physical examination is essential when evaluating individuals with psychiatric symptoms. Of particular importance in the physical examination is the assessment of neurological function, particularly of sensory systems like vision and hearing. In certain people, particularly the

THE PATIENT The wife of a retired 73-year-old man tells the doctor that her husband has been acting differently over the past few months. She reports that he no longer does the crossword puzzles he formerly enjoyed and shows little interest in the television shows he looked forward to weekly. His wife is convinced that he is depressed or is developing Alzheimer's disease. Physical and neurological examinations are essentially normal, but ocular examination reveals bilateral central lens opacities (cataracts).

COMMENT This case illustrates why physical examination is important for patients who are suspected of having a psychiatric illness. This patient shows symptoms of depression (e.g., decreased interest and lack of enjoyment in usual activities) in response to decreased sensory stimulation caused by his gradual loss of vision. In some patients, decreased vision or hearing can even result in symptoms resembling those of psychosis or dementia. For several reasons, including the fact that symptoms of sensory loss typically come on gradually, elderly patients may not identify the problem until it has caused significant social impairment.

TREATMENT When the cataracts are treated and his vision improves, the patient's interest in his environment and day-to-day activities should return. If there is no significant improvement, other reasons for the patient's depression, including the onset of dementia, should be identified and addressed.

elderly, sensory impairment can result in psychiatric symptoms like depression (see Chapter 4).

Physical abnormalities also can result from behavioral problems. For example, skin lesions identified in the physical examination can indicate illegal drug use or unreported domestic abuse.

■ LABORATORY STUDIES

Screening tests

Basic laboratory screening studies, such as urinalysis and blood studies, can help rule out physiological causes of psychiatric symptoms. Blood studies include complete blood count, erythrocyte sedimentation rate, and the **metabolic screening battery** (serum electrolyte level, glucose level and hepatic and renal function tests).

Tests of endocrine function are particularly important in patients with behavioral symptoms. Patients with depression may have endocrine irregularities, including abnormalities in growth hormone, melatonin, gonadotropin, and thyroid hormone. Abnormalities in gonadotropins are seen also in patients with schizophrenia. Patients with adrenal disorders like **Addison's disease** and **Cushing's syndrome** classically demonstrate psychiatric symptoms.

Thyroid function tests are used to screen for hypothyroidism and hyperthyroidism, which can mimic depression and anxiety, respectively.

THE PATIENT A 40-year-old female patient visits her family physician complaining of fatigue and feeling "cold all the time." Her symptoms started about one year ago. The interview reveals that the patient feels that her job as a schoolteacher has become too "draining" and she wants to give it up. She also relates that her marriage is in trouble because her husband does not understand why she is too tired to go out in the evenings or on weekends. The patient says that these problems have made her feel sad and hopeless and that she cries frequently.

Physical examination reveals that the patient has gained 8 pounds in the past year. Her skin and hair appear dry and her voice is hoarse. Otherwise, the physical exam is unremarkable.

Laboratory studies indicate that serum concentrations of thyroid stimulating hormone (TSH) are increased and triiodothyronine (T_3) and thyroxine (T_4) are decreased.

COMMENT Hypothyroid patients like this woman can present with symptoms of depression. Thyroid status therefore must be evaluated in patients who show depression along with classic symptoms of hypothyroidism like cold intolerance, weight gain, lethargy, and dryness of the skin and hair. Voice and hearing changes also may occur in hypothyroid patients because of edema of the larynx and middle ear. Other symptoms of hypothyroidism include constipation, menstrual irregularities, and slow return of deep tendon reflexes.

TREATMENT Treatment with l-thyroxine (Synthroid) starting with a low dose and titrating up to a maintenance dose of 0.1 to 0.15 mg/day is indicated for this patient. Within a few weeks, there should be normalization of serum thyroid hormone and TSH levels. Clinical improvement in her emotional and physical symptoms may take longer. Thyroid hormones also can be used to augment the effectiveness of antidepressant medication not only in hypothyroid patients like this one, but in euthyroid patients as well (see Chapter 19).

Although no clear association exists between primary depressive illness and abnormal thyroid function, about one third of depressed patients show decreased thyrotropin response to thyrotropin-releasing hormone. Clearly, thyroid function should be evaluated in depressed patients who also show physical symptoms of hypothyroidism. In a similar way, anxious, agitated patients who also show tremor and weight loss should be evaluated for hyperthyroidism.

Table 6–1 provides a summary of laboratory test results for patients with psychiatric symptoms that may be caused by physical illnesses. Analysis of blood **B$_{12}$** and **folate levels** and a **toxicology screen** to identify drug abuse (Table 6-2) should also be conducted for these patients.

Pharmacotherapy patients

Laboratory tests are used to monitor patients for biological complications of pharmacotherapy (see Chapter 19). Some psychoactive agents are more

TABLE 6-1	Laboratory Testing of Patients With Psychiatric Symptoms		
MAJOR PSYCHIATRIC SYMPTOM*	**SUSPECTED PHYSICAL CONDITION**	**PHYSICAL SYMPTOMS**	**LABORATORY TEST RESULTS**
Depression	Hypothyroidism (myxedema)	■ Fatigue ■ Weight gain ■ Constipation ■ Edema ■ Hair loss ■ Cold intolerance	■ Increased TSH ■ Decreased T_3 ■ Decreased free T_4
	Addison's disease (adrenocortical insufficiency)	■ Hyperpigmentation ■ Hypotension ■ Weakness/fatigue	■ Decreased Na^+ ■ Increased K^+ ■ Eosinophilia
	Cushing's syndrome (adrenocortical excess)	■ Purple stria ■ Central (abdominal) obesity ■ Bruising ■ Muscle weakness	■ Positive dexamethasone suppression test ■ Poor glucose tolerance
	Pancreatic carcinoma	■ Weight loss ■ Abdominal pain	■ Increased amylase
Anxiety	Hyperthyroidism (thyrotoxicosis)	■ Flushing, fever ■ Weight loss ■ Diarrhea	■ Decreased TSH ■ Increased T_3 ■ Increased free T_4
	Pheochromocytoma	■ Hypertension ■ Headache ■ Tachycardia ■ Tremor	■ Urinary metanephrine work-up: elevated VMA
	Hypoglycemia	■ Sweating ■ Tachycardia ■ Somnolence	■ Low blood sugar
	Hyperglycemia	■ Polyuria ■ Nausea and vomiting ■ Anorexia	■ High blood sugar ■ Ketones in blood and urine ■ Anion gap acidosis

TABLE 6-1	Laboratory Testing of Patients With Psychiatric Symptoms (Continued)		
MAJOR PSYCHIATRIC SYMPTOM*	SUSPECTED PHYSICAL CONDITION	PHYSICAL SYMPTOMS	LABORATORY TEST RESULTS
Psychosis or personality changes	■ AIDS dementia	■ Ataxia ■ Weight loss ■ Fever	■ Positive HIV test ■ Low B_{12} level
	Acute intermittent porphyria	■ Peripheral neuropathy ■ Abdominal pain, nausea and vomiting ■ Fever	■ Elevated d-aminolevulinic acid ■ Elevated porphobilinogen ■ Leukocytosis
	Connective tissue disorders (e.g., SLE, rheumatoid arthritis)	■ Skin, nail, and mucous membrane changes ■ Joint pain ■ Fever ■ Headache	■ Anemia ■ Positive antiphospholipid ■ Positive ANA ■ Positive rheumatoid factor
	Hypoparathyroidism	■ Muscle spasm ■ Laryngeal spasm ■ Headache ■ Tetany ■ Paresthesias	■ Decreased Ca^2
	Hyperparathyroidism	■ Bone pain ■ Polydipsia ■ Constipation ■ Nausea	■ Variable PTH levels ■ Increased Ca^2
	Wilson's disease	■ Gait abnormalities ■ Rigidity	■ Increased urinary copper ■ Decreased serum ceruloplasmin

*Note that almost any psychiatric symptom can occur in almost any physical illness. ANA, antinuclear antibody; CT, computed tomography; PTH, parathyroid hormone; SLE, systemic lupus erythematosus; TSH, thyrotropin-stimulating hormone; T_3, triiodothyronine; T_4, thyroxine; VMA, vanillylmandelic acid.

TABLE 6-2	Laboratory Findings for Selected Drugs of Abuse	
CLASS OF SUBSTANCE	ELEVATED LEVELS IN BODY FLUIDS	LENGTH OF TIME AFTER USE THAT SUBSTANCE CAN BE DETECTED
Sedatives	Alcohol (legal intoxication is 0.08%–0.15% BAC, depending on state laws; coma occurs at BAC of 0.40%–0.50% in nonalcoholics)	Hours
	Gamma-glutamyltransferase	Hours
	Specific barbiturate or benzodiazepine or its metabolite	7 days or less
Opioids	Opiate other than methadone	12–36 hours
	Methadone	2–3 days
Stimulants	Cotinine (nicotine metabolite)	1–2 days
	Amphetamine	1–2 days
	Benzoylecgonine (cocaine metabolite)	1–3 days in occasional users; longer in heavy users
Hallucinogens and related agents	Cannabinoid metabolites	7–28 days
	Serum glutamic-oxaloacetic transaminase level and creatinine phosphokinase (reflecting muscle damage associated with PCP use)	More than 7 days

BAC, blood alcohol concentration; PCP, phencyclidine.

likely to cause physical difficulties than others. Specifically, the **mood stabilizing agents,** carbamazepine (Tegretol) and valproic acid (Depakene, Depakote) are associated with abnormal liver function. Carbamazepine and the antipsychotic agent clozapine (Clozaril) are associated with blood abnormalities such as agranulocytosis (decreased number of granulocytic white blood cells). These abnormalities usually become apparent within the first few months of treatment.

Because they can develop hypothyroidism and kidney problems, patients being treated with the antimanic agent **lithium** should have regular thyroid (T_3, T_4, and TSH) and kidney function (blood urea nitrogen, creatinine, and urinanalysis) tests. Because of the drug's narrow therapeutic range, lithium levels also should be monitored regularly. Plasma concentrations of some antipsychotic and antidepressant agents also may be measured to evaluate patient compliance or to determine whether therapeutic blood levels of the agent have been reached in nonresponding patients.

Measurement of biogenic amines

Altered concentrations of monoamines in neural tissue are involved in the manifestations of major psychiatric disorders (see Chapter 5). Despite this close association, it is difficult to correlate directly or predict how changes in these concentrations are associated with changes in behavior. One reason for this is that for practical reasons, levels of monoamines cannot be measured in the brain tissue of living patients. Instead, metabolites of the monoamines, present in higher quantities than the actual monamines, are measured in body fluids like cerebrospinal fluid (CSF), blood, and urine. Although not commonly used in diagnosis, measurement of these metabolites can provide useful clinical and research information about the patient (Table 6–3).

TABLE 6-3	Monoamines: Metabolites, Brain Production, and Associated Psychopathology	
NEUROTRANSMITTER (PRIMARY SITE OF PRODUCTION IN BRAIN)	**CONCENTRATION OF METABOLITE IN BLOOD PLASMA, CEREBROSPINAL FLUID, OR URINE (INCREASED [↑] OR DECREASED [↓])**	**ASSOCIATED PSYCHOPATHOLOGY**
Dopamine (Substantia nigra, ventral tegmental area)	(↑) HVA	■ Schizophrenia ■ Other psychotic illnesses
	(↓) HVA	■ Parkinson's disease ■ Patients treated with antipsychotic agents ■ Depression
Norepinephrine (Locus ceruleus)	(↑) VMA	■ Adrenal medulla tumor (pheochromocytoma)
	(↓) MHPG	■ Severe depression ■ Attempted suicide
Serotonin (Raphe nuclei)	(↓) 5-HIAA	■ Severe depression ■ Attempted suicide ■ Aggressiveness and violence ■ Impulsiveness ■ Fire setting ■ Tourette's syndrome ■ Alcohol abuse ■ Bulimia

5-HIAA, 5-hydroxyindoleacetic acid; HVA, homovanillic acid; MHPG, 3-methoxy-4-hydroxyphenylglycol; VMA, vanillylmandelic acid.

◼ DIAGNOSTIC TESTS

Psychiatric diagnosis is mostly based on the clinical interview (see Chapter 24) and is augmented by standardized neuropsychological (see below) and psychological tests (see Chapter 10). However, diagnostic instruments, such as the **dexamethasone suppression test, drug-assisted interviewing, sodium lactate administration,** and **galvanic skin response,** can provide supplemental information when formulating psychiatric diagnoses.

Dexamethasone suppression test

In a person with a normal hypothalamic-adrenal-pituitary axis, administration of 1 mg of dexamethasone, a synthetic glucocorticoid equivalent to 25 mg of cortisol, suppresses the endogenous secretion of cortisol. In contrast, approximately one-half of patients with major depressive disorder have a positive dexamethasone suppression test (DST) (i.e., this suppression is limited or absent).

The DST has been used to predict responsiveness to biological therapies for depression because patients with a positive DST are more likely to respond to treatment with antidepressant agents or to electroconvulsive therapy (see Chapter 19). One reason for the limited clinical usefulness of the DST in the diagnosis of depression is that positive findings are not specific. False-positive results (nonsuppression) are associated with schizophrenia, dementia, pregnancy, anorexia nervosa, severe weight loss, and Cushing's disease, as well as abuse of alcohol and withdrawal from benzodiazepines. False-negative results on the DST are associated with Addison's disease and treatment with benzodiazepines or high doses of steroids.

Drug-assisted interviewing

Drug-assisted interviewing can be used to indicate whether organic pathology is responsible for a patient's psychiatric symptoms. This technique involves administration of a sedative agent prior to the clinical interview with the purpose of relaxing the patient and facilitating coherent verbal expression. Drug-assisted interviewing is particularly useful in identifying conditions involving high levels of anxiety like dissociative disorders, and conversion disorder as well as mute psychotic states, and malingering. Sedative agents that have been used for this purpose include amobarbital sodium (given intravenously, also known as **the Amytal interview**), other barbiturates, and benzodiazepines.

Sodium lactate administration

Because intravenous administration of sodium lactate can provoke a panic attack (see Chapter 15) in susceptible patients, this procedure can help to identify individuals with **panic disorder.** The simpler procedure of inhaling of carbon dioxide can produce the same effect.

Galvanic skin response

Galvanic skin response, a component of the **lie detector test,** uses the finding that the electric resistance of skin varies with a person's psychological state. Higher sweat gland activity, seen with sympathetic nervous system arousal (e.g., when lying), results in decreased skin resistance and a positive test. However, anxious people can have positive tests although they are not lying. Also, people who are not bothered by telling lies, such as those antisocial personality disorders, can have negative tests. In part because of the likelihood of such false positives and false negatives, the results of lie detector tests are not generally admissible as evidence in courts of law.

■ NEUROLOGICAL EVALUATION

Neuroimaging

Structural and physiological abnormalities in the brain can be identified using a variety of neurodiagnostic tests. Structural changes can be identified by **computed tomography (CT)** and magnetic resonance imaging (MRI) (Fig. 6–1). Physiological changes can be identified by **positron-emission tomography (PET)** (Fig. 6–2), **functional magnetic resonance imaging (fMRI)** (see Fig. 5–2), and **single photon emission computed tomography (SPECT).** Because activation of the anterior cingulate gyrus,

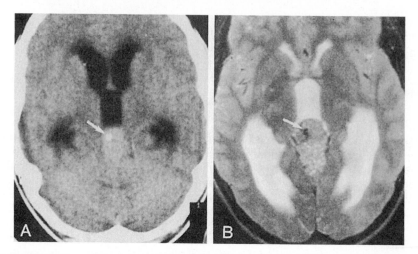

FIGURE 6-1.   Comparison of computed tomography **(A)** and magnetic resonance imaging **(B)** scans. The arrow identifies a calcified lesion (tumor) in the pineal gland. In **(A),** cerebrospinal fluid (CSF) appears black; brain tissue is gray (gray and white matter cannot be differentiated); and the skull is white. In **(B),** CSF appears white; gray and white brain matter can be distinguished as shades of gray; and the skull is black.

(Reprinted with permission from Grossman, C. B. (1996). Magnetic resonance imaging and computed tomography of the head and spine (2nd ed.). Baltimore: Williams & Wilkins.)

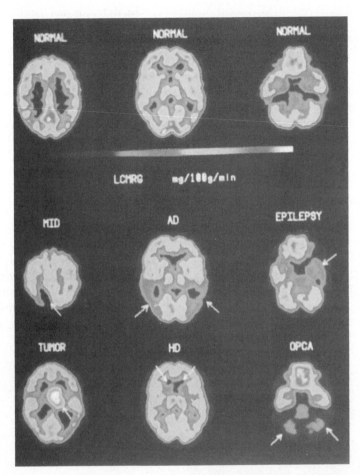

FIGURE 6-2. Positron-emission tomography scans at three different brain levels. From left to right: high level through the parietal lobes, intermediate level through the basal ganglia and low level through the base of the frontal lobes, temporal lobes and cerebellum) in a control patient and in six patients with neurological disorders: multi-infarct dementia (MID) (arrow points to area of absent glucose metabolism); Alzheimer's disease (AD) (arrows point to hypometabolism in both parietal lobes); temporal lobe epilepsy (arrow points to hypometabolism in the right temporal lobe); brain tumor (arrow points to hypermetabolism in the site of the tumor, thalamus); Huntington's disease (HD) (arrows point to bilateral hypometabolism in the caudate nuclei); and olivopontocerebellar atrophy (OPCA) (arrow points to hypometabolism in the cerebellum and brainstem).

(Reprinted with permission from Gilman, S. (1992). Advances in neurology. N Engl J Med, 326, 1610.)

TABLE 6-4	Neuroimaging in the Biological Evaluation of the Psychiatric Patient
TEST	**USES AND CHARACTERISTICS**
Computed tomography (CT)	▪ Identifies anatomically based brain changes (e.g., enlarged brain ventricles) in cognitive and psychotic disorders
Magnetic resonance imaging (MRI)	▪ Identifies demyelinating disease (e.g., multiple sclerosis) ▪ Shows the anatomic and biochemical condition of neural tissues without exposing the patient to ionizing radiation
Functional MRI (fMRI)	▪ Detects and visualizes rapid biochemical changes in neural tissue during specific tasks or as a result of trauma
Positron emission tomography (PET)	▪ Localizes areas of the brain that are physiologically active during specific tasks by characterizing and measuring metabolism of glucose in neural tissue ▪ Measures specific neurotransmitter receptors using positron-emitting compounds ▪ Requires availability of a cyclotron because of short half-life of such compounds
Single photon emission computed tomography (SPECT)	▪ Obtains similar data to PET but is more practical for clinical use because it uses a standard gamma camera rather than a cyclotron

a component of the limbic system (see Chapter 5), is seen in volunteers instructed to lie during a specific task (Langleben et al., 2002), neuroimaging may someday provide another tool for law enforcement to detect when a person is lying. Other specific uses for each of these tests can be found in Table 6–4.

Electroencephalogram

The electroencephalogram (EEG) measures electrical activity in the cortex. It is used in diagnosing epilepsy (sharp waves, spikes, and paroxysmal activity) and in differentiating delirium (slowing of the EEG) from dementia (often-normal EEG). Although the EEG is not particularly useful in clinical diagnosis, abnormalities in the EEG are seen in some psychiatric disorders. In schizophrenia, the EEG shows decreased alpha waves, increased theta and delta waves, and epileptiform activity.

Evoked EEG (evoked potentials) is a testing procedure that quantifies electrical activity in the cortex in response to tactile, auditory, or visual stimulation. This test is used to evaluate vision and hearing loss in infants and brain responses in comatose and suspected brain-dead patients (see Chapter 26).

Neuropsychological tests

Neuropsychological tests are designed to augment the clinical impression in patients with suspected neurologic problems. In particular, these tests assess general intelligence, memory, reasoning, orientation, perceptuomotor performance, language function, attention, and concentration. Tests that are used include the **Halstead-Reitan Battery** (to detect and localize brain lesions and determine their effects), the **Luria-Nebraska Neuropsychological Battery** (to determine left or right cerebral dominance and specific types of brain dysfunction, such as dyslexia), and the **Bender Visual Motor Gestalt Test** (to evaluate visual and motor ability in adults and children through the reproduction of designs) (Figs. 6–3, 6–4).

The **Folstein Mini-Mental State Examination** is a neuropsychological test commonly used at the bedside to follow improvement or deterioration in function in patients with suspected neurological dysfunction (Table 6–5). The **Glasgow Coma Scale** uses a point scale from 3 (total

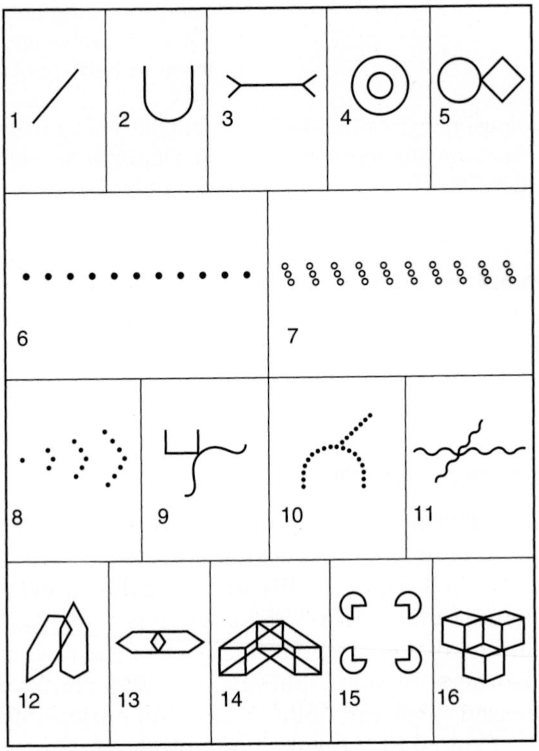

FIGURE 6-3. Bender Visual Motor Gestalt Test. The test consists of sixteen designs that are presented to the individual. Individuals are instructed to copy each design.

(Copyright (c) 2003 by The Riverside Publishing Company. All rights reserved. Published pursuant to the agreement with the American orthopsychiatric Association, Inc., and the Estate of Lauretta Bender)

unconsciousness or coma) to 15 (completely alert) to assess level of consciousness as measured by responsiveness to verbal commands and to painful stimuli in patients with suspected neurological impairment (Table 6–6).

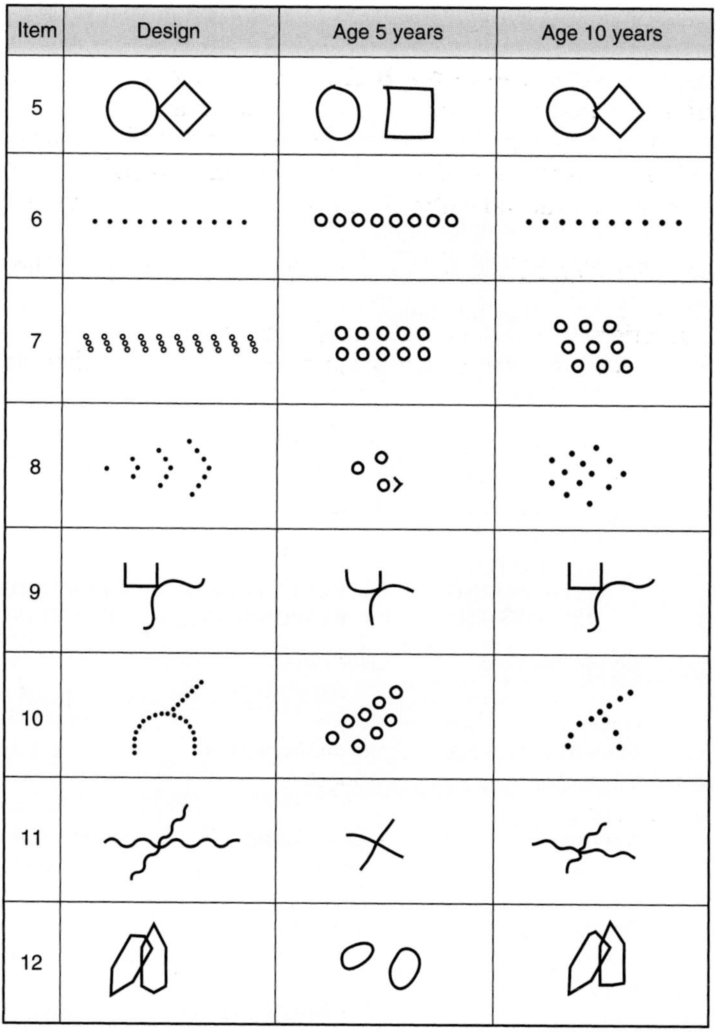

Item	Design	Age 5 years	Age 10 years
5			
6			
7			
8			
9			
10			
11			
12			

FIGURE 6-4. Responses of children 5 and 10 years of age to designs 5 through 12 of the Bender Visual Motor Gestalt Test.

(Adapted from Copyright (c) 2003 by The Riverside Publishing Company. All rights reserved. Published pursuant to the agreement with the American orthopsychiatric Association, Inc., and the Estate of Lauretta Bender.)

TABLE 6-5   Folstein Mini-Mental State Examination (MMSE)

SKILL EVALUATED	SAMPLE INSTRUCTIONS TO THE PATIENT	MAXIMUM SCORE*
Orientation	"Tell me where you are and what day it is."	10
Language	"Name the object that I am holding." (Present a common object, e.g., a pencil.)	8
Attention and calculation	"Subtract 7 from 100 and then continue to subtract 7s."	5
Registration	"Repeat the names of these three objects." (Present three common objects.)	3
Recall	Remove the objects and after 5 minutes, "Recall the names of the three objects I showed you."	3
Construction	"Copy this design."	1

*Maximum total score on the MMSE = 30; total score of less than 25 suggests cognitive problems; total score of less than 20 suggests significant impairment.

TABLE 6-6   Glasgow Coma Scale (GCS)*

NUMBER OF POINTS	BEST EYE-OPENING RESPONSE (E)	BEST VERBAL RESPONSE (V)	BEST MOTOR RESPONSE (M)
1	No eye opening	No verbal response	No motor response
2	Opens eyes in response to painful stimulus	Makes incomprehensible sounds	Shows extension to painful stimulus
3	Opens eyes in response to a verbal command	Speaks using inappropriate words	Shows flexion to painful stimulus
4	Opens eyes spontaneously	Makes confused verbal response	Withdraws from painful stimulus
5	—	Is oriented and can converse	Localizes a source of pain
6	—	—	Obeys commands

*Maximum total score on the GCS = 15, lowest possible score = 3; a GSC score of less than 12 indicates mild; 9 to 12 indicates moderate; and less than 9 indicates severe, neurological impairment. The reported score is commonly broken down into components (e.g., E3 V1 M4 = GCS 8).

REVIEW QUESTIONS

1. Five weeks after initiation of pharmacotherapy, a 34-year-old female psychiatric patient develops a fever and a sore throat. She reports feeling weak and lethargic. Blood studies reveal a white blood cell (WBC) count of less than 2,000. This patient is most likely to be taking which of the following agents?

   (A) l-thyroxine
   (B) Carbamazepine
   (C) Lithium
   (D) Dexamethasone
   (E) Sodium lactate

2. A 54-year-old man reports that he has been waking up before his alarm, has little appetite, and has lost interest in his normal activities. Which of the following is the most likely laboratory finding in this man?

   (A) Negative dexamethasone suppression test (DST)
   (B) Positive dexamethasone suppression test (DST)
   (C) Increased response to a challenge with thyrotropin-releasing hormone
   (D) Agranulocytosis
   (E) Hyperthyroidism

3. A formerly high-functioning 67-year-old male stroke patient has scored 18 on the Folstein Mini-Mental State Examination. From this score, the doctor can conclude that this patient probably

   (A) has a lower than normal IQ
   (B) cannot read
   (C) is cognitively impaired
   (D) is "faking bad"
   (E) is normal

Questions 4–6. For each of the following numbered questions, choose the lettered test with which it is most closely associated.

   (A) Positron emission tomography (PET)
   (B) Computed tomography (CT)
   (C) The Amytal interview
   (D) Electroencephalogram (EEG)
   (E) Evoked EEG
   (F) Sodium lactate administration

4. Determine which brain areas are physiologically active when a 44-year-old man is doing a mathematical calculation.

5. Determine whether a 5-month-old infant, who otherwise appears to be developing normally, is able to hear sounds.

6. Identify whether panic disorder should be diagnosed in a 28-year-old woman who has experienced three episodes over the last 2 weeks. These episodes include "palpitations," trouble breathing, and feelings of intense fear. The results of physical examination, ECG, and basic laboratory screening tests are unremarkable.

ANSWERS AND EXPLANATIONS

1-B. This patient's symptoms suggest that she has agranulocytosis, a disorder characterized by decreased granulocytes, fever, sore throat, weakness, and lethargy (see Chapter 19). This disorder is seen particularly in the first few months of treatment in patients taking clozapine, an antipsychotic, or carbamazepine, an anticonvulsant used to treat bipolar disorder. Lithium, l-thyroxine, dexamethasone, and sodium lactate are not specifically associated with agranulocytosis.

2-B. Poor appetite, early morning awakening, and lack of interest in normal activities characterize patients with major depression (see Chapter 13). In this depressed man, the dexamethasone suppression test is likely to be positive. A positive result is seen when the synthetic glucocorticoid dexamethasone fails to suppress the secretion of cortisol as it would in a normal patient. Also, depressed patients can experience a reduced response to a challenge with thyrotropin-releasing hormone. Hypothyroidism often results in symptoms of depression; hyperthyroidism is more commonly associated with symptoms of anxiety. Agranulocytosis is a blood disorder seen in patients taking clozapine or carbamazepine (see Question 1).

3-C. A scores of less than 20 on the Folstein Mini-Mental State Examination indicates significant cognitive impairment, and this patient had a score of 18. This test does not measure IQ, reading ability, or whether the patient is purposely trying to look more ill than he is ("faking bad").

4-A, 5-E, 6-F. Positron emission tomography (PET) localizes physiologically active brain areas by measuring glucose metabolism. Thus, this test can be used to determine which brain area is being used during a specific task, such as calculating.

The auditory evoked electroencephalogram (EEG) can be used to assess whether a 5-month-old child can hear. Evoked EEGs measure electrical activity in the cortex in response to sensory stimulation. The EEG, which measures electrical activity in the cortex, is useful in diagnosing epilepsy and in differentiating delirium from dementia.

Intravenous administration of sodium lactate can help identify individuals with panic disorder because it can provoke a panic attack in such patients. The sodium amobarbital (Amytal) interview is used to determine whether psychological factors are responsible for physical symptoms and computed tomography (CT) identifies anatomical brain changes.

REFERENCES

Cooper, J. R., Bloom, F. E., & Roth, R. H. (1996). *The biochemical basis of neuropharmacology* (7th ed.). New York: Oxford University Press.

Grant, I., & Adams, K. M. (1996). *Neuropsychological assessment of neuropsychiatric disorders* (2nd ed.). New York: Oxford University Press.

Langleben, D., Schroeder, L., Maldjian, J., Gur, R., McDonald, S., Ragland, J. D., et al. (2002). Brain activity during simulated deception: An event-related functional magnetic resonance study. *Neuroimage, 15,* 727–732.

Teasdale, G., & Jennett, B. (1974). The Glasgow coma scale. *Lancet, 2,* 81–83.

Sleep 7

On March 4, 1984, an 18-year-old woman named Libby Zion died at Cornell Medical Center's New York Hospital. The cause of death was a drug-drug interaction, which occurred when an opioid (Demerol) she was given in the emergency room interacted with the prescription and street drugs she had been taking. Her father, Sidney Zion, a writer for the New York Times, sued the hospital **(Zion vs. New York Hospital),** claiming that his daughter's medical care had been inadequate because she had been treated by unsupervised, sleep-deprived house officers. The grand jury for the case noted that medical residents at New York Hospital commonly worked more than 100 hours per week, including shifts of more than 24 hours each. The jury found that such physician-training methods, common across the United States at that time, were faulty and potentially dangerous to patients (Kwan, 2002). This case and subsequent responses to it by government agencies resulted in the **Bell Regulations: New York State Health Code** (DeBuono & Osten, 1998), considered a national model for residency training that led to reforms in graduate medical education nationwide. The Bell Regulations include:

1. 12-hour work limits for residents and attending physicians in emergency departments
2. Work periods not exceeding 24 hours consecutively in areas other than the emergency room
3. Scheduled work week for resident physicians not exceeding an average of 80 hours per week over a 4-week period
4. At least one 24-hour period of non-working time per week
5. 24-hour supervision of acute care inpatient units by experienced attending physicians
6. Improved working conditions and ancillary support for resident physicians

Although these regulations were an important step toward reform, many American hospitals do not observe these suggested guidelines, and the effects of sleep deprivation still have the potential to cause significant problems during residency training.

It may be difficult for those who do not have the opportunity to sleep to empathize with those who have the opportunity but are unable to sleep. However, insomnia is common, occurring in at least one third of all adults at some time in their lives. Insomnia and other sleep disorders may be early indications of physical or emotional illness. Understanding the requirements for and physiology of normal sleep enables physicians to provide effective interventions for their patients with sleep disturbances and helps ensure that they themselves obtain adequate, high-quality sleep.

■ NORMAL SLEEP

Some fortunate individuals can function well on 5 or 6 hours of sleep, while others need at least 9 or 10 hours. Most healthy people need about 8 hours of sleep per night. Human beings are not unique in their need for sleep—other mammals that have been studied, including nonhuman primates and rodents, sleep for some portion of their circadian period.

Over the last few decades, progress has been made in understanding the physiology of sleep, including its electroencephalographic characteristics, states, stages, and patterning or architecture. However, even after many years of study, it is still not clear how sleep restores function and preserves health.

The electroencephalogram in waking and sleeping

During the awake state, the electroencephalogram (EEG) shows characteristic brain waves. With active mental concentration, **beta waves** over the frontal lobes predominate. **Alpha waves** (8 to 12 cycles per second) over the occipital and parietal lobes are seen when an awake person relaxes with closed eyes and becomes drowsy (Fig. 7–1A).

The two major physiological states in normal sleep are rapid eye movement (**REM**) and **non-rapid eye movement (NREM).** The former is characterized by fast-wave EEG activity, and the latter includes a progression through four stages of increasing depth and slowing of the EEG.

Non-REM sleep. Non-REM sleep, which makes up approximately 75% of total sleep time, is identified by slow eye movements, high amplitude, low-frequency brain waves, and increased muscle tone. **Stage 1** takes up about 5% of total sleep time and is characterized by low-voltage theta wave activity at 3 to 7 cycles per second. Stage 1 quickly changes to stage 2, with spindle-shaped waves at 12 to 14 cycles per second (**sleep spindles**) and slow, high-amplitude groups of waves called **K-complexes.**

Stage 2 sleep makes up 45% of sleep time in young adults, more than any other one stage. This stage is associated with tooth grinding or **bruxism,** a chronic condition that can lead to tooth and gum problems, jaw pain, and headaches.

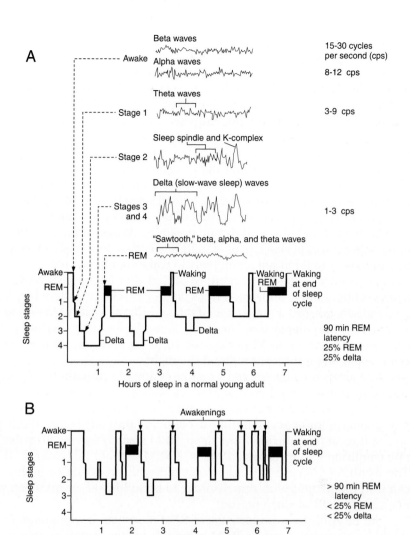

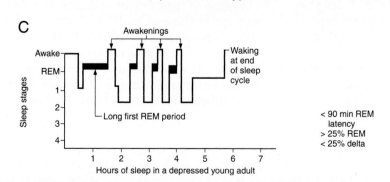

FIGURE 7-1. Electroencephalographic tracings and associated sleep architecture in normal young adult **(A)**, elderly **(B)**, and depressed **(C)** patients.

(Adapted from Wedding, D. (1995). Behavior and medicine. St. Louis: Mosby Year Book.)

Stages 3 and 4 sleep are collectively known as **slow-wave or delta sleep** characterized by high-voltage delta waves at 1–3 cycles per second. Delta sleep takes up about 25% of sleep time in young adults and occurs mainly during the first half of the sleep cycle. Delta is the deepest part of NREM sleep and is associated with unusual behavioral characteristics like **sleepwalking (somnambulism), enuresis,** and **night terrors.**

REM sleep. REM sleep is characterized by rapid eye movements; decreased muscle tone; and low-amplitude, high-frequency brain waves (including alpha and beta waves) that form a tracing resembling the teeth of a saw (**sawtooth waves**). It makes up about 25% of total sleep time in young adults, occurs primarily during the second half of the sleep cycle, and is associated with high levels of brain activity and dreaming. When compared with people in other stages of sleep, people in REM sleep are less likely to be woken by external stimuli but are more likely to wake spontaneously.

The average time to the first REM period after falling asleep (**REM latency**) is 90 minutes. Shortened REM latency is seen in patients with major depressive disorder and is one of the identifying signs of the sleep disorder called **narcolepsy** (see later text). After the first REM period, people normally experience REM periods of 10 to 40 minutes, each occurring about every 90 minutes throughout the night.

REM sleep is characterized by suppression of sympathetic activity as shown by miosis (pupil contraction), as well as penile and clitoral erection. However, except for skeletal muscles controlling respiration and movements of the eyes and middle ear ossicles, the body is essentially paralyzed (i.e., atonic) during REM sleep. **REM sleep behavior disorder** is a rare condition that includes episodes of REM without this muscle atonia. The resulting physical activity associated with dreaming or nightmares can lead the patient with this disorder to harm himself or his sleep partner during an REM sleep period.

The physiological importance of REM sleep can be demonstrated by the phenomenon known as **REM rebound.** In this situation, people deprived of sleep one night because of repeated awakenings or use of sedative agents experience a rebound or increase in REM sleep during the next sleep period. This rebound phenomenon, coupled with the findings of sleep studies conducted in conjunction with learning studies, have led to the hypothesis that REM sleep and dreaming are important in learning and memory consolidation. Recent research studies, however, fail to support this hypothesis, and the ultimate function of REM sleep remains unknown (Siegel, 2001).

Sleep architecture. Sleep progresses through the four stages of NREM, which then occur in reverse order back to stage 1, typically followed by a period of REM. Although NREM sleep stages and REM periods may be missed or repeated, five to six cycles of NREM sleep with a REM period occur per night, each cycle taking about 90 minutes. This produces a structure known as **sleep architecture** (Fig. 7-1). Aging, psychopathological states such as depression, and use of psychoactive agents can affect sleep architecture.

Neonates sleep about 16 hours per day, 50% of it in REM. By young adulthood, the percentage of REM sleep has decreased to 25%. The sleep architecture of the elderly is characterized by a combination of changes that often result in nonrestful sleep and daytime tiredness. These changes include

- Further reduction in REM sleep
- Decreased total sleep time
- Decreased delta sleep
- Increased nighttime awakenings (Fig. 7–1B)

Sleep architecture also changes in depression. Depressed patients characteristically show

- Short **sleep latency** (time from going to bed to falling asleep)
- Short **REM latency** (appearance of REM within about 45 minutes of falling asleep)
- Increased REM early in the sleep cycle
- Decreased REM later in the sleep cycle (may be associated with the early morning awakening [**terminal insomnia**] that specifically characterizes sleep in depression)
- Long first REM period
- Increased total REM
- Decreased delta sleep
- Increased nighttime awakenings (Fig. 7–1C)

Evidence suggests that increased REM sleep not only may result from depression, it may also be related to its pathophysiology. For example, drugs that increase the percentage of REM sleep (e.g., reserpine, an antihypertensive agent) or reduce the percentage of REM sleep (e.g., heterocyclic antidepressants) respectively exacerbate and improve depressive symptoms. Also, restriction or deprivation of REM and NREM sleep in depressed patients leads to temporary improvement in their depressive symptoms.

Sleep deprivation

As the Zion case demonstrated, normal individuals deprived of sleep experience impaired physical and mental performance. If the deprivation persists, they may show psychiatric symptoms such as confusion, agitation, and, ultimately, pathological anxiety and psychotic symptoms such as paranoid delusions and hallucinations (Case 7–1).

Sleep is required for optimal physical and mental performance but may also be necessary for life itself. **Fatal familial insomnia,** a rare disorder resulting from mutations in the prion protein gene, leads to degeneration of the thalamus, a brain region associated with arousal and consciousness (see

THE PATIENT During the 30th hour of a marathon radio program aimed at raising money for charity, the host, a 20-year-old college student who has no history of emotional or medical problems, begins to have difficulty concentrating and seems confused. By the 50th hour of the marathon, the student is agitated, refuses to eat anything his assistants bring him, and states, "I know you are all trying to poison me." His colleagues become alarmed at his behavior and call 911. On the way to the hospital, the student starts shouting that everyone is against him. He is restrained after punching the emergency medical technician.

COMMENT This student is showing the emotional effects of extended sleep deprivation. These effects include initial confusion and, with extended deprivation, symptoms suggesting a loss of touch with reality (e.g., intense agitation and uncharacteristic aggression) and delusional thinking (e.g., the belief that people are trying to harm him).

TREATMENT The obvious treatment for this student is to allow him to sleep. However, because he is agitated and has psychotic symptoms, he could injure himself or others before he is able to fall asleep. The antipsychotic agents chlorpromazine (Thorazine) or risperidone (Risperdal) are good choices to reduce the student's agitation and delusional thinking. Antipsychotics also have the beneficial side effect in this instance of causing general sedation. High-potency agents like haloperidol (Haldol) should be avoided in this case because young men are at particular risk for acute dystonic reactions when treated with these agents (see Chapter19).

Chapter 5). This degeneration results in the complete inability to sleep, followed by dementia. It is, as the name of the disorder implies, fatal within 1 to 2 years (Parchi et al., 1998).

SANDman: Serotonin, acetylcholine, norepinephrine, and dopamine and the production of sleep

Because the monoamines are closely involved in the production and maintenance of sleep, use of psychoactive medications that alter their availability results in alterations in sleep patterns and sleep quality.

Serotonin and **acetylcholine** promote sleep. Specifically, increased availability of serotonin is associated with increased total sleep time and increased delta sleep. In contrast, reduction in serotonin by events like damage to the neural structures that produce it (e.g., the dorsal raphe nuclei) decreases these measures. Although it is intuitive that ingestion of **melatonin,** a serotonin metabolite manufactured by the pineal gland during darkness, should improve sleep, such an effect has not been demonstrated in controlled clinical trials.

Acetylcholine (ACh) in the reticular formation is associated with inducing REM sleep. In patients with conditions associated with decreased ACh, such as normal aging and Alzheimer's disease, REM sleep, total sleep time, and delta sleep are decreased.

Norepinephrine and **dopamine** promote arousal and wakefulness. Increased levels of norepinephrine, present in anxious patients, may increase sleep latency and decrease both total sleep time and the percentage of time spent in REM sleep. Increased levels of dopamine seen in mania and other psychotic illnesses are associated with decreased total sleep time.

Psychoactive agents that alter neurotransmitter availability can have profound effects on sleep duration and sleep quality. For example, treatment with antipsychotics, which block dopamine receptors, and antidepressants, which increase serotonin availability, can improve sleep in patients with psychiatric disorders. In contrast, stimulant agents that increase dopamine and norepinephrine can cause wakefulness.

■ SLEEP DISORDERS

The Diagnostic and Statistical Manual of Mental Disorders, 4th edition-Text Revision (DSM-IV-TR) classifies sleep disorders into two major categories: the dyssomnias and the parasomnias. The most common sleep disorders are the **dyssomnias,** which are characterized by problems in the timing, quality, or amount of sleep. The dyssomnias include insomnia, breathing-related sleep disorder (sleep apnea), and narcolepsy, as well as the less common hypersomnias, circadian rhythm sleep disorder, restless leg syndrome, sleep drunkenness, and nocturnal myoclonus (Table 7–1).

The **parasomnias** are characterized by abnormalities in physiology or in behavior associated with sleep. They include bruxism, nightmare disorder, sleep terror disorder, sleepwalking disorder, and REM behavior disorder (Table 7–2). The characteristics of the most important sleep disorders—insomnia, sleep apnea, and narcolepsy—are discussed below.

Insomnia

Insomnia is identified as difficulty falling asleep or staying asleep that occurs three times per week for at least 1 month and leads to sleepiness during the day or causes problems fulfilling social or occupational obligations. Insomnia resulting from all causes is a common complaint in at least 30% of the population.

Caffeine use is a common cause of insomnia. Other physiological causes include use of other central nervous system stimulants and withdrawal of drugs with sedating action, such as alcohol, benzodiazepines, and opioids. Medical conditions that cause pain also result in insomnia, as do endocrine and metabolic disorders.

Common psychological causes of insomnia include mood (Chapter 13) and anxiety (Chapter 15) disorders. Although some patients with major depressive disorder sleep excessively, most have difficulty maintaining sleep. In contrast to depressed patients who typically show normal sleep latencies, manic or hypomanic bipolar patients and anxious patients commonly have trouble falling asleep.

TABLE 7-1	Characteristics and Treatment of Dyssomnias	
SLEEP DISORDER	**CHARACTERISTICS**	**TREATMENT**
Insomnia	■ Difficulty falling asleep or staying asleep that occurs 3 times weekly for at least 1 month; leads to daytime sleepiness or problems fulfilling social or occupational obligations	■ Avoidance of caffeine ■ Development of a sleep ritual ■ Maintaining a fixed sleep and wake schedule ■ Relaxation techniques
Breathing-related sleep disorder	■ Cessation of breathing for periods during sleep; leads to anoxia and nighttime awakenings and results in chronic daytime sleepiness	■ Weight loss (if overweight) ■ Continuous positive airway pressure ■ Surgery to enlarge the airway
Narcolepsy	■ Episodes of sudden daytime sleepiness that occur daily for at least 3 months despite a normal amount of sleep at night ■ Sleepiness is relieved by daytime naps	■ Stimulant agents (e.g., methylphenidate) ■ Planned, timed daytime naps
Primary hypersomnias (e.g., Kleine-Levin syndrome and menstrual-associated syndrome [symptoms only in the premenstruum])	■ Recurrent bouts of excessive sleepiness occurring almost daily for at least 1 month ■ Sleepiness is not relieved by daytime naps ■ Often accompanied by hyperphagia (overeating) ■ Sleepiness is not better accounted for by narcolepsy or other sleep disorder	■ Stimulant agents (e.g., methylphenidate) and stimulating antidepressants (e.g., fluoxetine [Prozac])

| TABLE 7-1 | Characteristics and Treatment of Dyssomnias (Continued) |

SLEEP DISORDER	CHARACTERISTICS	TREATMENT
Circadian rhythm sleep disorder	■ Sleepiness at inappropriate times during the day because of inability to sleep at appropriate times ■ Three types: *delayed sleep phase type* involves falling asleep and waking later than desired; *jet lag type* lasts 2–7 days after a change in time zones; and *shift work type* involves changes in scheduled work hours that cause mixed insomnia and sleepiness, leading to errors in performance at work and home	■ *Delayed sleep phase type:* Gradually (over days) push back the hour of going to sleep ■ *Jet lag type:* Change sleep and meal times prior to travel to conform to those of the destination ■ *Shift work type:* Bright light therapy during "daytime" and consistent observation of new bedtime hours
Restless legs syndrome	■ Uncomfortable sensation in the legs (and sometimes arms) necessitating frequent motion and causing insomnia and repetitive (every 25–40 sec) limb jerking during sleep ■ More common with aging, pregnancy, and kidney disease ■ Associated with: *dopamine deficiency* in subcortical brain areas; *iron deficiency,* which disrupts dopamine production in brain; and *low levels of magnesium*	■ L-dopa ■ Iron supplements ■ Magnesium supplements
Sleep drunkenness	■ Difficulty awakening fully after adequate sleep ■ Rare, associated with genetic factors ■ Must be differentiated from substance abuse or other sleep disorder	■ Stimulant agents (e.g., methylphenidate)
Nocturnal myoclonus	■ Repetitive, abrupt muscular contractions in the legs from toes to hips causing nighttime awakenings ■ More common in the elderly	■ Benzodiazepines ■ Quinine ■ L-dopa ■ Opioids (rarely used)

TABLE 7-2	Characteristics and Treatment of Parasomnias		
SLEEP DISORDER	**CHARACTERISTICS**	**TREATMENT**
Bruxism	■ Tooth grinding ■ Occurs primarily in stage 2 sleep ■ Can lead to tooth damage and jaw pain	■ Dental appliance worn at night ■ Corrective orthodontia
Nightmare disorder	■ Repetitive, frightening dreams that occur during REM sleep and are recalled on nighttime awakenings	■ Pharmacologic agents that suppress REM sleep (e.g., tricyclic antidepressants and benzodiazepines)
Sleep terror (pavor nocturnus) disorder	■ Repetitive experiences of fright in which a person (usually a child) screams in fear but cannot be awakened and has no memory of having a dream ■ Occur during delta (slow-wave) sleep ■ Onset in adolescence may presage temporal lobe epilepsy	■ Pharmacologic agents that suppress delta sleep (e.g., benzodiazepines)
Sleepwalking disorder	■ Repetitive walking during sleep ■ No memory of the episode on awakening ■ Occurs during delta sleep ■ Begins in childhood (usually at 4–8 years of age) ■ Has a genetic component ■ Is associated with enuresis	■ Pharmacologic agents that suppress delta sleep (e.g., benzodiazepines)
REM sleep behavior disorder	■ REM sleep and dreaming without skeletal muscle atonia ■ Highly active sleeping patients can harm themselves and their sleeping partners	■ Anticonvulsants (e.g., carbamazepine [Tegretol]) ■ Pharmacologic agents that suppress REM sleep (e.g., benzodiazepines)

Treatment of insomnia

Patients with insomnia often request prescriptions for sleep medication from their physicians. However, although they are effective initially, **sedative agents** such as alcohol, barbiturates, and, to a lesser extent, benzodiazepines are associated with changes in sleep architecture, such as reduced REM sleep and delta sleep. These changes, and the tendency of these agents to cause daytime sedation, dependence, and tolerance, can ultimately exacerbate the patients' sleep problems. Newer, **nonbenzodiazepine** sleep agents such as zolpidem (Ambien) and zaleplon (Sonata) cause fewer changes in sleep architecture and are less likely to cause dependence and tolerance (see Chapter 19).

Benzodiazepines are useful for treating delta sleep disorders such as night terrors and bedwetting because they reduce the likelihood of delta sleep. Also, because benzodiazepines coincidentally reduce core body temperature, they may improve sleep disorders associated with elevated core body temperature, such as certain types of insomnia and frequent nighttime awakenings.

In patients without significant psychopathology, the initial treatment strategy for insomnia is avoidance of caffeine, especially before bedtime. Treatment also involves developing a set of behaviors that become associated with bedtime. This **sleep ritual** or **sleep hygiene** includes behaviors such as taking a warm bath, listening to music, and developing and following a fixed sleeping and waking schedule. Daily exercise, preferably performed early in the day and not immediately before sleep, and relaxation techniques are other aspects of sleep hygiene.

Breathing-related sleep disorder (sleep apnea)

Patients with **sleep apnea** stop breathing for brief intervals, sometimes as many as 500 times, during the night. Low oxygen and high carbon dioxide levels in the blood awaken them each time they stop breathing, resulting in daytime sleepiness. This condition occurs in at least 10% of middle-aged and older persons and, in some patients, is related to the occurrence of depression, headaches, or pulmonary hypertension (Dart et al., 2003). Sleep apnea also can result in sudden death during sleep, particularly when it occurs in older persons and in infants.

The two basic types of sleep apnea are central and obstructive. In patients with **central sleep apnea** (more common in the elderly), the airway is open but little or no respiratory effort occurs. In patients with **obstructive sleep apnea,** respiratory effort occurs, but an airway obstruction prevents air from reaching the lungs. The usual result in both conditions is that less oxygen reaches the lungs and the patient awakens. Obstructive sleep apnea is the more common type. It occurs most often in people 40 to 60 years of age and is found more often in men (8:1 male-to-female ratio) and in the obese. Patients with obstructive sleep apnea are sometimes first identified by a sleep partner's complaints of loud snoring. **Pickwickian**

syndrome is a related condition in which daytime sleepiness results from airway obstruction. It is seen primarily in people who have central obesity and a short, fat neck, a body habitus that leads to mechanical obstruction of diaphragmatic movement.

Treatment of breathing-related sleep disorder

In overweight patients, obstructive breathing-related sleep disorder is treated initially with weight loss. If the problem does not remit, the next step in treatment is to provide persistent, gentle pressure to keep the airway open using a **continuous positive airway pressure** device applied to the face at night. Surgical procedures, such as **uvulopalatoplasty** to remove the uvula and associated mucoid and lymphoid tissue, and even permanent **tracheostomy,** are last-resort treatments. Recently, sleep apnea patients with cardiac pacemakers showed improvement in their sleep when their heart rates were increased (Gottlieb, 2002), although the mechanism of this effect is not known.

Narcolepsy

Patients with **narcolepsy** have sleep attacks during which they fall asleep suddenly during the daytime. When compared with normal individuals, narcoleptics experience the same amount of total nighttime sleep but demonstrate a decreased sleep latency (less than 2 minutes) and abnormalities in REM sleep, such as a short REM latency (less than 10 minutes), reduced total REM, and interrupted REM periods or **sleep fragmentation.** Narcolepsy occurs in 0.04 to 0.9% of the population and may be underdiagnosed or misdiagnosed as laziness. It occurs most frequently in adolescents and young adults and has a strong genetic component. The differential diagnosis of narcolepsy includes sleep deprivation, abuse of sedative agents, withdrawal from stimulant drugs, and sleep apnea leading to daytime sleepiness.

Narcolepsy is characterized by **hypnagogic** (upon falling asleep) or **hypnopompic** (upon awakening) **hallucinations.** These strange perceptual experiences occur in 20 to 40% of patients with the disorder.

Cataplexy and sleep paralysis are seen in 30 to 70% of narcoleptic patients and occur while the patient is awake. **Cataplexy** is characterized by a sudden physical collapse caused by the loss of all muscle tone after a strong emotional stimulus, such as anger, laughter, or sexual stimulation. **Sleep paralysis** is an alarming symptom identified by the inability to move the body for a few seconds after waking. As in REM sleep, the eye muscles are active during cataplectic or sleep paralysis attacks in narcoleptic patients.

Treatment of narcolepsy

Narcolepsy is treated prophylactically with stimulant agents such as methylphenidate (Ritalin). Antidepressants are helpful if cataplexy is part

THE PATIENT A 26-year-old graduate student in microbiology visits his school health service with the complaint of excessive daytime sleepiness. Despite the fact that he goes to bed at about 11:00 PM and wakes up at 7:30 AM, he has difficulty staying awake during lectures and has had a few minor car accidents when he fell asleep while driving. He also reports that he recently had an "episode" during which he fell to the ground when a friend surprised him on the street. The student also tells the physician that he is frightened because sometimes he cannot move his arms or legs for a brief period after awakening. The student appears appropriately enthusiastic and animated when discussing his dissertation project, and he denies being anxious or depressed. Physical examination is unremarkable.

COMMENT This student is showing the characteristic symptoms of narcolepsy. He has daytime sleepiness despite a normal amount of sleep at night, cataplexy (loss of muscle tone with an emotional surprise), and sleep paralysis (inability to move immediately after awakening). In the sleep laboratory, rapid sleep onset and short REM latency (less than 15 minutes) would characterize the sleep of this patient.

TREATMENT Laboratory sleep studies are needed to confirm the diagnosis of narcolepsy. Once diagnosed, narcolepsy is treated with stimulant agents such as dextroamphetamine (Dexedrine) or methylphenidate (Ritalin). Because this patient also shows cataplexy, a nonsedating antidepressant such as fluoxetine (Prozac) should be added to the protocol. This patient should also be encouraged to take at least two 10- to 20-minute naps each day, particularly before driving.

of the clinical picture, but they are less useful in preventing the sleepiness. Timed daytime naps provide refreshment and can help avoid the sudden sleepiness that is troublesome and even dangerous (e.g., if it occurs while driving) in patients with this disorder.

REVIEW QUESTIONS

1. A 45-year-old man reports that over the past 9 months he has lost interest in activities he formerly enjoyed and has little appetite for food or sex. He then states that "my family would be better off it I weren't around." Physical examination is unremarkable. Which of the following is most likely to characterize the sleep of this patient?

(A) Shift in REM from the last part to the first part of the sleep cycle

(B) Short first REM period

(C) Increased slow-wave sleep

(D) Lengthened REM latency

(E) Reduced percentage of REM sleep

2. A 35-year-old female patient is being monitored in a sleep laboratory. When her electroencephalogram (EEG) shows primarily delta waves, which of the following is most likely to characterize this patient?

(A) Clitoral erection

(B) Paralysis of skeletal muscles

(C) Episodic body movements

(D) Nightmares

(E) Increased brain oxygen use

3. An 85-year-old patient reports that he is often tired during the day-time. His mood is normal and his general health is good. Sleep in this patient is most likely to be characterized by increased

(A) stage 3 sleep

(B) stage 4 sleep

(C) total sleep time

(D) REM sleep

(E) nighttime awakenings

4. A 28-year-old student asks his doctor for "sleeping pills" because he often has lain awake in bed for more than 2 hours before falling asleep. He cannot wake up in time for class, is often tired and forget-ful, and makes mistakes on exams. When questioned, the student re-lates that although he goes to bed at 11 PM on weeknights, he com-monly stays up until 3 AM on weekends. What is the doctor's most appropriate recommendation?

(A) A glass of milk before bedtime

(B) A fixed wake-up and bedtime schedule

(C) A short-acting benzodiazepine at bedtime

(D) One hour of exercise before bedtime

(E) A large meal before bedtime

5. A 5-year-old child often screams during the night. When this hap-pens, his parents report that he sits up, opens his eyes, and "looks right through them," but they cannot awaken him. He has no memory of these experiences in the morning. Which of the following sleep dis-orders best matches this clinical picture?

(A) Kleine-Levin syndrome

(B) Nightmare disorder

(C) Sleep terror disorder

(D) Sleep drunkenness

(E) Circadian rhythm sleep disorder

ANSWERS AND EXPLANATIONS

1-A. This man has a dysphoric mood (loss of interest in activities and decreased interest in food and sexual activity) as well as suicidal ideation, and he is therefore probably experiencing a major depressive episode (see Chapter 13). Sleep in major depression is associated with a shift in REM from the last to the first part of the sleep cycle, long first REM period, reduced slow-wave sleep, shortened REM latency, and greater percentage of REM.

2-C. Delta waves characterize sleep stages 3 and 4 (slow-wave sleep), which is also associated with episodic body movements, somnambulism, night terrors, and enuresis. Delta sleep is the deepest, most relaxed stage of sleep. Clitoral erection, paralysis of skeletal muscles, nightmares, and increased brain oxygen use occur during REM sleep.

3-E. Sleep in elderly patients, like this 85-year-old, is characterized by increased nighttime awakenings, decreased REM sleep, decreased delta sleep (stages 3 and 4), and decreased total sleep time. All of these changes could result in the daytime sleepiness that this patient demonstrates.

4-B. The most appropriate intervention for this student who is having problems falling asleep is to recommend a fixed wake-up and bedtime schedule; that is, he should go to sleep at about the same time on weekdays and weekends. Late bedtimes on weekends can make it difficult to fall asleep earlier on weekdays, leading to daytime sleepiness and impairment in functioning. Benzodiazepines are not appropriate for this student because of their high abuse potential and possibility of causing daytime sedation. These agents also decrease sleep quality by reducing REM and delta sleep. Exercise should be done early in the day; if done before bedtime, it can be stimulating and cause wakefulness. A large meal before bedtime is more likely to interfere with sleep than to help sleep. Although many lay people believe that milk helps induce sleep, this effect has never been proved scientifically.

5-C. This child demonstrates sleep terror disorder, which occurs in delta sleep and is characterized by screaming during the night and the inability to be awakened or to remember these experiences in the morning. In contrast, nightmare disorder occurs during REM sleep and the child wakes up and can relate the nature of his frightening dreams. Kleine-Levin syndrome is usually seen in adolescents and involves recurrent periods of hypersomnia and hyperphagia, each lasting 1 to 3 weeks. In sleep drunkenness, a patient cannot come fully awake after sleep. In circadian rhythm sleep disorder, sleeping and waking occur at inappropriate times.

REFERENCES

Brody, J. E. (2001, November 27). Restless legs: Treatable if recognized. *The New York Times.*

Dart, R. A., Gregoire, J. R., Gutterman, D. D., & Woolf, S. H. (2003). The association of hypertension and secondary cardiovascular disease with sleep-disordered breathing. *Chest, 123,* 244–260.

DeBuono, B. A., & Osten, W.M. (1998). The medical resident workload: the case of New York State. *JAMA, 280,* 1882–1883.

Gottlieb, D. J. (2002). Cardiac pacing—a novel therapy for sleep apnea? *N Engl J Med, 346,* 34.

Kandel, E. R., Schwartz, J. H., & Jessell, T. M. (2000). Principles of neural science (4th ed.). New York: Elsevier.

Kaplan, H. I., & Sadock, B. J. (2003). Normal sleep and sleep disorders. *Synopsis of psychiatry* (9th ed.). Baltimore: Lippincott, Williams & Wilkins.

Kwan, R. 2002. *A primer on resident work hours* (2nd ed.). Reston, VA: American Medical Student Association.

Parchi, P., Petersen, R. B., Chen, S. S. G., Autilio-Gambetti, L., Capellari, S., Monari, L., et al. (1998). Molecular pathology of fatal familial insomnia. *Brain Pathol, 8,* 539–548.

Siegel, J. M. (2001). The REM sleep-memory consolidation hypothesis. *Science, 294,* 1058–1063.

8

Psychodynamic Theory in Medical Practice

P sychodynamic theory is based on the idea, cast by Sigmund Freud and modified later by others, that behavior is influenced by forces derived from processes of which individuals are not aware. While these unconscious forces keep thoughts and emotions out of consciousness, they are at the same time dynamic and affect peoples' choices, emotions, and behavior throughout life. Psychotherapeutic treatments, such as psychoanalysis and related therapies (see Chapter 11), are based on this concept of the **dynamic unconscious.**

This chapter introduces and explains the language of psychodynamic theory. The discussion focuses on the concepts of individual defense mechanisms and transference reactions between doctor and patient. At first glance, the relationship between these intellectual constructs and everyday medical practice may seem obscure. However, understanding these ideas can help physicians decipher and respond to seemingly inconsistent, hostile, or even self-destructive behavior in their patients.

■ FREUD'S THEORIES OF THE MIND

Early in his career, Freud developed the topographic theory of the mind to explain his ideas about behavior. Later in his career, he developed the structural theory.

Topographic theory

In the topographic theory, the mind contains three levels: the unconscious, preconscious, and conscious. The **unconscious mind** contains repressed thoughts and feelings that are not available to the conscious mind. The unconscious employs **primary process thinking,** a type of thinking associated with primitive drives, wish fulfillment, immediate gratification, and pleasure seeking. It has no logic or concept of time. Primary process thinking is seen in young children and in adults with psychotic illnesses (see Chapter 12).

The **preconscious mind** contains memories that are not immediately available but can be accessed easily. The names of the cranial nerves, not on the tip of a medical student's tongue but accessible for exams, are examples of preconscious material. The **conscious mind** contains thoughts that a person is currently aware of. It operates in close conjunction with the preconscious mind but, unlike the preconscious mind, does not have access to the unconscious mind. The conscious mind uses **secondary process thinking** (logical, mature, and time-oriented) and can delay gratification.

One question that the topographic theory raises is whether it can be known that the unconscious mind really exists. Freud suggested that one piece of evidence for the existence of the unconscious is the presence of **dreams,** which represent gratification of unconscious instinctive impulses and wish fulfillment. Other examples of the unconscious are the phenomena of **parapraxes** or Freudian slips—errors of speech (or of hearing) that reveal one's true but unconscious feelings, and **hypnosis**—a psychotherapeutic technique that bypasses the conscious mind to reveal material in the unconscious (Table 8–1).

Structural theory

In Freud's structural theory, the mind contains three parts: the id, ego, and superego. The **id,** present at birth, contains instinctive sexual and aggres-

TABLE 8-1	Freud's Proofs of the Unconscious
PROOF	**EXAMPLE**
Dreams	A man who has personally unacceptable sexual feelings for his therapist, Dr. Freud, dreams that he is walking down a street named "Sigmund Road," naked.
Parapraxes	A woman who unconsciously fears the responsibilities of her new and lucrative position states, "My new job is a landmine . . . I mean a goldmine."
Hypnosis	Under hypnosis, a woman who has no conscious memory of the event reveals that she was sexually abused as a child by her father.

sive drives. It is controlled by primary process thinking and is not influenced by external reality. The **ego** controls the expression of the id and adapts it to the requirements of the external world primarily through defense mechanisms (see later text). The ego enables one to sustain satisfying interpersonal relationships and, through reality testing (i.e., constantly evaluating what is valid and then adapting that to real life), enables a person to maintain a sense of reality about his or her own body and the external world. The **superego,** which also controls id impulses, represents moral values and conscience.

Conflict arises when the drives of the id threaten to overwhelm the control of the ego and superego. When this situation occurs, the ego pushes the id impulses and unacceptable emotions deeper into the unconscious by the active defense mechanism of repression. Unfortunately, material pushed into the unconscious does not sit quietly. Although the person may be unaware of its content, this material affects his or her emotional state, causing psychiatric symptoms (such as anxiety and depression) and dissociative and somatic symptoms. Freud developed a treatment technique, psychoanalysis, to recover and consciously address this repressed material (see Chapter 11). He observed that when patients were treated with psychoanalysis, their distressing psychological symptoms dissipated. Freud strongly suspected that psychotic illnesses such as schizophrenia were not caused by unconscious conflicts. He surmised, correctly as subsequent investigation confirmed, that psychotic illnesses were organic and, as such, could not be helped by psychoanalytic treatment.

■ DEFENSE MECHANISMS

Like defending themselves against physical pain, people protect themselves, albeit unconsciously, from emotional pain. The techniques they use to do this, which Freud called defense mechanisms, work by keeping conflict out of the conscious mind. This protection serves to decrease anxiety and thereby helps the individual maintain a sense of safety, equilibrium, and self-esteem.

People in need of medical and psychiatric care commonly use defense mechanisms to deal with the fear and pain associated with their illnesses. As such, these mechanisms can serve a useful purpose for the patient. However, defense mechanisms that prevent a patient from seeking care or complying with treatment recommendations can ultimately be harmful.

Mature and less mature defense mechanisms

The type of defense mechanism used by an individual is closely associated with that person's coping style and personality (see Chapter 24). For example, a person who tends to become childlike and demanding when stressed by illness is coping by using the defense mechanism of regression (see later text).

Defense mechanisms can be less mature or more mature. Less mature defense mechanisms protect the person from anxiety and negative personal feelings, but at significant social cost. Mature defense mechanisms serve the same function but without important social cost. For example, using the less mature defense mechanism of **displacement,** a man deals with his unacknowledged anger toward his employer by verbally abusing his office assistant. In contrast, using the mature defense mechanism of **sublimation,** the same man could deal with his anger by engaging in a strenuous game of racquetball.

Mature defense mechanisms may even have social benefits. When a man with low self-esteem donates time to visit patients in the hospital, he is using the defense mechanism of **altruism** to feel better about himself. Other mature defense mechanisms in addition to sublimation and altruism are humor and suppression.

Humor involves expressing personally uncomfortable feelings without causing emotional discomfort. For example, a patient who is uncomfortable about his erectile problems makes jokes about Viagra (sildenafil citrate). Using **suppression,** a defense mechanism that includes some aspects of consciousness, a person deliberately pushes anxiety-provoking or personally unacceptable emotions out of conscious awareness. For example, a prostate cancer patient who mentally changes the subject when his mind wanders to the possibility of relapse, yet seeks appropriate treatment for his illness, is using suppression as a defense mechanism.

Common defense mechanisms in medical patients: Repression, denial, undoing, and regression

Repression is the most basic defense mechanism; the other defense mechanisms are used only when repression fails. Repression is closely related to the defense mechanism of denial, and both are commonly used by medical patients. In **repression,** a patient unconsciously refuses to believe an aspect of internal reality. In **denial,** he unconsciously refuses to believe an aspect of external reality. For example, using repression, a cocaine abuser does not feel bad about the addiction because he fails to remember, or admit to himself, that the length of his drug use spans years rather than months. Using **denial,** he believes (although there is evidence to the contrary) that he can stop using the drug at any time.

Undoing and regression are other defense mechanisms often seen in medically ill patients. In **undoing,** a patient believes that she can magically reverse past events caused by "incorrect" behavior by now adopting "correct" behavior. For example, a woman who is terminally ill with AIDS caused by intravenous drug abuse decides to stop using the drug and start an exercise and healthful diet program. When she is hospitalized for complications of her illness, this same woman may show **regression** by reverting to childlike behavior patterns like whining, pouting, and insisting that relatives pay more attention to her.

Rationalization, intellectualization, and isolation of affect

Educated and uneducated people use defense mechanisms to avoid negative emotions. However, educated people tend to use defense mechanisms that employ the mind's higher functions. These mechanisms include rationalization, intellectualization, and isolation of affect. In **rationalization,** an individual unconsciously distorts his or her perception of an event so that its negative outcome seems reasonable. A blind person who believes that he now has supernormal hearing is using this defense mechanism. **Intellectualization** involves using cognition to avoid negative emotions. The pilot of a doomed flight who explains the technical details of the engine failure to the passengers is using this defense mechanism. Using **isolation of affect,** an individual does not consciously experience any emotion when thinking about or describing an emotional event. The person who expresses no emotion when talking about the loss of a loved one has isolated his emotions from the sad event.

Somatization and dissociation

Somatization and dissociation are dramatic defense mechanisms that characterize somatoform (Chapter 16) and dissociative (Chapter 18) disorders.

CASE 8-1

THE PATIENT A 35-year-old surgeon loses his left arm above the elbow in an automobile accident. During his recovery, the surgeon tells visitors and colleagues that the loss of his arm was unfortunate but ultimately beneficial to his medical practice. He says that it helps him understand the experience of his amputee patients. The surgeon also frequently explains in detail the technical aspects of the accident and surgery to others. The surgeon states, seemingly without emotion, that he understands that the loss of his arm means that he can no longer practice surgery.

COMMENT This surgeon is dealing with the devastating loss of his arm by using several defense mechanisms. Using rationalization, he gives a seemingly reasonable explanation (i.e., the loss was ultimately beneficial for his practice) for his personally unacceptable feelings of grief at the loss of his arm. He also avoids unacceptable emotions by focusing on the technical and medical aspects of the accident and surgery using intellectualization. Finally, although he says that he understands the significance of the loss of his arm, the doctor does not show and in fact does not consciously experience any emotion (isolation of affect) when stating that he can no longer practice surgery.

TREATMENT These defense mechanisms have probably served the doctor well in his work by allowing him to perform his job during stressful emergencies. They may also have helped him in the short term to cope with the loss of his arm. However, their excessive long-term use can prevent him from dealing with his real feelings about the loss of his arm. Failure to deal with his true feelings can ultimately hamper his full recovery (see Chapter 25).

Using **somatization,** a person unconsciously deals with negative emotions by experiencing and expressing physical symptoms. The somatoform disorders are a group of conditions that present with physical symptoms without sufficient biological basis. In **dissociation,** the individual mentally separates part of his or her consciousness from reality, sometimes even "forgetting" that certain events have in fact occurred. For example, a teenager with the dissociative disorder **dissociative amnesia** has no conscious memory of a car accident in which he was driving and his girlfriend was killed.

Defense mechanisms and psychopathology

Some defense mechanisms can explain aspects of psychopathology. For example, one explanation for the tendency of some abused children to grow into abusers is that the person has unconsciously patterned himself after a powerful figure from his past using the defense mechanism of **identification** (in this case **identification with the aggressor**). Although that example shows a negative outcome, identification can have a positive outcome if the individual uses a supportive, loving figure from the past as a model for his own behavior.

Use of the **projection** defense mechanism (attributing one's own personally unacceptable feelings to others) can be associated with psychopathology such as paranoia or even with common prejudice. The man with unconscious homosexual impulses who begins to believe, erroneously, that his male boss is making sexual advances toward him is using projection to protect himself from recognizing his own personally unacceptable homosexual feelings.

Certain individuals tend to place people or situations into categories of either wonderful or dreadful. This use of the defense mechanism of **splitting** relieves the person of having to confront the uncertainty engendered by the fact that people have both bad and good qualities. Splitting is a common defense mechanism used by patients with borderline personality disorder (Chapter 18).

Acting out refers to avoiding personally unacceptable emotions by behaving in an attention-getting, often socially inappropriate manner. It is more commonly seen in teenagers and can result in academic and social dysfunction. A 14-year-old boy with no history of disruptive behavior who begins to talk back to the teacher and to fail classes when his parents divorce may be acting out his depressed and anxious emotions over his parents' break-up.

When a person purposely behaves in a friendly fashion toward someone he does not like, we call it hypocrisy. If done unconsciously because disliking that individual is personally unacceptable, it is an example of the defense mechanism of **reaction formation.** A woman who spends excessively on expensive gifts and clothing for her children because she is unconsciously resentful of the responsibilities of childrearing is using reaction formation. Other examples of defense mechanisms are listed in Table 8–2.

TABLE 8-2	Commonly Used Defense Mechanisms	
DEFENSE MECHANISM	**EXPLANATION**	**CLINICAL EXAMPLE**
MORE MATURE DEFENSE MECHANISMS		
Altruism	Unselfishly assisting others to avoid negative personal feelings	A woman with a poor self-image volunteers in a soup kitchen on her day off from work.
Humor	Expression of feeling without causing discomfort	A man who has had a leg amputated makes jokes about one-legged people.
Sublimation	Rerouting an unacceptable drive in a socially acceptable way	A man whose son was killed by a drunk driver regularly speaks to high school students about the dangers of drinking and driving.
Suppression	Consciously putting aside but not repressing unwanted feelings	A breast cancer patient decides that she will worry about her illness for only 10 minutes per day.
LESS MATURE DEFENSE MECHANISMS		
Acting out	Avoiding personally unacceptable feelings by behaving in an attention-getting, often socially inappropriate manner	A teenager with a terminally ill younger sibling begins to do badly at school and argues with her parents at home.
Denial	Not believing personally intolerable facts about reality	An accountant who had a myocardial infarction (MI) 2 days ago is found doing push-ups on the floor of the coronary care unit. The patient, who exercised regularly prior to the MI, states that his heart attack was not serious and that he does not want to fall behind in his fitness program.

| TABLE 8-2 | Commonly Used Defense Mechanisms (Continued) |

DEFENSE MECHANISM	EXPLANATION	CLINICAL EXAMPLE
Displacement	Transfer of emotions from an unacceptable to acceptable person or object	A man whose son was killed by a drunk driver attacks and seriously injures a drunken street-person.
Dissociation	Separation of function of mental processes	A woman who was sexually abused as a child has two distinct personalities in adulthood.
Identification	Unconsciously patterning one's behavior after that of someone who is more powerful	A man who had a critical, punitive father berates and verbally insults his own son.
Intellectualization	Using the mind's higher functions to avoid experiencing uncomfortable emotions	A physician who has received a diagnosis of pancreatic cancer excessively discusses the statistics of the illness with his colleagues and family.
Isolation of affect	Failing to experience the feelings associated with a stressful life event, although logically understanding the significance of the event	Without showing any emotion, a woman tells her husband the results of tests that show that her cancer has metastasized.
Projection	Attributing one's own personally unacceptable feelings to others	A man who has sexual feelings for his brother's wife begins to believe that his own wife is cheating on him.
Rationalization	Giving seemingly reasonable explanations for unacceptable or irrational feelings	A medical student who fails the final genetics exam says that it does not matter because it was not an important course.

TABLE 8-2	Commonly Used Defense Mechanisms (Continued)	
DEFENSE MECHANISM	EXPLANATION	CLINICAL EXAMPLE
Reaction formation	Denying unacceptable feelings and adopting opposite attitudes	A man who is unconsciously attracted to a coworker frequently picks fights with her.
Regression	Appearance of childlike patterns of behavior during stressful situations	A hospitalized 48-year-old patient insists on only eating hot dogs, french fries, and ice cream.
Somatization	Turning an unacceptable impulse or feeling into a physical symptom	A man who is anxious about a new job develops a headache the morning of the first day of work.
Splitting	Believing people or events are either all bad or all good because of intolerance of ambiguity	A woman who believed her physician was godlike begins to think he is a terrible physician after he is late for an appointment with her.
Undoing	Erasing an unacceptable event in the past by adopting acceptable behavior in the present (superstitious behavior)	A woman who was robbed when she went out the door on the right side of her office building now will only use the door on the left side of the building.

Adapted from Fadem, B. 2001. *High yield behavioral science* (2nd ed.). Baltimore: Lippincott, Williams & Wilkins.

■ TRANSFERENCE REACTIONS

The relationships and attitudes that individuals form as adults are unconsciously modeled on relationships that they had with important people, such as their parents, early in life. This modeling, called **transference,** is particularly strong in relationships formed with people who have functions that initially were performed by parents. People commonly show intense transference reactions in their relationships with caregivers, such as doctors, psychotherapists, and teachers. Analysis of these reactions is used in certain types of psychotherapy to provide information to the therapist about a patient's past important relationships.

THE PATIENT A 19-year-old male patient is brought to the emergency room after having a grand mal seizure at a college football game. The patient, who has a history of epilepsy, has been under the care of the same physician for the past 5 years. The patient is stabilized and resting comfortably when his doctor arrives in the emergency room. The doctor becomes very agitated when the patient tells her that he has not been taking his medication regularly because "I don't think I need it anymore." She then loudly berates the patient for his poor judgment and immaturity in not taking his medication. In a subsequent discussion with a colleague, the doctor reveals that she is having a great deal of difficulty with her 17-year-old son who is doing badly in school and has been arrested for drunk driving.

COMMENT The doctor-patient relationship is a professional one. Although patient noncompliance can be frustrating, this doctor's intense emotional reaction to her patient's noncompliant behavior is excessive. It most likely results from countertransference because the doctor has unwittingly and unconsciously transferred her feelings about her own son to her patient.

TREATMENT It is important for the doctor to identify this countertransference reaction because it can interfere with her medical judgment. It can also result in patient anger and, ultimately, noncompliance. The doctor needs to explore her feelings about her son as they apply to her relationships with patients. When she recognizes her own countertransference reactions, she can deal more effectively with her patients.

Because transference increases emotionality, its presence may alter judgment and behavior in patients' relationships with their doctors. This alteration can be positive or negative. In **positive transference,** the patient may have unrealistic confidence in the doctor. If intense, the patient may overidealize or even develop sexual feelings for the doctor. In contrast, in **negative transference,** patients may become resentful or angry toward the doctor if the patient's desires and expectations are not realized. This unconscious resentment can result in noncompliance with medical advice.

Doctors also experience transference reactions toward patients. These reactions stem from the doctor's own important past relationships, a phenomenon known as **countertransference.** Countertransference reactions can occur when a patient reminds the doctor of a close friend or relative. They also commonly occur when a doctor is treating a colleague, friend, or relative. In both instances, countertransference can cloud medical judgment and cause an inappropriate reaction to a patient.

REVIEW QUESTIONS

1. According to Freudian theory, which of the following structures of the mind are completely developed in a normal 1-year-old child?

(A) The id only

(B) The id and the ego only

(C) The id, ego, and superego

(D) The superego only

(E) Neither the id, ego, nor superego

2. A 10-year-old boy is frequently truant from school. When he does go to school, he is often sent to the principal's office for hitting other children. At home, he has had pet fish and birds, but none of them have survived for more than a few weeks. Which aspect of the mind is probably deficient in this child?

(A) The id only

(B) The id and the ego only

(C) The id, ego, and superego

(D) The superego only

(E) Neither the id, ego, nor superego

Questions 3–5. For each of the numbered patients, choose the correct defense mechanism that he or she is using.

(A) Regression

(B) Acting out

(C) Denial

(D) Splitting

(E) Projection

(F) Dissociation

(G) Reaction formation

(H) Intellectualization

(I) Sublimation

(J) Displacement

3. A 34-year-old woman states that she cannot remember buying a dress that is hanging in her closet. The dress is low-cut and bright red and is unlike the type of clothing that she usually wears. The woman also relates that at least twice a week she wakes up on the living room sofa fully dressed, although she remembers going to sleep in a nightgown in her own bed.

4. A 28-year-old medical student who has unconscious, violent feelings decides to apply for a residency in surgery.

5. A 14-year-old girl who has never had a sexual relationship and has no psychiatric history has sexual encounters with multiple partners in the months after her mother's death.

ANSWERS AND EXPLANATIONS

1-A. Only the id is completely developed in a 1-year-old child. In Freud's structural theory, the mind is divided into the id, ego, and superego. The id operates completely on an unconscious level while the ego and super-ego operate partly on an unconscious and partly on preconscious and conscious levels. The id is present at birth. The ego begins to develop immediately after birth, and the superego is developed by about age 6 years.

2-D. The superego is associated with moral values and conscience, and it controls impulses of the id. This boy, who hits other children, is truant, and most likely kills his pets is showing deficiencies in his superego. Children over age 6 years and under age 18 years who have poor superego development may have conduct disorder (see Chapter 2). The id contains instinctive sexual and aggressive drives and is not influenced by external reality. The ego also controls the expression of the id, sustains satisfying interpersonal relationships, and, through reality testing, maintains a sense of reality about the body and the external world.

3-F. This patient who relates that she wakes up fully dressed at least twice a week and cannot remember buying something in her closet is exhibiting dissociative identity disorder (multiple personality disorder). Dissociation, separating part of one's consciousness from real-life events, is the defense mechanism used by individuals with this disorder. This patient is likely going out at night but does not remember doing so because she was experiencing another personality at that time (see Chapter 18).

4-I. In sublimation, the medical student reroutes his unconscious, unacceptable wish for committing a violent act to a socially acceptable route (cutting people during surgery). Other mature defense mechanisms include suppression, altruism, and humor.

5-B. This teenager is acting out her depression and anxiety over the loss of her mother in socially unacceptable behavior.

REFERENCES

Brenner, C. (1973). *An elementary textbook of psychoanalysis.* New York: International Universities Press.

Chodoff, P. (2000). The changing role of dynamic psychotherapy in psychiatric practice. *Psychiatr Serv, 51,* 1404–1407.

Despland, J. N., de Roten, Y., Despars, J., Stigler, M., & Perry, J. C. (2001). Contribution of patient defense mechanisms and therapist interventions to the development of early therapeutic alliance in a brief psychodynamic investigation. *J Psychother Pract Res, 10,* 155–164.

Freud, A. (1966). *The ego and the mechanisms of defense* (Rev. ed.). New York: International Universities Press.

Gabbard, G. O. (1999). *Countertransference issues in psychiatric treatment.* Washington, DC: American Psychiatric Press.

Glucksman, M. L. (2001). The dream: A psychodynamically informative instrument. *J Psychother Pract Res, 10,* 223–230.

Vaillant, G. E. (1971). Theoretical hierarchy of adaptive ego mechanisms. *Arch Gen Psychiatry, 24,* 107–118.

Chapter

Learning Theory   **9**

In Freudian theory, normal and abnormal human behavior results from conscious and unconscious mental forces (see Chapter 8). In the **behaviorist** view, behavior results from adaptive and maladaptive learning. For example, the psychoanalyst believes that a 35-year-old woman's unexplained, disabling fear (**phobia**) of animals is caused by a repressed frightening experience. The behaviorist claims that the woman simply made an exaggerated association in childhood between animals and pain and now experiences mental pain and fear in the presence of animals.

The idea that behavior is acquired by learning is more optimistic than the Freudian view. Because behavior that has been learned can be "unlearned," it is more easily modified and improved than behavior that is due to unconscious and hence obscure mental forces.

Mechanisms of learning include simple forms, such as habituation and sensitization, and more complex types, including classical conditioning, operant conditioning, and modeling. These mechanisms form the basis of treatment techniques (see Chapter 11) aimed at increasing the frequency of desired behavior and decreasing the frequency of unwanted behavior.

■ HABITUATION AND SENSITIZATION

Habituation and **sensitization** are the simplest forms of learning. In habituation, repeated stimulation results in a decreased response; in sensitization, repeated stimulation results in an increased response. Eric

Kandel received the Nobel Prize in 2000 for research that showed that habituation and sensitization can be demonstrated even in a relatively uncomplicated organism, the marine snail *Aplysia.* A touch to the snail's siphon caused a withdrawal response; with repeated touching, the withdrawal response decreased. If the snail's siphon was initially stimulated with a strong electric shock, only very slight stimulation was subsequently needed to elicit a withdrawal response. A clinical parallel of this experiment can be seen in young children who receive weekly allergy injections. Almost all children cry at the first injection, but with repeated injections, crying decreases in some children. Other children, particularly those whose first injection was very uncomfortable, show more fearfulness and crying with each ensuing injection.

CLASSICAL CONDITIONING

In **classical** or **respondent conditioning,** a natural, reflexive, or unconditioned response (a behavior) is elicited by a learned or conditioned stimulus (a cue from an internal or external event). Classical conditioning can explain both negative and positive emotional responses. For example, because of a prior stressful medical event, a man experiences a negative emotional response (fear) when he hears his doctor's voice. In contrast, a positive emotion, pleasure, is elicited when the same man hears his lover's voice.

Elements of classical conditioning

The four elements of classical conditioning are the unconditioned stimulus, the unconditioned response, the conditioned stimulus, and the conditioned response. Pavlov's classic study illustrates these elements—dogs learned that the sound of a bell, rung in conjunction with presentation of food in the past, meant that food would appear in the present.

An **unconditioned stimulus** (e.g., the odor of food) automatically produces a reflexive, natural, unlearned, or **unconditioned response** (e.g., salivation). A **conditioned stimulus** is something that produces a response following learning (e.g., the sound of the bell). A **conditioned response** is a behavior that is learned by an association made between a conditioned stimulus and an unconditioned stimulus (e.g., salivation in response to the bell).

Characteristics of classical conditioning

Response acquisition, extinction, spontaneous recovery, and stimulus generalization are characteristics of classical conditioning. In **acquisition,** the conditioned response (salivation in response to the bell) is acquired or learned. After learning has occurred, if the conditioned stimulus (the sound of the bell) is never again paired with the unconditioned stimulus (the presence of food), the conditioned response (salivation) decreases. This decrease and ultimate disappearance of the conditioned response is known as **extinction.** Sometimes, after extinction, the sound of the bell again generates salivation. This unexpected reoccurrence is called **spontaneous recovery.** Sometimes, a new stimulus, such as a buzzer that resembles a conditioned stimulus (the bell), causes the conditioned response (salivation). This phenomenon is called **stimulus generalization.** A 2-year-old child who is afraid of nurses in white uniforms and cries when his grandmother comes to visit wearing a white jacket is an example of stimulus generalization.

Learned helplessness and imprinting

When an animal receives a series of painful electric shocks from which it is unable to escape, it learns, by classical conditioning, to make an association between the aversive stimulus (e.g., electric shock) and the inability to escape. Subsequently, the animal makes no attempt to escape when shocked or in fact when faced with any new aversive stimulus. Instead, the animal becomes hopeless and apathetic. This phenomenon has been termed **learned helplessness.**

Learned helplessness in animals has been proposed as a model system for depression in humans. In this model, the person who has repeatedly tried and failed to control external events becomes hopeless, apathetic, and depressed (like the shocked animal) when faced with a new life stressor. Learned helplessness can help explain why children who repeatedly fail in school despite their best efforts eventually stop trying to do well and give up.

Imprinting is another phenomenon that has been observed in animal models. It is based on the concept of **critical periods,** limited intervals during which a developing animal is more sensitive to certain stimuli than at other times in its development. During the critical period for imprinting, the animal makes an association with and then follows the first thing it sees after birth or hatching. Although seen mainly in birds, imprinting has applications to human development, particularly for the critical period of attachment between an infant and its mother (see Chapter 1).

■ OPERANT CONDITIONING

In **operant conditioning** or **trial and error learning,** learning occurs because of the consequences to the individual of a previous behavior. Although the previous behavior may have occurred randomly at first, the consequence, occurring immediately after the behavior, determines whether the behavior continues.

Reinforcement and punishment

The likelihood that a behavior will occur is increased by reinforcement and decreased by punishment. Reinforcement can be positive or negative. **Positive reinforcement** is the introduction of a stimulus that results in an increase in the rate of a behavior. For example, if a child increases her studying behavior to earn money by receiving good grades in math, money is the reinforcer or reward that increases the desired studying behavior. Reinforcement can be praise, attention, or a tangible reward such as money.

Negative reinforcement is the removal of an aversive stimulus that results in an increase in the rate of behavior. For example, if a child increases her studying behavior to avoid being scolded, active avoidance of an aversive stimulus (being scolded) increases the desired studying behavior.

Clinically, negative reinforcement is a major factor in **compliance** with medical advice. Patients rarely comply with a doctor's advice to get a reward, but they often comply to avoid illness (a negative consequence). A patient who walks more to decrease the amount of antihypertensive medication that she requires is exercising because of negative reinforcement.

Punishment is the introduction of an aversive stimulus aimed at reducing the rate of an unwanted behavior. For example, if a child decreases her "fooling around" behavior after her mother scolds her, the scolding can be considered a punishment.

The introduction of a stimulus that seems aversive can actually increase the rate of unwanted behavior. For example, if a child increases her "fooling around" behavior after her mother scolds her, the scolding can be considered a positive reinforcer rather than a punishment because it increases the rate of the problematic behavior.

Extinction in operant conditioning is the gradual disappearance of a learned behavior when reinforcement (reward) is withheld. For example, if the mother's attention is a reinforcer, the child stops "fooling around" when that behavior is ignored by her mother. Characteristically, an initial increase in "fooling around" behavior occurs before it finally disappears.

Punishment versus extinction

Behavior is changed more effectively over the long term by rewarding or reinforcing individuals for desired behavior (positive reinforcement) or by not rewarding them for unwanted behavior (extinction), than by punishing unwanted behavior. Also, in contrast to extinction, which reduces behavior for a long time, the behavioral effects of punishment are more likely to be temporary.

One strategy that encourages extinction is **time out.** In this technique, an individual (usually a child) is temporarily removed from the social situation each time he or she misbehaves. Because during each time-out period the child receives no positive reinforcement (attention) for the undesirable behavior, that behavior ultimately becomes extinct.

Schedules of reinforcement

The pattern, or schedule, of reinforcement affects how quickly a behavior is learned and how quickly a behavior becomes extinct (i.e., disappears)

THE PATIENT The mother of a 4-year-old boy tells the pediatrician that the child frequently makes his 2-year-old brother cry when she is out of the room. She relates that sometimes she scolds the older child but sometimes she just ignores this behavior. No matter what she does, his negative behavior toward the 2-year-old persists and is getting worse. When the mother is present, the boy behaves appropriately and even affectionately toward the younger child. The 4-year-old shows no developmental delay and gets along well with children his own age. The mother asks the doctor what she should do to improve the older child's poor behavior toward the younger child.

COMMENT The negative behavior that this child shows toward his brother has been learned through operant conditioning. A likely scenario for how it was learned follows: A bored 4-year-old is in the living room with his 2-year-old brother while his mother prepares dinner in the kitchen. While playing, he accidentally kicks his little brother who starts to cry. The mother comes in, scolds the 4-year-old, and goes back to the kitchen. The older child's hitting behavior has elicited a response from the mother and the child has received attention, a positive reinforcer. Subsequently, he purposely kicks the 2-year-old to elicit the reinforcement, a return visit by the mother.

TREATMENT The mother should be advised to avoid giving the older child attention for his unacceptable behavior toward the 2-year-old. Rather than scolding him, she should quietly separate the children by putting the older child in another room ("time out"). In addition, the mother should reinforce the 4-year-old's good behavior by giving him attention and praise when he is kind toward his brother. It is also appropriate that the mother avoid leaving the children alone in a room together and that she set aside time when she can play just with the older child to give him the attention from her that he clearly craves.

---

when it is not rewarded. Schedules of reinforcement include continuous, fixed ratio, fixed interval, variable ratio, and variable interval. **Continuous reinforcement,** in which an individual is rewarded each time he shows a desired behavior, is particularly useful for the rapid establishment of new behavior patterns (see Question 1). For example, if a child receives money every time he walks the dog (continuous reinforcement), his dog-walking behavior is learned quickly. In **ratio schedules** of reinforcement, a reward is given after a set number (fixed ratio) or changeable number (**variable ratio**) of responses. Continuous reinforcement is a type of **fixed ratio** reinforcement. In **interval schedules** of reinforcement, reward is given after a set amount of time (**fixed interval**) or variable amount of time (**variable interval**) passes. Whether or not ratio or interval schedules are used, learning takes longer with variable rather than fixed schedules of reinforcement. For example, if a child only occasionally receives money for walking the dog (variable ratio reinforcement), his dog-walking behavior takes longer to learn. Table 9-1 lists more examples of schedules of reinforcement.

Resistance to extinction is the force that prevents a behavior from disappearing when the reward is withheld. Behavior learned using variable ratio and variable interval reinforcement is more resistant to extinction (persists without reward) than behavior learned by continuous or fixed reinforcement schedules. In the previous example, if the child is paid only occasionally for walking the dog, he will continue to walk the dog for a period of time even without payment. In contrast, if the child is paid each time he walks the dog, his dog-walking behavior will stop almost immediately if he is not paid.

In real life, reinforcement commonly occurs unpredictably; that is, on a variable reinforcement schedule rather than on a continuous or fixed reinforcement schedule. For example, people are rarely rewarded for every good deed they do. Rather, they are sometimes praised but more often ignored when they show helpful behavior.

Shaping

Reinforcement can increase the rate of behavior once the behavior occurs. However, if the desired behavior is not shown in the first place, it cannot be reinforced. To achieve behavior by **shaping,** a person is rewarded or reinforced when he or she randomly (by trial and error) shows something like the desired behavior. Closer and closer approximations of the wanted behavior are then reinforced until the correct behavior is achieved. Thus, the parents of an autistic child who does not speak are told to reward him with a treat each time he makes any sound. After he has learned to make sounds to get the reward, they require him to use words that resemble the desired word. Finally, they require actual words before dispensing the treat.

■ MODELING

Modeling is a type of observational learning. Using modeling, an individual observes others and imitates their behavior. This type of learning is more efficient and faster than operant learning and is particularly useful in acquiring skills like driving a car. Like the well-known description of learning in medicine, "see one, do one, teach one," modeling can be used to learn a medical procedure and to then teach it to others. Although learning by modeling is often a positive way to learn, it can have a negative outcome (Case 9–2).

Studies have shown that modeling can be used to ease fear in people undergoing medical procedures. For example, before having an endoscopy, a patient is instructed to view a videotape of another patient comfortably undergoing the same procedure while successfully using relaxation and other coping strategies. When the patient herself then undergoes the procedure, she is relaxed and comfortable.

TABLE 9-1   Schedules of Reinforcement

SCHEDULE	REINFORCEMENT	EXAMPLE	EFFECT ON BEHAVIOR
Continuous	Presented after every response	A teenager receives a candy bar each time she puts a dollar into a vending machine. One time she puts a dollar in and nothing comes out. She never buys candy from the machine again.	Putting money in the machine to receive candy is rapidly learned, but it disappears rapidly (has low resistance to extinction) when not reinforced (no candy comes out).
Fixed ratio	Presented after a designated number of responses	A man is paid $10 for every five hats he makes.	Fast response rate (many hats are made quickly). He makes as many hats as he can during his shift.
Fixed interval	Presented after a designated amount of time	A student has an anatomy test every Friday. He does not study Saturday through Tuesday but studies for 10 minutes on Wednesday nights and for 2 hours on Thursday nights.	The response rate (studying) increases toward the end of the interval (week). When graphed, the response rate forms a scalloped curve; it decreases just after a reinforcement (the first test) and increases just before the next reinforcement (the next test).
Variable ratio	Presented after a random and unpredictable number of responses	After a slot machine pays off $5 for a single quarter, a woman plays $50 in quarters despite the fact that she receives no further payoffs.	The behavior (playing the slot machine) continues (is highly resistant to extinction) despite the fact that it is only reinforced (winning money) after a large but variable number of responses.
Variable interval	Presented after a random and unpredictable amount of time	After 5 minutes of fishing at a lake, a man catches a large fish. He then spends many hours waiting for another bite.	The behavior (fishing) continues (is highly resistant to extinction) despite the fact that it is only reinforced (a fish is caught) after varying time intervals.

Adapted from Fadem, B. (1999). *Behavioral science* (3rd ed.). Baltimore: Lippincott, Williams & Wilkins.

THE PATIENT A 7-year-old child is referred to the school physician because he shows a disabling fear of cats. The teacher reports that the child's fear is so intense that even when the class is shown a photograph or drawing of a cat, the child screams and runs out of the classroom. The teacher has removed all books about cats from the class library but fears that another child will inadvertently expose the fearful child to cats. The child also seems tense when he must go outside at the end of the school day. When questioned about this he says, "How do I know there are no cats outside?" The child is working at the age-appropriate level in school and interacts well with other children. The physician calls a conference with the teacher and the child's mother.

COMMENT At the conference, the physician notes that the mother seems uncomfortable. She states that she is upset because she saw a kitten near the school door when she entered the building. The mother says that although she is afraid of cats, she knows that cats are harmless and has tried not to show her fear in the child's presence. Although the mother has tried to hide her fear, the child has learned to be afraid of cats after observing his mother show anxiety in their presence. Thus, the child has learned his fear of cats by modeling his mother's behavior.

TREATMENT The physician's first suggestion is to help the mother deal with her own fear. Several treatment techniques can be used based on learning theory, like systematic desensitization, flooding, and implosion (see Chapter 11). When the mother's fear subsides, the child's symptoms will likely improve. In addition (or alternatively), the child himself can receive behavioral treatment to deal with his own fear.

REVIEW QUESTIONS

1. Over the past year, an obese patient on a calorie-restricted diet has been visiting her physician weekly to be weighed. In the first 6 months of the diet, the physician praised the patient each time she lost weight, and she lost a total of 20 pounds. In the second 6 months of the diet, the doctor rarely praised the patient when she lost weight and she lost only 3 pounds. This patient's dieting and weight loss behavior is most likely to have been learned using which of the following methods?

   (A) Continuous reinforcement

   (B) Variable interval reinforcement

   (C) Fixed interval reinforcement

   (D) Variable ratio reinforcement

   (E) Punishment

2. When a 46-year-old man visited his physician for a check-up in 2003, he was diagnosed with atrial fibrillation. His blood pressure at the time was high normal at 130/85. The patient's father, who also had atrial fibrillation, died of a stroke at age 47. In addition to taking medication for the arrhythmia, the patient buys a blood pressure machine and carefully watches his diet. When taken at home, the patient's blood pressure varies from 120–130/80–90 throughout the year. However, when he visits the doctor in 2004, his blood pressure is 150/92. The doctor says that although other tests need to be done, the patient is probably showing "white-coat hypertension." For this scenario, which element represents the conditioned response?

(A) Elevated blood pressure during the 2003 visit

(B) Elevated blood pressure during the 2004 visit

(C) The presence of the doctor in 2003

(D) The presence of the doctor in 2004

(E) Pairing the doctor with bad news

3. A political prisoner has received beatings in the past and could never escape. He no longer tries to escape new beatings. This behavior by the prisoner is an example of

(A) stimulus generalization

(B) modeling

(C) shaping

(D) imprinting

(E) learned helplessness

4. A 50-year-old man with diabetes is told that the more time he spends on his treadmill, the fewer insulin injections he will need to control his blood sugar. Subsequently, he increases his time on the treadmill. This man's increased exercising behavior is a result of

(A) punishment

(B) negative reinforcement

(C) positive reinforcement

(D) shaping

(E) classical conditioning

5. A 62-year-old man has undergone three sessions of chemotherapy in a hospital. Before the fourth session, he becomes nauseated when the needle is put into his vein even though the medication has not yet begun to flow. This patient's reaction is a result of the type of learning best described as

(A) operant conditioning

(B) classical conditioning

(C) modeling

(D) imprinting

(E) biofeedback

ANSWERS AND EXPLANATIONS

1-A. This patient learned to diet and lose weight by continuous reinforce-ment (i.e., the doctor's praise each time she lost weight). Behavior learned in this way is acquired quickly but also ceases quickly (extinction) when it is not reinforced—her rate of dieting and weight loss decreased when the doctor stopped praising her. Behavior learned by variable schedules of re-inforcement is learned more slowly but is more resistant to extinction than that learned by continuous reinforcement. If the doctor had praised this pa-tient only at some visits for her dieting and weight loss, she would have lost weight more slowly at first, but it would have continued longer in the absence of praise (i.e., been more resistant to extinction). Punishment is aversive and is aimed at suppressing an undesirable behavior.

2-B. The conditioned response is the elevated blood pressure in 2004 that results from an association made between anticipation of danger (death from the arrhythmia) and a prior visit to the doctor in 2003. This reaction is commonly called "white-coat hypertension." The cue that this response is learned is that the patient's blood pressure is relatively normal when taken at home. The presence of the doctor in 2003 and 2004 represent the unconditioned and conditioned stimuli, respectively. The patient's blood pressure in 2003 is the unconditioned (unlearned) response.

3-E. In learned helplessness, an association is made between an aversive stimulus and the inability to escape. Subsequently, the prisoner makes no attempt to escape; instead, he becomes hopeless and apathetic when faced with any new aversive stimulus. Learned helplessness may be a model paradigm for the development of depression. In contrast, modeling is a type of observational learning. In stimulus generalization, a new stimulus that resembles a conditioned stimulus causes a conditioned response. Shaping involves rewarding closer and closer approximations of the wanted behavior until the correct behavior is achieved. Imprinting is the tendency of organisms to make an association with and then follow the first thing they see after birth or hatching.

4-B. Because the behavior (exercise) is increased to avoid something neg-ative (insulin injections), this is an example of negative reinforcement. Both negative and positive reinforcement increase behavior. Punishment decreases or suppresses behavior. In classical conditioning, a natural, or reflexive, response (behavior) is elicited by a learned stimulus (a cue from an internal or external event).

5-B. This common clinical phenomenon is an example of classical conditioning (learning by association). In this example, a man comes into the hospital for an intravenous chemotherapy treatment (unconditioned stimulus). The chemotherapy drug is toxic and he becomes nauseated after the treatment (unconditioned response). The next month, when the needle enters his arm (conditioned stimulus), he becomes nauseated (conditioned response). Thus, the needle (the conditioned stimulus) has become paired with chemotherapy (the unconditioned stimulus), which elicited nausea. Now, nausea (unconditioned response) can be elicited by the needle alone (conditioned stimulus). In operant conditioning, behavior is determined by its consequences. Modeling is a type of observational learning. Biofeedback is a treatment technique based on operant conditioning (see Chapter 11).

REFERENCES

Kandel, E. R., & Hawkins, R. D. (1992). The biological basis of learning and individuality. *Sci Am, 267* (3), 78–86.

Pavlov, I. (1927). *Conditioned reflexes.* London: Oxford University Press.

Peterson, C., Maier, S., & Seligman, M. E. P. (1995). *Learned helplessness: A theory for the age of personal control.* New York: Oxford University Press.

Rescorla, R. A., & Holland, P. C. (1982). Behavioral studies of associative learning in animals. *Annu Rev Psychol, 33,* 265–308.

Skinner, B. F. (1938). *The behavior of organisms. An experimental analysis.* New York: Appeleton.

Skinner, B. F. (1979). *The shaping of a behaviorist.* New York: Knopf.

Walker, S. (1984). *Learning theory and behavior modification.* London: Methuen.

Psychological **10** Assessment of Patients With Behavioral Symptoms

T he evaluation of patients who show abnormal behavior normally occurs in the context of the clinical interview (see Chapter 24). The psychiatric history and structured instruments, such as the Mental Status Examination (MSE) and Beck Depression Inventory (BDI), are also used in the evaluation of such patients. Helpful adjuncts to these methods include psychological tools like intelligence, achievement, and personality tests.

Evaluation instruments can be administered to an individual or to a group of individuals at one time. Individually administered tests allow careful observation and evaluation of that person. Tests given to a group of people simultaneously have the advantages of efficient administration, grading, and statistical analysis. Tests commonly used in the psychological evaluation of patients fall into three main categories: intelligence, achievement, and personality/psychopathology (Table 10–1).

TABLE 10-1	Commonly Used Intelligence, Achievement, and Personality/Psychopathology Tests

TYPE OF TEST	SPECIFIC TEST
Intelligence	Wechsler Adult Intelligence Scale-Revised (WAIS-R) Wechsler Intelligence Scale for Children-Revised (WISC-R) Wechsler Preschool and Primary Scale of Intelligence (WPPSI) Stanford-Binet Intelligence Scale
Achievement	Scholastic Aptitude test (SAT) Medical College Admissions Test (MCAT) United States Medical Licensing Examination (USMLE) Wide-Range Achievement Test (WRAT) California, Iowa, Stanford, and Peabody Achievement Tests
Personality and psychopathology	Minnesota Multiphasic Personality Inventory (MMPI) Rorschach Inkblot Test Sentence Completion Test (SCT) Thematic Apperception Test (TAT) Mental Status Examination (MSE) Beck Depression Inventory-II (BDI-II) Zung Self-Rating Depression Scale Hamilton Rating Scale for Depression (HAM-D) Raskin Depression Scale

■ PSYCHIATRIC EVALUATION

The psychiatric history

A patient's **psychiatric history** is taken as part of the medical history. Although both histories focus on gathering factual information to define the chief complaint and determine the background of the current illness, the psychiatric history also investigates the patient's personality characteristics, relationships with others, and sources of stress. Aspects of the psychiatric history are summarized in Table 10–2.

The mental status examination and related instruments

The **mental status examination (MSE)** is a comprehensive survey used to evaluate an individual's current state of mental functioning. The MSE assesses a variety of characteristics, including general presentation (appearance, behavior, attitude toward the examiner, and level of consciousness); cognition (orientation, memory, attention and concentration, cognitive ability, and speech); emotional state (mood and affect); thought and perception (form or process, content, and perception); judgment and insight; and reliability and impulse control (Table 10–3). Terms used to describe psychophysiologic symptoms and mood in patients with psychiatric illness are listed in Table 10–4.

TABLE 10-2   Areas Addressed in the Psychiatric History

EARLY CHILDHOOD (0–3 YEARS)	CHILDHOOD (3–11 YEARS)	ADOLESCENCE (11–20 YEARS) AND ADULTHOOD (>20 YEARS)
BACKGROUND		
■ Normal pregnancy and delivery? ■ Wanted child? ■ Feeding, sleep, and toilet training? ■ Timely development of motor and social skills? ■ Caretakers other than mother?	■ School history and skill development? ■ Learning disabilities? ■ Punishment methods used in the home? ■ Response to first separation from mother?	■ Employment history? ■ Legal history? ■ Psychiatric history of family members? ■ Military service? ■ Level of education achieved? ■ Religious activities? ■ Current living situation?
PERSONAL CHARACTERISTICS		
■ Parental and sibling relationships? ■ Personality (e.g., shy or outgoing, active or passive)? ■ Temperment (e.g., easy, difficult, slow to warm up)?	■ Peer relationships (e.g., follower, leader, popular)? ■ Personality (e.g., assertive, anxious)? ■ Presence of unrealistic fears? ■ Cruelty to animals, bed wetting?	■ Emotional problems? ■ Drug and alcohol use? ■ Role models? ■ Social relationships? ■ Sexuality?

Rating scales for depression

The **Beck Depression Inventory-II (BDI-II)** is a commonly used self-rating scale containing 21 items (Table 10–5). Each item on the BDI-II has four possible answers scored from 0 to 3 (lowest to highest level of depression); 63 is the highest total score. For example, for item #5, guilt, the patient must choose one of the following four choices:

■ I don't feel particularly guilty = 0 points
■ I feel bad or unworthy a good part of the time = 1 point
■ I feel quite guilty = 2 points
■ I feel as though I am very bad or worthless = 3 points

Because the BDI-II asks about the presence of depression directly and is easy to administer, it is particularly useful for primary care physicians.

Other rating scales of depression include the Zung, Hamilton, and Raskin scales. Using the **Zung Self-Rating Depression Scale,** the patient rates

TABLE 10-3   The Mental Status Examination

CATEGORY	CHARACTERISTIC	EXAMPLE INDICATING NEED FOR FURTHER EVALUATION
PRESENTATION		
Appearance	Posture	Has a hunched-over posture while standing
	Grooming	Is unshaven
	Appearance for age	Appears older than his chronological age
	Clothing	Is wearing a heavy coat on a hot day
Behavior	Mannerisms	Shows unusual facial expressions or hand movements
	Psychomotor behavior	Seems physically speeded up (agitated) or slowed down (retarded)
	Tics	Uses repetitive, nonproductive movements
Attitude toward the examiner	Cooperative	Is not helpful
	Seductive	Behaves in a sexually provocative fashion
	Hostile	Seems angry
	Defensive	Seems to take remarks personally
Level of consciousness	Consciousness	Has a Glasgow Coma Scale of 10 (see Chapter 6)
	Lethargy	Seems mentally slowed down
	Sleepiness	Dozes off repeatedly
COGNITION		
Orientation	Person	Does not know her name or with whom she lives
	Place	Does not know where she is
	Time	Does not know the year, day, or time
Memory	Immediate	Cannot remember three words when questioned after 5 minutes
	Recent	Cannot remember her activities during the last 12 hours (verify information to rule out confabulation, i.e., filling in memory gaps with false information)
	Remote	Cannot remember where she was born
Attention and concentration	Attention	Cannot pay attention to you without being distracted by other stimuli
	Concentration	Cannot repeat a string of three to six numbers forward and backward (digit span) or spell the word "world" backward

TABLE 10-3   The Mental Status Examination (Continued)

CATEGORY	CHARACTERISTIC	EXAMPLE INDICATING NEED FOR FURTHER EVALUATION
Cognitive ability	Verbal ability	Cannot read a simple paragraph of text; cannot tell you how many states make up the United States Cannot compute 4 times 6
	Spatial ability	Cannot copy a simple drawing
	Abstraction ability	Cannot describe how a pear and an apple are alike Cannot explain the meaning of the proverb, "People who live in glass houses should not throw stones"
Speech	Timbre	Speaks too softly
	Speed	Speech is pressured (seems compelled to speak quickly)
	Articulation	Speech is not readily understandable
	Deficiencies in language	Uses words poorly or has a poor vocabulary
EMOTIONAL STATE		
	Mood	Describes feeling depressed (low, hopeless, helpless, suicidal) or manic (high, euphoric, irritable)
	Affect	Shows decreased (blunted, restricted, or flat) external expression of mood
	Congruence	Described mood and visible affect are dissimilar
	Appropriateness	Mood and affect are not appropriate to the current situation
THOUGHT AND PERCEPTION		
Form or process (associations between thoughts)	Flight of ideas	Has thoughts that move rapidly from one to the other
	Perseveration	Repeats thoughts over and over
	Echolalia	Responds to the rhyming sounds rather than to the meaning of a word
Content	Compulsions	Cannot refrain from performing an act (e.g., washing his hands)
	Obsessions	Cannot get a thought out of his head
	Phobias	Has irrational fears (e.g., is afraid to eat in a public place)
	Delusions	Has a false belief (e.g., is convinced that spies are after him)

TABLE 10-3	The Mental Status Examination (Continued)	
CATEGORY	CHARACTERISTIC	EXAMPLE INDICATING NEED FOR FURTHER EVALUATION
	Idea of reference	Believes that an actor in a movie is talking about him
Perception	Illusions	Misinterprets reality (e.g., thinks that a toy on the floor in a dark room is a live pet)
	Hallucinations	Has false sensory perceptions (e.g., feels insects crawling on his skin)
	Depersonalization and derealization	Has a feeling of being outside of himself or the environment
JUDGMENT AND INSIGHT		
Judgment and insight	Judgment	Gives an unusual response to a hypothetical situation (e.g., says she would discard a stamped, addressed letter found on the sidewalk)
	Insight	Does not realize that her thoughts and perceptions are not rational (e.g., says that she washes her hands excessively because they have "germs all over them")
Reliability and impulse control	Truthfulness	Provides incorrect information about previous hospitalizations (based on information from family or friends as well as clinical judgment)
	Aggressive and sexual impulses	Cannot control impulses (based on the history and current behavior)

herself with respect to symptom severity. With the **Hamilton Rating Scale for Depression (HAM-D),** the examiner interviews and rates the patient from 0 to 4 on characteristics such as work and activities, anxiety and somatic symptoms, and feelings of guilt, helplessness, hopelessness, and worthlessness. On the **Raskin Depression Scale,** the patient is rated using his or her own verbal report and on displayed behavior and secondary symptoms.

■ INTELLIGENCE AND INTELLIGENCE TESTS

Intelligence versus achievement

Intelligence and achievement, although related, are different entities. **Achievement** is a culture-specific measure of knowledge and skills acquired from education and experience. In contrast, **intelligence** is a meas-

TABLE 10-4	Glossary of Psychophysiologic States

MOOD
Euphoric mood: strong feelings of elation
Expansive mood: feelings of self-importance and generosity
Irritable mood: easily annoyed and quick to anger
Euthymic mood: normal mood, with no significant depression or elevation of mood
Dysphoric mood: subjectively unpleasant feeling
Anhedonic mood: inability to feel pleasure
Labile mood (mood swings): alternations between euphoric and dysphoric moods

AFFECT
Restricted affect: decreased display of emotional responses
Blunted affect: strongly decreased display of emotional responses
Flat affect: complete lack of emotional responses
Labile affect: sudden alterations in emotional responses not related to environmental events

FEAR AND ANXIETY
Fear: fright caused by real danger
Anxiety: fright caused by imagined danger
Free-floating anxiety: fright not associated with any specific cause

CONSCIOUSNESS AND ATTENTION
Normal: alert, can follow commands, normal verbal responses
Clouding of consciousness: inability to respond normally to external events
Somnolence: abnormal sleepiness
Stupor: responds only to shaking, shouting, and prodding
Coma: total unresponsiveness to stimuli

ure of an individual's innate potential for learning. Intelligence is quantified by the ability to reason: to think logically and come to a conclusion; to understand abstract concepts; to assimilate, recall, analyze, and organize information; and to meet the special needs of new situations.

Determinants of intelligence

Intelligence is determined largely by genetic factors. Monozygotic twins tend to have equivalent intelligence even if they are raised in separate households. Approximately one half of the difference between one person's intelligence test score and the scores of others (**the variance**) can be explained by genetic factors (Bouchard et al., 1990; Plomin et al., 1994; Weiss, 1992). Biological factors that negatively affect intelligence include poor nutrition and illness early in life. Environmental factors (such as exposure to educational enrichment), social factors (such as a good parent-child relationship), and emotional factors (such as a positive response to a testing situation) can influence performance on intelligence tests.

THE PATIENT A 25-year-old medical student is brought to the hospital by his brother after he accused his parents of trying to kill him. The brother says that the patient has been behaving strangely for the past 2 weeks, ever since he failed a microbiology examination. The patient is unkempt, unshaven and agitated, but shows no evidence of drug or alcohol abuse. When given the MSE (see Table 10–5), the patient listens and responds to the examiner with understandable speech. He is oriented times 3 (to person, place, and time) and, although he seems distracted, shows immediate, recent, and remote memory function. Although he cannot spell the word "world" backwards, he reads a paragraph clearly and is able to multiply 3 times 8. When asked how an apple and an orange are alike he says that they are both full of poison fluid and that a voice in his head told him not to eat anything cold.

COMMENT This student is showing evidence of psychotic thinking, such as paranoia (belief that he will be killed), hearing voices, inability to concentrate (inability to spell the word "world" backward), and poor abstraction ability (inability to explain how an apple and an orange are alike) despite normal consciousness and memory. Because the symptoms have been present for only 2 weeks and began after a stressful life event (the exam failure), the best diagnosis at this time is brief psychotic disorder. If the symptoms persist for 1 to 6 months, the diagnosis changes to schizophreniform disorder. Persistence longer than 6 months suggests schizophrenia (see Chapter 12).

TREATMENT The emergency room treatment of psychotic patients like this young man involves use of antipsychotic medication. Although high-potency dopamine-2 receptor antagonists like haloperidol (Haldol) work quickly, atypical agents such as risperidone (Risperdal) and olanzapine (Zyprexa) have better side effect profiles, particularly in young men, than haloperidol (see Chapter 19).

TABLE 10-5 Items in the Beck Depression Inventory-II (BDI-II)

1. Sadness	12. Social withdrawal
2. Pessimism	13. Indecisiveness
3. Sense of failure	14. Negative body image
4. Dissatisfaction	15. Inability to work
5. Guilt	16. Insomnia
6. Expectation of punishment	17. Fatigueability
7. Dislike of self	18. Loss of appetite
8. Self-blame	19. Loss of weight
9. Suicidal ideation	20. Preoccupation with health
10. Episodes of crying	21. Low level of sexual interest
11. Irritability	

Each of the 21 items can be scored from 0 to 3. Total scores of 30 to 63 indicate severe depression, and total scores of 5 to 9 indicate no or little depression. Very low total BDI scores (e.g., <4) may indicate that the patient is "faking good" because even normal people sometimes have sad feelings. Conversely, very high scores (e.g., >40) may suggest "faking bad."

Ethnic differences can affect performance on intelligence tests. Comparisons between the two largest ethnic groups suggest that white Americans tend to score higher than African Americans. Because intelligence tests use culture-specific language and tend to reflect the values and knowledge of American middle-class white culture, this difference in test performance has been attributed primarily to cultural and socioeconomic factors (Helms, 1992).

In the absence of brain pathology, intelligence is relatively stable throughout life. Although an individual's intelligence is essentially the same in old age as in childhood, a characteristic decrease in processing speed with age can affect performance on timed aspects of standardized intelligence tests.

Mental age, chronological age, and IQ

Many instruments have been developed to assess intelligence. One of the first, devised by Alfred Binet, presented the construct of **mental age (MA).** In this view, mental age reflects a person's level of intellectual functioning. For example, a child with a test score that reveals an MA of 8 is functioning like an average 8 year old. Because mental age has an obvious relationship with actual or **chronological age (CA),** Binet's scale was later adapted to include the age variable, and the concept of intelligence quotient (IQ) was produced. Operationally, IQ is the ratio of MA to CA times 100; an equation expressed as $MA/CA \times 100 = IQ$. Because an equal numerator and denominator result in 1, an IQ of 100 means that the person's mental and chronological ages are equivalent. A 10-year-old child with an MA of 10 years thus has an IQ of 100. A 10-year-old child with an MA of 9 has an IQ of 90. Because normal IQ varies within the range of 90 to 109, both of these children are considered average or normal. A child age 10 years with an MA of 12 has an above-normal IQ at 120.

Because MA does not increase measurably after age 15 years, 15 is usually the highest number used in the denominator of the IQ formula. For example, a 20-year-old man with an MA of 10 years has an IQ of $10/15 \times 100 = 67$ (not $10/20 = 50$).

The standard deviation (see Appendix) in IQ scores is about 15 points. Although other factors such as level of social functioning are considered, a person with an IQ that is more than two standard deviations below the mean (IQ = 70) fits into the category of mental retardation (see Chapter 2). An IQ score between 71 and 84 indicates borderline intellectual function, and a person with an IQ more than two standard deviations above the mean (IQ >130) has superior intelligence. DSM-IV-TR classifications of mental retardation are

- Mild (IQ 50–70): Function at about sixth grade level
- Moderate (IQ 35–55): Function at about second grade level
- Severe (IQ 20–40): Function below grade school level
- Profound (IQ <20): Function significantly below grade school level

The overlap or gap in IQ in these categories is related to differences in testing instruments.

Intelligence tests

The Wechsler intelligence tests, each taking about 2 hours to administer to one subject, are commonly used in the clinical setting. The **Wechsler Adult Intelligence Scale-Revised (WAIS-R)** is given to adults aged 16 to 75 years. It has six verbal and five performance subtests (Table 10–6).

TABLE 10-6	Subtests of the Wechsler Adult Intelligence Scale-Revised (WAIS-R)	
SUBTESTS	WHAT IS MEASURED	SCORE CLOSELY INFLUENCED BY:
VERBAL		
General information	Knowledge that a person has amassed	Education and culture
Comprehension	Understanding and social judgment	Culture
Arithmetic	Competence to do simple calculations	Ability to concentrate
Similarities	Ability to identify likenesses between two objects	Intellectual ability
Digit span	Ability to remember a string of numbers	Neurological function
Vocabulary	Ability to define vocabulary words	Educational level
PERFORMANCE		
Picture completion	Ability to finish a drawing that is incomplete	Vision and perception
Block design	Ability to replicate a visual design with blocks	Left-right dominance
Picture arrangement	Ability to arrange drawings in proper order to tell a story	Thinking style
Object assembly	Ability to put disjointed figures in the proper arrangement	Perception and manual dexterity
Digit symbol	Ability to quickly match numbers with corresponding characters	Speed of new learning and problem solving

THE PATIENT A 6-year-old girl who has been in kindergarten for 2 months is referred by her teacher to the school's child study team. The child cannot sit still in class and annoys the other children. Her speech is not clear and she does not seem to understand the teacher's instructions. The child seems appropriately interactive and friendly. The school physician finds that the child's hearing and vision are within the normal range. When the psychologist on the team administers the WPPSI, she finds that the child has an MA of 4 years. The Vineland Social Maturity Scale reveals that the child cannot dress herself or tie her shoes.

COMMENT With a CA of 6 years and an MA of 4 years, this child's IQ is 4/6 × 100 = 67. The results of the Vineland scale indicate that the child shows social maturity more appropriate to a 3 or 4 year old than a 6 year old. With no evidence of sensory deficits or interactional problems, these findings suggest that this child is mildly mentally retarded.

TREATMENT Many school systems "mainstream" mildly mentally retarded students. If mainstreamed, the child will continue to be in a regular classroom but will receive extra assistance with academic subjects like mathematics and reading from teachers who have been specially trained to deal with children with special needs. Alternatively, the child will be placed in "special education" classes with other children who have similar learning difficulties.

From these subtests, a verbal IQ, performance IQ, and full-scale IQ are derived. Although the WAIS-R is not specifically designed as a neuropsychological test, large differences between verbal and performance IQs suggest that the person has cerebral impairment. Specifically, patients with right-hemisphere lesions show better verbal than performance IQ scores, whereas those with left-hemisphere lesions show better performance than verbal IQ scores. The **Wechsler Intelligence Scale for Children-Revised (WISC-R)** is used to test intelligence in children 6 to 16½ years of age, and the **Wechsler Preschool and Primary Scale of Intelligence (WPPSI)** is used to test intelligence in children 4 to 6½ years of age.

Related tests include the **Vineland Social Maturity Scale** (Table 10–7), which is used to evaluate skills for daily living in mentally retarded (see Chapter 2) and other challenged people (e.g., those with impaired vision or hearing).

Giftedness

Clearly, high IQ as measured by standard tests is one aspect of a gifted child. However, most educators agree that gifted children not only have outstanding intellectual abilities, they are also capable of outstanding performance in other areas. These areas can be academic, such as mathematics, or creative, such as dance, music, or art. In contrast to common beliefs, gifted children are more likely than nongifted children to be well adjusted emotionally and to demonstrate social and educational achievement.

TABLE 10-7	Examples from the Vineland Social Maturity Scale	
EXPECTED AGE OF ACQUISITION	MOTOR ABILITY	COGNITIVE/VERBAL ABILITY
2 years	Removes clothing without assistance	Says at least 50 words
5 years	Ties shoelaces	Tells stories, jokes, and plots of television shows
8 years	Engages in sports	Can keep a secret for at least 1 day
11 years	Uses the telephone without assistance	Shows interest in gaining new information
16 years	Takes care of own health	Responds to indirect cues in conversation

■ ACHIEVEMENT TESTS

Achievement tests evaluate how well an individual has mastered specific subject areas such as reading and mathematics. These tests are used for career counseling in schools and industry. They are used also to evaluate performance in areas in which an individual has been specifically instructed. Achievement tests include the **Scholastic Aptitude Test (SAT), Medical College Admissions Test (MCAT),** and **United States Medical Licensing Examination (USMLE).**

Achievement tests such as the **Wide-Range Achievement Test (WRAT)** are used clinically to evaluate arithmetic, reading, and spelling skills in patients. Achievement tests used by school systems include the **California, Iowa, Stanford,** and **Peabody Achievement Tests.** A school system uses these test results not only to evaluate individual student performance, but also to monitor the effectiveness of its teaching program, teachers, and administrators and to compare itself with other school systems.

■ PERSONALITY TESTS

Personality tests are used to evaluate psychopathology and personality characteristics in patients in whom a behavioral disorder is suspected. These tests can help distinguish between a personality trait and a personality disorder, a point at which that trait has become maladaptive (see Chapter 18).

Personality tests are classified as either objective or projective. An **objective personality test** is based on questions that are easily scored and statistically analyzed. Because of this characteristic, objective tests can be administered by individuals with no special training. Thus, although these tests are usually interpreted by a psychologist, a family physician can administer the Minnesota Multiphasic Personality Inventory or the Million Clinical Multiaxial Inventory-II, which contain objective true or false questions (see later text) and are scored by machine.

A **projective personality test** requires the subject to interpret the questions by projecting his or her emotions, conflicts, and defense mechanisms into the answers. An examiner must have special training in interpreting the subject's responses in a projective test. Commonly used projective personality tests include the Rorschach Test and the Thematic Apperception Test and the Sentence Completion Test.

Objective personality tests

The Minnesota Multiphasic Personality Inventory (MMPI) is the most commonly used objective personality test. Patients answer 566 true (T) or false (F) items about themselves (for example, "My mother is (was) a good person," "I never do anything for the thrill of it," and "My work is very tension-provoking"). Clinical scales include depression, paranoia, schizophrenia, and hypochondriasis. Validity scales identify trying to look ill ("**faking bad**") or trying to look well ("**faking good**") (Fig. 10–1).

The Million Clinical Multiaxial Inventory-II (MCMI-II) generates scores that are directly compatible with personality disorders (pds) (see Chapter 24) and other diagnoses in the DSM-IV-TR. For example, a person who scores high on the borderline scale would be diagnosed as a borderline pd. The MCMI-II contains 175 items and, like the MMPI, these items are answered true or false. Scoring on the pds section of the MCMI-II is broken down into **basic personality pattern** and **pathological personality disorder.** The former includes 10 less severe pds (e.g., schizoid, avoidant, dependent, histrionic, narcissistic, antisocial, compulsive, and passive aggressive). The latter includes the three most severe pds: borderline, schizotypal, and paranoid disorders (see Chapter 24). Another section of the MCMI-II separates clinical syndromes into less severe (e.g., anxiety, somatoform, hypomania, dysthymia, alcohol abuse, and drug abuse) and more severe (e.g., psychotic thinking, psychotic depression, and psychotic delusion sections) (see Chapters 12–18).

Projective personality tests

The **Rorschach Test** is the most commonly used projective personality test. It is used primarily to identify thought disorders and defense mechanisms. In the Rorschach, patients are asked to interpret 10 bilaterally symmetrical inkblot designs (Fig. 10–2A). Five of the designs are in black and white, two are in black and red, and three are in pastel colors. The patient is first told to view the figures and, without any direction, is told to "Describe what you see in this figure." The patient is then asked why he

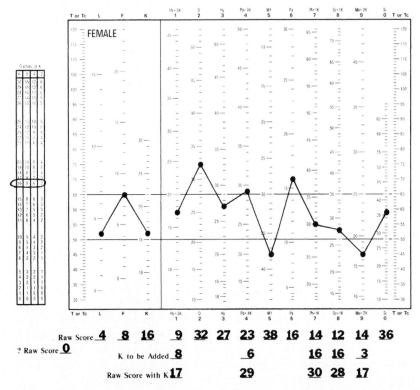

Raw Score **4** **8** **16** **9** **32** **27** **23** **38** **16** **14** **12** **14** **36**

? Raw Score **0**

K to be Added **8** **6** **16** **16** **3**

Raw Score with K **17** **29** **30** **28** **17**

FIGURE 10-1. Example of a Minnesota Multiphasic Personality Inventory (MMPI) personality profile obtained from a depressed, anxious man. Scores at the level of about 50 are average and scores above 70 are considered high. "L" is the lie scale, "F" is the infrequency scale, and "K" is the "suppressor" or correction scale that is added to some clinical scales to correct for "faking good." The clinical scales seen on the X axis in the example are as follows:
1 Hs - Hypochondriasis: Excessive concern about physical well-being
2 D - Depression: Feelings of hopelessness and helplessness
3 Hy - Hysteria: Unexplained physical symptoms
4 Pd - Psychopathic deviance: Lack of morality and concern for others
5 Mf - Masculinity-Femininity: Behavior typical of either gender
6 Pa - Paranoia: Suspicious about the motivation of others
7 Pt - Psychasthenia: Anxious and worried
8 Sc - Schizophrenia: Bizarre ideas and false beliefs (delusions)
9 Ma - Hypomania: Elevated mood and high energy
0 Si - Social Introversion: Shyness and lacks of self-confidence

(Reprinted with permission from Rathus, S. A. (1996). Psychology in the new millennium (6th ed.). Forth Worth, TX: Harcourt Brace.)

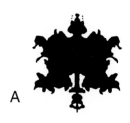 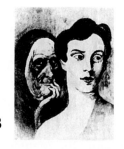

A   B

FIGURE 10-2.   Rorschach Ink Blot **(A)** and Thematic Apperception Test Card **(B).**

(Original source of Rorschach illustration: Kleinmuntz, B. (1974). Essentials of abnormal psychology. New York: Harper & Row. Original source of TAT illustration: Phares, E. J. (1984). Clinical psychology: Concepts, methods, and profession (2nd ed.). Homewood, IL: Dorsey. Both illustrations from Krebs, D., & Blackman, R. (1988). Psychology: A first encounter. Fort Worth, TX: Harcourt Brace. Used by permission of the publisher.)

responded the way that he did. Scoring is based on the content of and explanation for the response.

In the projective **Thematic Apperception Test (TAT),** stories are used to evaluate patients' unconscious emotions and conflicts. The patient can be shown a series of 30 cards, although sometimes only a few cards are used. Each card depicts an ambiguous social situation that can be interpreted in several ways (Fig. 10–2B). The subject is then told, "Using this picture, make up a story that has a beginning, a middle, and an end." The examiner interprets the subject's responses, which are believed to reflect basic personality characteristics and motivation.

The **Sentence Completion Test (SCT)** is used to identify a patient's worries and problems by verbal associations. In the SCT, the patient is told to complete nonstructured sentences started by the examiner; for example: "My father . . ." "I wish . . ." "Most people . . . ," and so on. The examiner then analyzes the responses to the sentence completions with respect to the patient's motivation and conflicts.

REVIEW QUESTIONS

1. A 12-year-old girl has an IQ of 25. The mental ability of this child is equivalent to that of a child aged

   (A) 2 years

   (B) 3 years

   (C) 4 years

   (D) 5 years

   (E) 6 years

2. A primary care doctor is evaluating a 20-year-old female patient for depression. Of the following, which is the most appropriate test for the doctor to use?

(A) Thematic Apperception Test (TAT)

(B) The Beck Depression Inventory

(C) Wechsler Intelligence Scale for Adults-Revised (WAIS-R)

(D) Rorschach Test

(E) Folstein Mini-Mental State Examination

3. A physician is asked to examine an 85-year-old woman who has been a nursing home patient for the past 2 years. Despite diabetes and some loss of vision, the patient's physical condition is good. During the interview, the patient tells the doctor that she does not enjoy anything anymore, even the desserts that she used to like, and that she no longer looks forward to visits with her family. She says that she cannot imagine that anything would make her feel better and that she just wants to die. The best description of this patient's mood is

(A) euphoric

(B) dysphoric

(C) euthymic

(D) labile

(E) anhedonic

4. For evaluating the self-care skills of a 44-year-old man with an IQ of 60 for placement in a group home, what is the most appropriate test?

(A) Rorschach Test

(B) Vineland Social Maturity Scale

(C) Wide Range Achievement Test (WRAT)

(D) Folstein Mini-Mental State Examination

(E) Glasgow Coma Scale

ANSWERS AND EXPLANATIONS

1-B. The mental age of a 12-year-old child with an IQ of 25 is 3 years. The MA is calculated using the IQ formula: $IQ = MA/CA \times 100$; that is, $25 = x/12$, $x = 3$. Thus, this child may be severely mentally retarded.

2-B. The Beck Depression Inventory is an objective test that can be used by primary care physicians. Primary care physicians probably cannot administer and interpret the results of projective personality tests, such as the Thematic Apperception Test (TAT) and Rorschach Test. Intelligence, including general information and reading comprehension, can be tested using the Wechsler Adult Intelligence Scale- Revised (WAIS-R). The Folstein Mini-Mental State Examination is used to evaluate a person's current state of mental functioning.

3-E. This severely depressed woman is showing anhedonia (the inability to feel pleasure) and suicidality. Both are characteristics of severe depression. Despite her placement in a nursing home, she should be able to enjoy some aspects of her life. Antidepressant medication and counseling can help this woman to enjoy the remainder of her life. Euphoric mood is an elated mood, and euthymic mood is a normal mood with no significant depression or elevation. Dysphoric mood is a subjectively unpleasant feeling. Labile moods (mood swings) are alterations between euphoric and dysthymic moods.

4-B. The Vineland Social Maturity Scale is the most appropriate test for evaluating the self-care skills of mentally retarded individuals like this man.

REFERENCES

Bouchard, T. J., Jr., Lykken, D. T, McGue, M., Segal, N. L., & Tellegen, A. (1990). Sources of human psychological differences: The Minnesota study of twins reared apart. *Science, 250,* 223–228.

Bouchard, T. J., & McGue, M. (1981). Familial studies of intelligence: A review. *Science, 212,* 1055–1059.

Cohen, R., Duncan, M., & Cohen, S. L. (1994). Classroom peer relations of children participating in a pull-out enrichment program. *Gifted Child Q, 38,* 33–37.

Graham, J. R. (1993). MMPI-2: *Assessing personality and psychopathology.* New York: Oxford University Press.

Hamilton, M. (1960). A rating scale for depression. *J Neurol Neurosurg Psychiatry, 23,* 56.

Helms, J. E. (1992). Why is there no study of cultural equivalence of standardized cognitive ability testing? *Am Psychol, 47,* 1083–1101.

Magruder-Habib, K., Zung, W. K, & Feussner, J. R. (1990). Improving physicians' recognition and treatment of depression in general medical care. *Med Care, 28,* 239–250

Matarazzo, J. D. (1972). *Wechsler's measurement and appraisal of adult intelligence* (5th ed.). New York: Oxford University Press.

Plomin, R., McClearn, G. E., Smith, D. L., Vignetti, S., Chorney, M. J., Chorney, K., et al. (1994). DNA markers associated with high versus low IQ: The IQ quantitative trait loci (QTL) project. *Behav Genet, 24,* 107–118.

Schaie, K. W. (1994). The course of adult intellectual development. *Am Psychol, 49,* 304–313.

Sparrow, S. S., Ballo, D. A., & Cicchetti, D. V. (1984). Vineland adaptive behavior scales. Circle Pines, MN: American Guidance Service.

Steer, R. A., Rissmiller, D. J., & Beck, A. T. (2000). Use of the Beck Depression Inventory -2 with depressed geriatric patients. *Behav Res Ther, 38* (3), 311–318.

Steinberg, L., Lamborn, S. D., Dornbusch, S. M., & Darling, N. (1992). Impact of parenting practices on adolescent achievement: Authoritative parenting, school involvement and encouragement to succeed. *Child Dev, 63,* 1266–1281.

Teasdale, G., & Jennet, B. (1974). Assessment of coma and impaired consciousness: A practical scale. *Lancet, 2,* 81–84.

Weiss, V. (1992). Major genes of general intelligence. *Personality and Individual Differences, 13,* 1115–1134.

Wortham, S. C. (1990). *Tests and measurement in early childhood education.* Columbus: Merrill Publishing.

11

Psychological Therapies

Psychological therapy or **psychotherapy** describes any interaction between a patient (i.e. client) and a trained individual in which specific techniques are used to help the patient overcome psychological problems such as depression, adjust to life situations like divorce, increase individual development (e.g., achieve career success), or improve compliance with clinical recommendations (McDonald et al., 2002).

The most familiar models of psychotherapy are the psychoanalytic and behavioral models. In **psychoanalysis and related therapies,** treatment focuses on understanding the underlying, intrapsychic, and unconscious reasons for a person's problematic emotions and behavior. The expectation of this type of therapy is that once the person understands the basis of the feelings and behavior, he will be able to change them. In **behavioral therapy,** the actions of the person are the focus of treatment. The expectation of behavioral therapy is that by learning adaptive behavior and unlearning maladaptive behavior, a person can change his or her problematic behavior. In a related way, **cognitive-behavioral therapy** attempts to identify and then change problematic cognitions; that is, ideas patients have about themselves that ultimately affect their behavior. These ideas include erroneous interpretations of life events and unrealistic expectations of themselves. These and other commonly used types of psychotherapy are summarized in Table 11-1 and are discussed later in this chapter.

TABLE 11-1 Models of Psychotherapy and Major Uses

MODEL	TYPE	MAJOR USES
Psychoanalytical	Psychoanalysis and psychoanalytically oriented psychotherapy	To treat emotional problems (e.g., conversion disorder, obsessive-compulsive disorder, moderate to severe personality disorders, dysthymic disorder) resulting primarily from childhood conflict
	Brief dynamic therapy	To improve coping with current life stressors
	Interpersonal therapy	To gain insight into the causes of one's difficulties with others
Behavioral	Systematic desensitization	To treat phobias
	Aversive conditioning	To treat addictions (e.g., smoking), paraphilias (e.g., pedophilia), and maladaptive habits (e.g., nail biting)
	Flooding and implosion	To treat phobias
	Token economy	To increase positive behavior in autistic or mentally retarded persons
	Biofeedback	To treat chronic physical disorders
	Cognitive-behavioral therapy	To treat mild to moderate, unipolar, nonpsychotic depression
Other	Group therapy	To improve interpersonal relationships and treat personality disorders
	Leaderless group therapy	To provide support during stressful life experiences (e.g., cancer survivors' or ostomy groups) and to deal with addictions (e.g., Alcoholics Anonymous)
	Family therapy Marital/couples therapy Sex therapy	To treat family, relationship, or sexual problems
	Supportive therapy	To sustain people during stressful life experiences or chronic mental illness
	Stress management	To help people deal with chronic emotional stress

■ PSYCHOANALYSIS AND RELATED THERAPIES

Psychoanalysis and related therapies are based on Freud's psychodynamic concepts of the unconscious mind, transference reactions, and defense mechanisms (see Chapter 8). These therapies are insight-oriented. They aim to understand the underlying, unconscious basis of current conflicts and behaviors by recovering repressed experiences and integrating them into the patient's personality. Techniques that are used include free association, dream interpretation, analysis of transference reactions, and analysis of resistance (Table 11-2). These techniques can be useful not only in insight-oriented therapies, but also to enhance physician-patient relationships in primary care settings (Goldberg, 2000).

Types of therapy

The central strategy of classic **psychoanalysis** is to slowly uncover experiences that are repressed in the unconscious mind. To accomplish this goal, psychoanalytic patients receive extended treatment, often 4 to 5 ses-

TABLE 11-2	Techniques Used in Psychoanalysis	
TECHNIQUE	**DESCRIPTION**	**USE IN TREATMENT**
Free association	The patient says whatever comes to mind.	Layer by layer, unconscious memories are revealed and interpreted by the therapist; to do this, the patient must be as honest as possible with the therapist.
Interpretation of dreams	The patient reports her unedited dreams to the therapist.	The therapist interprets the dreams to examine the patient's unconscious conflicts and impulses.
Analysis of transference reactions	The patient's unconscious feelings (e.g., anger, disappointment) stirred up by physical or behavioral characteristics of the therapist are expressed toward the therapist.	These expressions are used by the therapist to understand the significance of the patient's important past relationships (see Chapter 8).
Analysis of resistance	The patient blocks unconscious thoughts from consciousness (resistance) because he or she finds them uncomfortable or unacceptable.	The therapist evaluates this unconscious editing of thoughts to identify the patient's painful or conflicted ideas, memories, or wishes.

sions weekly over 3 to 6 years. Typically, the patient reclines on a couch facing away from the therapist during treatment.

In contrast to psychoanalysis, **psychoanalytically oriented psychotherapy** has the patient sitting in a chair and facing the therapist. Also, psychoanalytically oriented psychotherapy is briefer and more direct.

Brief or short-term dynamic psychotherapy is designed to help people deal with current life problems or crises. It includes a lengthy first interview in which the patient is helped to quickly unlock the unconscious mind and focus on the present problem. Subsequently, the patient is confronted with his or her transference reactions and use of defense mechanisms during 12 to 40 weekly sessions.

Interpersonal therapy is based on the notion that psychiatric problems, specifically depression, result from difficulties in dealing with other people. In 12 to 16 structured weekly sessions, patients gain insight into how their interpersonal interactions and patterns of behavior lead to self-isolation. Positive transference with a consistently empathic and supportive therapist is facilitated; however, unlike psychoanalysis, interpersonal therapy focuses on present rather than past experiences.

Appropriate patients for psychoanalysis and related therapies

Certain patients are better suited to psychoanalysis and related therapies than others. The most appropriate patient for these therapies is intelligent, flexible, and not psychotic. He or she is also able to tolerate the negative emotions, such as anger and guilt, that can surface during this type of treatment. The patient must also be able to maintain an ongoing relationship with a therapist and, importantly, desire not only to relieve psychological symptoms but also to gain insight into and understanding of the problem. Additional characteristics are desirable for traditional psychoanalytic patients. Namely, they should be young (usually less than age 40 years) and not be dishonest or have an antisocial personality disorder. In addition, patients should have a stable life situation and, perhaps most significantly and practically, have the time and money to spend on this time-consuming and expensive form of treatment.

■ BEHAVIORAL AND COGNITIVE-BEHAVIORAL THERAPIES

Behavioral and cognitive-behavioral therapies are based on learning theory, including both classical and operant conditioning (see Chapter 9). In contrast to psychoanalysis and related therapies, the person's history and unconscious conflicts are considered irrelevant in these therapies and thus are not examined. Rather, the aim of these therapies is to relieve the person's symptoms by unlearning maladaptive behavior and altering negative thinking patterns. Therapies based on classical conditioning include systematic desensitization and aversive conditioning. Those based on operant conditioning include flooding and implosion, token economy, and biofeedback.

Systematic desensitization

Systematic desensitization is a technique used primarily in the treatment of phobias (i.e., irrational fears) (see Chapter 15). The theory behind this treatment is that in the past, through the process of classical conditioning, the phobic person associated an innocuous stimulus with a fear-provoking stimulus. Eventually, the innocuous stimulus became frightening. The treatment involves exposure to increasing doses of the fear-provoking stimulus while pairing it with a relaxing stimulus to induce a relaxation response. Because one cannot simultaneously be fearful and relaxed (**reciprocal inhibition**), the person shows less anxiety when exposed to the fear-provoking stimulus in the future. Case 11-1 demonstrates the use of systematic desensitization in the treatment of a phobia.

CASE 11-1

THE PATIENT A 35-year-old man asks his physician for help. He has recently been offered a job on the 30th floor of a high-rise building and, although it is a good career opportunity, the patient cannot take it because of his intense fear of elevators. The patient tells the doctor that he never had a bad experience in an elevator but was told that, as a child, he accidentally locked himself in a closet in his home and remained there for 2 hours before he was discovered.

COMMENT In the behaviorist view, this man made an unfortunate association in childhood between enclosed places, inability to escape, and fear. Although he is now an adult and can easily escape from most difficult situations, he now experiences mental pain and fear when anticipating being in such a place. The physician could refer the patient to a psychoanalyst to uncover and treat the repressed frightening memories of confinement. For practical reasons (the patient must accept or refuse the new job within the next month), the physician decides to treat him using the behavioral technique of systematic desensitization.

TREATMENT The doctor teaches the patient to relax using progressive muscle relaxation techniques. After 2 weeks of training, the patient is able to put himself into a relaxed state at will. On each of his four subsequent visits to the doctor, the patient first puts himself into this state. On the first visit after the patient is relaxed, the doctor shows him a photograph of people entering an elevator. On the second visit he is shown a video of office workers going into an elevator. On the third visit, the relaxed patient and the doctor enter and then leave a stationary elevator. On the fourth visit, the patient and the doctor take a ride in the elevator. The patient is then instructed to take an elevator ride without the doctor present. The patient is able to do this, takes the new job, and comfortably rides the elevator to work every day.

Aversive conditioning

Aversive conditioning is used mainly in the treatment of unwanted behavior such as paraphilias or addictions. Here, using classical conditioning, a personally pleasurable but maladaptive behavior like smoking or sexual interest in children is paired with an aversive or painful stimulus like an electric shock, so that the two become associated. Subsequently, the person stops engaging in the maladaptive behavior because it automatically provokes an unpleasant response. For example, a 35-year-old smoker is given an electric shock each time he is shown a videotape of a group of people smoking. Later he feels uncomfortable when he sees a package of cigarettes and avoids smoking.

Flooding and implosion

Flooding and **implosion** are operant conditioning techniques used primarily to treat phobias. The strategy of these techniques involves direct exposure (without the possibility of avoidance or escape) to the actual (flooding) or imagined (implosion) feared stimulus. For example, a woman who is afraid of riding in cars takes a long road trip (flooding) or imagines being in a car (implosion) on a long road trip. The theoretical basis of flooding and implosion is that by preventing avoidant/escape behavior, the conditioned response (avoidance of the feared stimulus) becomes extinct. Clearly, this dramatic form of treatment is best handled by a therapist well trained in these techniques.

Token economy

Token economy is a strategy used to increase positive behavior in persons who are severely disorganized (e.g., psychotic), autistic, or mentally retarded. Through the process of operant conditioning, desirable behavior (e.g., tooth brushing and hair combing) is reinforced by a reward or positive reinforcement (a token). Subsequently, the person increases the desirable behavior to gain the reward. For example, a 24-year-old poorly groomed female inpatient with disorganized schizophrenia is given a token when she takes a shower. She can exchange the tokens for privileges like visiting the snack bar or watching a movie. She then takes a shower every day.

Biofeedback

Biofeedback gained popularity in the 1970s as a noninvasive alternative to medication for treating physiological disorders. It has been effective in treating disorders such as hypertension, Raynaud's disease, migraine and tension headaches, chronic pain, fecal incontinence, and temporomandibular joint pain. Biofeedback is based on operant conditioning. A patient is given ongoing physiological information, and this information in turn acts as a reinforcer. The patient then uses this reinforcement in conjunction with relaxation techniques to control visceral changes.

The following is an example of how biofeedback can work in the clinical setting.

- A 60-year-old hypertensive woman has her blood pressure measured regularly and the readings are projected to her on her computer screen.
- She is then instructed to use a relaxing mental technique or image to reduce her blood pressure.
- By trial and error, the patient finds that when she imagines herself at the beach, the screen shows that her blood pressure decreases.
- This observed blood pressure decrease acts as positive reinforcement, and the patient increases her relaxation behavior.
- After a few weeks, the patient's beach image reduces her blood pressure even when she is not looking at the computer screen.

Cognitive-behavioral therapy

Cognitive-behavioral therapy, developed by Aaron Beck, Albert Ellis, and others, works on the premise that emotional problems like depression result from errors in thinking or cognition. Negative interpretations of the world and of oneself, as well as negative expectations for the future, are the **cognitive triad** that forms part of this cognitive model of depression. The learned helplessness model of depression (see Chapter 9) is closely related to this framework. The goal of cognitive therapy is to correct these errors in logic, which are also called **automatic thoughts.** Common automatic thoughts include **catastrophic thinking** (believing only the worst can happen, such as "I know that I will lose my job") and **overgeneralization** (making an unwarranted conclusion from one or a few experiences, such as "I can't do anything right"). Cognitive therapy is used primarily to treat mild to moderate depression and anxiety disorders and may be useful, in conjunction with antidepressants, for patients with major depression (Paykel et al., 1999). Operationally, the therapist and patient meet weekly, for 15 to 25 weeks. During these sessions, the patient is helped to identify distorted, negative, automatic thoughts about himself. He is told to replace these negative thoughts with positive, self-assuring thoughts. For example, a 25-year-old man who feels depressed, useless, and unappreciated by others is taught to examine the evidence for these feelings. As he rejects each negative, inaccurate, automatic thought, he replaces it with a mental image of an occasion or experience when he felt successful and valued. Even though the patient has not examined the underlying basis of these abnormal cognitions, his symptoms ultimately improve.

■ OTHER THERAPIES

Other therapies include group, family, marital, and supportive therapy as well as stress management techniques. Each of these therapies is particularly useful for certain populations.

Group therapy

In **group therapy,** people with a common negative life experience (e.g., rape victims), with particular disorders like anxiety or personality disorders, or with interpersonal problems such as trouble interacting with individual therapists as authority figures, get together with a therapist. Groups of about eight people usually meet weekly for 1 to 2 hours. The group provides members with an opportunity to express feelings as well as give feedback, support, and empathy. The therapist facilitates, observes, and comments on the members' interpersonal interactions.

In a related type of treatment, **leaderless group therapy,** no one person is in authority. Rather, members of the group provide each other with support and practical help for a shared problem like alcoholism, loss of a loved one, or a specific disorder. **Twelve-step groups** such as Narcotics Anonymous (NA) and Overeaters Anonymous (OA) are based on the original Alcoholics Anonymous (AA) leaderless group model (see Chapter 23).

Family therapy

In family systems theory, psychopathology in one family member, the identified patient, reflects dysfunction of the entire family system. Because all members of the family cause behavioral changes in other members, the entire family (not necessarily just one person) is really the patient in **family therapy.**

In family therapy, as many involved family members as possible meet with a therapist. In the initial sessions, the therapist identifies dyads, triangles, and boundaries within the family system. **Dyads** are subsystems between two family members. For example, the executive dyad should include only the two parents. Children should not be included in the executive dyad. **Boundaries** are barriers between subsystems; for example, a generational boundary should exist between the executive dyad and the children. Abnormal boundaries are defined as too rigid (e.g., the parents never consider how the children feel about family decisions) or too permeable (e.g., the parents talk to the children about their marital relationship). **Triangles** are dysfunctional alliances between two family members against a third member (e.g., a mother and son forming an alliance against the father).

Specific techniques used in family therapy include **normalizing boundaries** between subsystems and reducing the likelihood of triangles. **Redefining blame** (e.g., encouraging family members to reconsider their own responsibility for problems) is another important technique that is used. Another mechanism, **mutual accommodation,** is a process in which family members are encouraged to work toward meeting each other's needs. Family therapy is particularly effective as a treatment for children with behavioral problems, families in conflict, and people with eating disorders or substance abuse (Case 11-2).

THE PATIENT A physician conducts a yearly school physical on a 15-year-old girl. The physical examination is otherwise unremarkable, but the patient has lost 25 pounds since the previous year. The patient, who had been of normal weight, is now significantly underweight. The teenager explains that she has been dieting because she is "fat," and she needs to lose yet another 10 pounds to qualify for the gymnastics team at school. The doctor diagnoses anorexia nervosa (see Chapter 17), hospitalizes the patient, and calls a consult with a family therapist.

COMMENT Eating disorders such as anorexia nervosa are complex problems with many contributing factors. In addition to cultural beliefs that favor thin people, family conflicts like marital problems or overcontrolling parents are often involved in the etiology of such disorders. Because of this, the most effective form of psychotherapy for patients is family therapy. In this case, the therapist discovers in the first session that the parents have a poor marital relationship. At the same time, he discovers that the girl and her father spend more time together in recreational activities and conversation than the mother and father do. This situation between family members is best described as a triangle (an abnormal relationship between family members) that, in this case, crosses generational boundaries. In this triangle, the girl and her father are closer than the mother and the father, a situation that fosters instability in the family system and contributes to symptoms (in this case anorexia nervosa) in at least one family member.

TREATMENT After the patient is assessed and medically stabilized (see Case 17-1), the family therapist arranges to meet with the girl, her mother, her father, and her siblings at the hospital two times a week. The aim of therapy is to normalize the boundaries between the child and parental subsystems by strengthening the bond between the parents and, in the process, weakening the overly close bond between father and daughter. The family members will also be encouraged to reconsider their own responsibility for the girl's eating disorder, a process known as redefining blame.

Marital/couples therapy

Marital/couples therapy is related to family therapy in that the relationship—the couple in this case—is really the patient. Heterosexual or homosexual couples work together with a therapist on problems like communication, psychosexual issues, or differences in value systems. Types of marital/couples therapy include conjoint therapy, in which one therapist sees the couple together, and concurrent therapy, in which the therapist sees both members of the couple individually. Other types include collaborative therapy, in which two therapists see both members of the couple individually, and four-way therapy, in which two therapists see both members of the couple together. The latter type of marital/couples therapy is used commonly to deal with sexual problems.

Supportive psychotherapy

Supportive psychotherapy is based on the premise that "well-adjusted" individuals as well as those with mental disorders can benefit from support and reassurance. In supportive therapy, emotionally well people who are experiencing a life crisis (e.g., living with metastatic cancer; Classen et al., 2001) or chronically mentally ill people dealing with ordinary life situations are seen regularly by a therapist. For the latter, therapy may be used over many years along with medication. This type of therapy is not aimed at insight into problems, but it is not just "handholding" and sympathy. Rather, true supportive therapy is a methodical process aimed at raising self-esteem and providing support, and it requires professional training similar to that of other types of psychotherapy. The techniques used in supportive psychotherapy may also be used in the context of psychodynamic psychotherapy, specifically during times of crisis.

Stress management

Stress management techniques are used to relieve symptoms in patients with anxiety disorders and stress-related illnesses, such as headaches, hypertension, and irritable bowel syndrome (see Chapter 25). Although many techniques have been used to achieve the goal of stress management, most include some type of relaxation training, such as meditation, or progressive muscle relaxation. Time management training and exercise, particularly aerobic training, are other useful stress management techniques.

REVIEW QUESTIONS

1. A 23-year-old woman joins eight other women who have run up large gambling debts. The women meet weekly and are led by a psychotherapist who is trained in treating compulsive gamblers. This type of therapy is best described as

   (A) supportive therapy

   (B) implosion

   (C) brief dynamic psychotherapy

   (D) systematic desensitization

   (E) group therapy

2. A 30-year-old female patient who has tension headaches is provided with ongoing measurement of the tension in her frontalis muscle as she uses mental relaxation techniques to decrease this tension. This method of pain relief is based primarily on

   (A) reciprocal inhibition

   (B) classical conditioning

(C) aversive conditioning

(D) operant conditioning

(E) stimulus generalization

3. A 35-year-old man with sexual interest in children (pedophilia) is given an electric shock each time he is shown a videotape of children. Later, he feels tense around children and avoids them. Which of the following treatment techniques does this example illustrate?

(A) Implosion

(B) Biofeedback

(C) Aversive conditioning

(D) Token economy

(E) Flooding

(F) Systematic desensitization

(G) Cognitive-behavioral therapy

4. A 28-year-old female patient tells her therapist that she wants to take a new job but is afraid that she will not be able to do the work, will be humiliated, and then will be fired. The therapist tells her that each time she has this negative thought she should imagine a situation in her current job in which she solved a problem or completed a difficult assignment. This treatment technique is most closely related to which of the following types of therapy?

(A) Implosion

(B) Biofeedback

(C) Aversive conditioning

(D) Token economy

(E) Flooding

(F) Systematic desensitization

(G) Cognitive-behavioral therapy

5. A 10-year-old boy, his mother, father, and siblings visit a family therapist. The parents relate that for the past 6 months the boy has been truant from school, has been fighting with his siblings, and has been defying his parents' rules. They say that their family had been happy but that the child's bad behavior has "ruined" their family life. During the first session, the therapist discovers that the boy's symptoms started when he found out by chance that his father had a life-threatening illness. She explains that the boy is "using" bad behavior to avoid dealing directly with his depression and fear resulting from the father's illness. She also notes that the family should work toward meeting each others needs and deal with family crises more openly

and with all family members. The family therapy technique used by the therapist is best described as

(A) redefining blame
(B) a subsystem
(C) a triangle
(D) mutual accommodation
(E) normalizing boundaries

ANSWERS AND EXPLANATIONS

1-E. This type of therapy is best described as group therapy, a treatment technique in which people with a common problem (e.g., gamblers) meet with a psychotherapist. In supportive therapy, a therapist helps a person feel protected and supported during a specific life crisis, such as a job loss. Implosion is a behavioral therapy technique in which a person is exposed to an imagined overwhelming dose of a feared stimulus or situation. Brief dynamic psychotherapy is a form of psychoanalytically oriented therapy in which a person works with a therapist to gain insight into the cause of his problems. In systematic desensitization, increasing doses of the frightening stimulus are paired with a relaxing stimulus to provoke a relaxation response in situations involving the frightening stimulus.

2-D. The treatment technique described here is biofeedback, a technique based primarily on operant conditioning (see Chapter 9 for a discussion of operant conditioning, classical conditioning, and stimulus generalization). Reciprocal inhibition is the mechanism that prevents one from feeling two opposing emotions at the same time (e.g., relaxation and fear) and is associated with systematic desensitization. In aversive conditioning, classical conditioning is used to pair a maladaptive but pleasurable stimulus with an aversive or painful stimulus so that the two become associated and the person stops engaging in the maladaptive behavior.

3-C. The treatment technique described here is aversive conditioning, in which a maladaptive but pleasurable stimulus (for this man, sexual interest in children) is paired with a painful stimulus (e.g., a shock) so that the two become associated. The man then associates sexual interest in children with pain and stops this maladaptive behavior. In flooding, a treatment technique used primarily to treat phobias, a person is exposed to an overwhelming dose of the feared stimulus or situation. In implosion, a person is exposed to an imagined, rather than actual, overwhelming dose of a feared stimulus or situation. In systematic desensitization, increasing doses of the frightening stimulus are paired with a relaxing stimulus to provoke a relaxation response in situations involving the frightening stimulus. In cognitive-behavioral therapy, a person is helped to identify distorted, negative thoughts and to replace them with positive, self-assuring thoughts. In token economy, a person's desired behavior is reinforced by a reward or positive reinforcement; the person then increases the desired behavior to get the reward. See Question 2 for a description of biofeedback.

4-G. The treatment technique described here is most closely related to cognitive-behavioral therapy. In this short-term behavioral treatment technique, the patient is instructed to replace each negative thought with a positive mental image. Here, the patient is helped to identify her expectation of failure as an automatic thought that, when it surfaces, is replaced with a mental image of success and praise. See also answers to Question 3.

5-D. This family therapist is using the technique known as mutual accommodation. This technique encourages family members to try to meet the needs of other family members. A triangle is an abnormal relationship between family members that crosses boundaries; normalizing boundaries between subsystems is another technique used in family therapy. In redefining blame, family members review their own responsibility for another member's (the boy in this case) behavioral problems.

REFERENCES

Beck, A. T. (1976). *Cognitive therapy and the emotional disorders.* New York: International Universities Press.

Beck, A. T. (1991). Cognitive therapy: A 30 year retrospective. *Am Psychol, 46,* 368–375.

Bowen, M. (1978). *Family theory in clinical practice.* New York: Aronson.

Classen, C., Butler, L. D., Koopman, C., Miller, E., DiMiceli, S., Giese-Davis, J., et al. (2001). Supportive-expressive group therapy and distress in patients with metastatic breast cancer: A randomized clinical intervention trial. *Arch Gen Psychiatry, 58,* 494–501.

Gaarder, K. R., & Montgomery, S. (1981). *Clinical biofeedback: A procedural manual for behavioral medicine.* Baltimore: Williams & Wilkins.

Goldberg, P. E. (2000). The physician-patient relationship: Three psychodynamic concepts that can be applied to primary care *Arch Fam Med, 9,* 1164–1168

Kaplan, H. I., & Sadock, B. J. (Eds.). (1993). *Comprehensive group psychotherapy* (3rd ed.). Baltimore: Williams & Wilkins.

Klerman, G. L., Weissman, M. M., & Rounsaville, B. J. (1984). *Interpersonal psychotherapy of depression.* New York: Basic Books.

Liberman, R. P. (1972). *A guide to behavioral analysis and therapy.* New York: Pergamon Press.

McDonald, H. P., Garg, A. X., & Haynes, R. B. (2002). Interventions to enhance patient adherence to medication prescriptions: Scientific review. *JAMA, 288,* 2868–2879.

Minuchin, S. (1974). *Families and family therapy.* Cambridge: Harvard University Press.

Paykel, E. S., Scott, J., Teasdale, J. D., Johnson, A. L., Garland, A., Moore, R., et al. (1999). Prevention of relapse in residual depression by cognitive therapy: A controlled trial. *Arch Gen Psychiatry, 6,* 829–835

Scott, J. (1996). Cognitive therapy of affective disorders: A review. *J Affect Dis, 37,* 1–11.

Selye, H. (1976). *The stress of life, revised.* New York: McGraw-Hill.

Sifneos, P. E. (1987). *Short-term dynamic psychotherapy evaluation and technique* (2nd ed.). New York: Plenum.

12

Schizophrenia and Other Psychotic Disorders

■ INTRODUCTION TO THE DSM-IV-TR

This and the next six chapters of the book focus on mental disorders. Inclusion and diagnostic criteria for these disorders are based on a consensus of current opinions and concepts in psychiatry as described in the **Diagnostic and Statistical Manual of Mental Disorders, Fourth Edition-Text Revision (DSM-IV-TR),** a classification scheme devised by the American Psychiatric Association. The DSM-IV-TR is compatible with the other major psychiatric classification scheme, the **Tenth Revision of the International Statistical Classification of Diseases and Related Health Problems (ICD-10),** developed by the World Health Organization and used mainly in Europe and other areas outside of the United States.

The DSM-IV-TR includes 15 major diagnostic groupings, plus a grouping called "other conditions that may be a focus of clinical attention" (Table 12-1). The DSM-IV-TR uses a **multiaxial system** that codes a patient's condition along five axes (a definitive diagnosis can be made using only the first three axes):

- Axis I: Clinical disorders
- Axis II: Personality disorders and mental retardation
- Axis III: General medical conditions

TABLE 12-1	Diagnostic and Statistical Manual of Mental Disorders, 4th Edition, Text Revision: Disorders in Adults	
CONDITION	**EXAMPLES**	
Delirium, dementia, and amnestic and other cognitive disorders	Delirium caused by congestive heart failure, Alzheimer's dementia	
Mental disorders caused by a general medical condition not otherwise classified	Personality change caused by systemic lupus erythematosus	
Substance-related disorders	Alcohol-related disorders, sedative-related disorders	
Schizophrenia and other psychotic disorders	Schizophrenia, schizophreniform disorder	
Mood disorders	Major depressive disorder, bipolar I disorder	
Anxiety disorders	Panic disorder, specific phobia, posttraumatic stress disorder	
Somatoform disorders	Conversion disorder, hypochondriasis	
Factitious disorders	Factitious disorder with predominantly psychological or predominantly physical signs and symptoms	
Dissociative disorders	Dissociative amnesia, depersonalization disorder, dissociative fugue	
Sexual and gender identity disorders	Secondary erectile dysfunction, gender identity disorders	
Eating disorders	Anorexia nervosa, bulimia nervosa	
Sleep disorders	Primary sleep disorders, sleep disorders related to another mental disorder	
Impulse-control disorders not elsewhere classified	Intermittent explosive disorder, kleptomania, compulsive gambling	
Adjustment disorders	Adjustment disorder with depressed mood, anxiety, mixed anxiety and depressed mood, and disturbance of conduct	
Personality disorders	Paranoid personality disorder, antisocial personality disorder	
Other conditions that may be a focus of clinical attention	Medication-induced movement disorders, problems relating to abuse or neglect, malingering	

- Axis IV: Psychosocial and environmental problems
- Axis V: The **global assessment of functioning (GAF) scale,** which quantifies a patient's level of function in daily life and emotional symptomology on a continuum that ranges from 1 (inability to maintain minimal personal hygiene, danger to self) to 100 (superior social and occupational functioning, no emotional symptoms)

Psychiatric disorders in the DSM-IV-TR can be separated into **subtypes** or have **specifiers.** The subtypes are based on the presentation of symptoms (e.g., schizophrenia, catatonic type). The specifiers denote the features and severity of the illness and describe whether the illness is in partial or full remission (e.g., major depressive disorder with atypical features). Specifiers also disclose the patient's history of the disorder and can be provisional if the practitioner believes that the full criteria for the disorder will be met over time. The specifier can also be "**not otherwise specified (NOS)**" for the following reasons:

- The illness does not meet the full criteria for a specific DSM-IV-TR disorder
- The disorder conforms to a symptom pattern that is included in the DSM-IV-TR
- The disorder has an uncertain etiology
- There is inconsistent or insufficient information available to allow classification of the disorder

SCHIZOPHRENIA

Schizophrenia is a chronic, debilitating psychotic disorder, usually starting in young adulthood, that is associated with rapid deterioration in mental function and behavior. Gross impairment in reality testing **(psychosis)** is the nucleus of the illness and is expressed by alterations in sensory perceptions, such as **hallucinations** (false perceptions), and abnormalities in thought processes, such as **delusions** (false beliefs) (see Table 10-3). Because the term "schizophrenia" literally means "split mind," lay people commonly but erroneously mistake schizophrenia for **multiple personality disorder.** The latter disorder, now called **dissociative identity disorder,** is an uncommon illness in which a person's consciousness is divided through unconscious processes into several different but nonpsychotic personalities (see Chapter 18). In contrast, the split mind of schizophrenia refers to the nonrational divergence between behavior and thought content that patients typically demonstrate (e.g., laughing while verbally expressing fear).

Schizophrenia is a biological illness that, although exacerbated by social stress, is not caused by any known social or environmental factor. The illness itself does, however, have serious social consequences. Theoretically, patients with schizophrenia are often found in lower socioeconomic groups (e.g., homeless people) because they drift down the socioeconomic scale because of their social deficits (the **"downward drift" hypothesis**).

Characteristics

Schizophrenia is characterized by at least one episode of psychosis and persistent disturbances of thought, behavior, appearance, speech, and affect, as well as impairment in occupational and social functioning (e.g., withdrawal). The DSM-IV-TR diagnostic criteria for schizophrenia indicate that these symptoms must persist for at least 6 months (Table 12-2). Despite their debilitating symptoms and in contrast to patients with delirium or substance abuse patients, schizophrenic patients do not have clouding of consciousness. Also, their memory capacity is typically intact and they are oriented to person, place, and time.

Positive and negative symptoms

The symptoms of schizophrenia are classified as **positive** or **negative.** These classifications help describe the characteristics of the disorder and predict the effects of antipsychotic medication. Positive symptoms are those additional to expected behavior (i.e., "excessive" function) and include delusions, hallucinations, agitation, and talkativeness. Negative (deficit) symptoms are those missing from expected behavior (i.e., decreased function) and include lack of motivation, social withdrawal, flattened affect, cognitive disturbances, poor grooming, and poor or impoverished speech content. Positive symptoms respond well to most traditional and atypical antipsychotic agents. Negative symptoms respond better to atypical than to traditional antipsychotics (see also Chapter 19).

TABLE 12-2 **DSM-IV-TR Diagnostic Criteria for Schizophrenia**

Criterion A. Symptoms: At least two of the following, each present for a significant portion of a 1-month period:
1. Delusions
2. Hallucinations
3. Disorganized speech
4. Grossly disorganized or catatonic behavior
5. Negative symptoms

Criterion B. Social/occupational dysfunction: Present for a significant portion of the time since the onset of illness
Decreased level of achievement (in adults)
Failure to achieve expected level of achievement (in children and adolescents)

Criterion C. Duration: Continuous signs of disturbance for at least 6 months
At least 1 month of symptoms that meet Criterion A (less if successfully treated)
Prodromal or residual symptoms (negative symptoms or attenuated forms of Criterion A symptoms) for the rest of the 6-month period

THE PATIENT A 28-year-old man who has lived in a group home for 5 years says that his roommates have begun to spy on him by listening to his thoughts through the television set. He is dressed strangely, shows poor grooming, and seems preoccupied. He reports that he has trouble paying attention to the doctor's questions because he says, "I am listening to the President talking to me in my head." Physical examination is normal. Neuropsychological evaluation reveals normal memory function; orientation to person, place, and time; and no evidence of mental retardation. Positron emission tomography scans of the brain reveal decreased activity in the prefrontal cortex.

COMMENT This schizophrenic man shows a variety of behavioral abnormalities, as well as paranoid delusions (his belief that roommates are spying on him) and auditory hallucinations (hearing the voice of the President). Decreased prefrontal cortical activity is also characteristic of schizophrenia but is not diagnostic. Schizophrenic patients usually show intact memory; orientation to person, place, and time; and normal intelligence. The fact that this patient's symptoms recently worsened suggest that he has stopped taking his antipsychotic medication.

TREATMENT The primary treatment for schizophrenia is antipsychotic medication. Atypical agents with improved side effect profiles rather than traditional agents have recently become first-line pharmacologic treatments. As seen in this patient, relapse is rapid when patients do not take their medication. In addition to resuming his antipsychotic medication, supportive psychotherapy (see Chapter 11) can help this patient comply with future treatment recommendations and can provide emotional support and help with practical matters, such as finding housing and employment.

Course

The course of schizophrenia can be divided into three phases: prodromal, psychotic, and residual. In the **psychotic phase** of the illness, the patient loses touch with reality. This loss is commonly manifested as hallucinations and delusions. **Prodromal** signs and symptoms occur before the first psychotic episode. Typically, in the prodrome, the patient avoids social activities and is quiet and passive. However, he also can be quite irritable. The patient may have physical complaints and show a sudden interest in religion, the occult, or philosophy. In contrast to the psychotic phase of the illness, in the prodromal phase the patient is in touch with reality. In the **residual phase** (the period between psychotic episodes) of schizophrenia, the patient is in touch with reality but does not behave normally. Rather, he or she shows flat or inappropriate affect (e.g., a bland reaction to disturbing news), peculiar thinking, and eccentric behavior (e.g., reading personal meaning into natural phenomena), and withdrawal from social interactions (e.g., choosing to be alone rather than with others). These and other symptoms of schizophrenia can be categorized into disorders of perception, thought content, thought processes, and form of thought (Table 12-3).

TABLE 12-3 **Selected Symptoms of Psychosis: Disorders of Perception, Thought Content, Thought Processes, and Form of Thought**

SYMPTOM	COMMENTS	EXAMPLES
Disorders of Perception		
Illusions	Misperception of real external stimuli	A woman interprets the appearance of a dress in a dark closet as a person.
Hallucinations	False sensory perceptions (auditory hallucinations are the most common); visual, tactile, gustatory, olfactory, and cenesthetic (visceral sensation) hallucinations are also seen	A patient hears two voices talking about her when she is alone in a room. Sometimes she smells nonexistent odors.
Disorders of Thought Content		
Ideas of reference	False conviction that one is the subject of attention by other people or the media	A patient believes that she is being discussed on a national television program.
Delusions	False beliefs not correctable by logic or reason, not based on simple ignorance, and not shared by a culture or subculture; delusions of persecution are most common	A woman believes that she is being followed by government agents who want her to spy on her neighbors.
Disorders of Thought Processes		
Loss of ego boundaries	Not knowing where one's mind and body end and those of others begin	A patient feels she is "merged" into others.
Impaired abstraction ability	Difficulty in discerning the essential qualities of objects or relationships despite normal intelligence	When asked what brought him to the hospital, a patient says "a bus."
Magical thinking	The idea that thoughts cause or prevent external events from happening (the defense mechanism of undoing is seen also in normal people as superstitious behavior)	A person knocks on wood after saying something positive about his health.

TABLE 12-3	Selected Symptoms of Psychosis: Disorders of Perception, Thought Content, Thought Processes, and Form of Thought (Continued)	
SYMPTOM	**COMMENTS**	**EXAMPLES**
Disorders of Form of Thought		
Echolalia	Associating words by their sounds, not by their logical meanings	A patient says, "I'm very sure I've got a cure and I'm not pure. . . . "
Loose associations	Ideas shift from one subject to another in an unrelated or partially related fashion	A patient begins to answer a question about her parents, then launches into a diatribe about world hunger.
Neologisms	Inventing new words	A patient refers to a restaurant as an "automatic automat."
Perseveration	Repeating the same word or phrase over and over	A patient says, "I'm bad . . . I'm bad . . . I'm bad . . . that I'm bad."
Tangentiality	Beginning a response in a logical fashion but then getting further and further from the point	A patient says, "I'll tell you about my thoughts, but let me tell you about other things in my head, like brains and blood."
Thought blocking	Abrupt halt in the train of thinking, often because of hallucinations	A patient suddenly stops talking even though her lips are moving and she seems to be concentrating on an inner stimulus.
Word salad	Uttering unrelated combinations of words or phrases	A patient says, "I'm not so utterly pure that I'm going away anyway to break it."

Adapted from Fadem, B., & Simring, S. S. (2003). *High-yield psychiatry.* Baltimore: Lippincott Williams & Wilkins, Table 11–1.

Etiology

Adoption and twin studies support the role of genetic factors in the etiology of schizophrenia (see also Chapter 5); the concordance rate in monozygotic twins is close to 50% versus 10% for dizygotic twins. De novo mutations arising in paternal germ cells could explain the recent intriguing finding that advanced paternal age is more commonly seen in the history of schizophrenic patients than of normal patients (Malaspina et al., 2001). Gender differences also occur in schizophrenia. Although schizophrenia occurs equally in men and women, the peak age of onset differs between the sexes (i.e., 15 to 25 years of age in men and 25 to 35 years of age in women). Also, women tend to respond better to antipsychotic medications than men.

Environmental factors during development, such as viral infection and exposure to drugs, have been implicated in the etiology of schizophrenia. The finding that more people with schizophrenia are born during cold-weather months (i.e., January through April in the northern hemisphere and July through September in the southern hemisphere) than during warm-weather months (Mortensen et al., 1999) has been attributed to viral infections that occur seasonally. Specifically, viral infection of the mother during the second trimester of pregnancy may negatively affect the developing fetal brain. Third-trimester maternal exposure to diuretics or, alternatively, severe maternal hypertension that requires use of these agents has recently been implicated in schizophrenia (Sørensen et al., 2003).

Neurological and neurotransmitter abnormalities

Specific pathology has been demonstrated in the brains of schizophrenic patients. Abnormalities of the frontal lobes, as demonstrated by decreased use of glucose in the prefrontal cortex; lateral and third ventricle enlargement; abnormal cerebral symmetry; and changes in brain density as well as decreased volume of the hippocampus, amygdala, and parahippocampal gyrus are seen in schizophrenic patients (see also Chapter 5). Other abnormal findings include decreased alpha waves, increased theta and delta waves, and epileptiform activity on the **electroencephalogram,** and abnormalities in eye movements, such as poor smooth visual pursuit.

Neurotransmitter abnormalities (specifically, increased dopaminergic, serotonergic, and noradrenergic activity and abnormal transmission of glutamate) appear to be involved in the pathophysiology of schizophrenia (see Chapter 5). The **dopamine hypothesis** states that schizophrenia results from excessive dopaminergic activity (e.g., excessive number of dopamine receptors, excessive concentration of dopamine or hypersensitivity of receptors to dopamine). As evidence for this notion, use of stimulant drugs that increase dopamine availability (e.g., amphetamines and cocaine) can cause psychotic symptoms (see Chapter 23). Laboratory tests of body fluids of patients with schizophrenia may also show elevated levels of homovanillic acid, a metabolite of dopamine (see Chapter 5).

Serotonin hyperactivity is implicated in schizophrenia because hallucinogens such as LSD that increase serotonin availability cause psychotic symptoms. Also, some new, effective antipsychotics such as clozapine (see Chapter 19) have anti-serotonergic-2 (5-HT$_2$) activity. **Norepinephrine hyperactivity** may be involved, particularly in the paranoid subtype of schizophrenia. Glutamate is also implicated for several reasons (see Chapter 5), including the fact that antagonists of the **N-methyl-D-aspartate (NMDA)** subtype of glutamate receptors (e.g., phencyclidine) increase and agonists of NMDA receptors (e.g., glycine, D-serine, and cycloserine) alleviate some symptoms of schizophrenia (Sawa & Snyder, 2002).

Subtypes of schizophrenia

The DSM-IV-TR lists five subtypes of schizophrenia: **undifferentiated, paranoid, residual, disorganized (previously hebephrenic),** and **catatonic.** Each subtype is associated with characteristic symptoms and prognosis (Table 12-4).

DSM-IV-TR criteria and differential diagnosis

Because they can also cause psychotic symptoms, certain medical and psychiatric illnesses can be misidentified as schizophrenia (Table 12-5). Medical illnesses that cause psychotic symptoms are referred to as **psychotic disorders caused by a general medical condition** (PDMC). PDMCs include neurological disorders, such as multiple sclerosis, Parkinson's disease, Huntington's disease, neoplasms, neurological infections, temporal lobe epilepsy, and cerebrovascular disease. They also include endocrine disturbances such as thyroid disease, Cushing's disease, and Addison's diseases; connective tissue diseases such as systemic lupus erythematosus; metabolic disorders such as porphyria; and vitamin deficiencies. Because schizophrenia itself is characterized by psychotic symptoms occurring concurrently with clear consciousness, the diagnosis of PDMC can be made only in the absence of delirium or dementia.

Some pharmacological agents cause psychotic symptoms that can lead to the mistaken diagnosis of schizophrenia. These medications include analgesic, antibiotic, anticholinergic, antihistaminergic, antineoplastic, antituberculosis, antiparkinson, and antihypertensive agents, as well as stimulants, cardiac glycosides (e.g., digitalis), and steroid hormones. Typically, and in contrast to the flat affect of schizophrenia, patients with medically caused psychotic symptoms usually show preservation of affect.

Psychiatric illnesses associated with psychotic symptoms are also mistaken for schizophrenia. These illnesses include:

- Other psychotic disorders (see later text)
- The **manic phase of bipolar disorder** (see Chapter 13)
- **Cognitive disorders** (see Chapter 18)
- **Substance-related disorders** (see Chapter 23)

Schizotypal, paranoid, and **borderline personality disorders** are not characterized by psychotic symptoms but have other characteristics of schizophrenia (see Chapter 24). Figure 12-1 provides a diagnostic flow chart for a psychotic patient after medical and pharmacological causes of the symptoms have been ruled out.

TABLE 12-4   DSM-IV-TR Subtypes of Schizophrenia

SUBTYPE*	CHARACTERISTICS	EXAMPLE
Undifferentiated	Characteristics of more than one subtype	A 21-year-old disheveled patient tells the doctor that she hears voices in her head. Although she has no systematized delusions, the patient believes that she can communicate with animals. Her affect is blunted but not flat, and she shows no catatonic features.
Paranoid	■ Systematized delusions of persecution ■ Older age of onset and better functioning than other subtypes	A 34-year-old patient seems fearful when she tells the doctor that the government has been listening in on all of her phone conversations for the past 2 years (see Case 12-1).
Residual	■ At least one previous psychotic episode ■ Subsequent negative symptoms and mild positive symptoms ■ No current frank psychotic symptoms	A 30-year-old man who was hospitalized five years previously with auditory hallucinations has since shown flat affect, social withdrawal, and strange behavior but no delusions or hallucinations.
Disorganized (hebephrenic)	■ Incoherent speech ■ Mirror gazing ■ Facial grimacing ■ Poor grooming ■ Inappropriate emotional responses (silliness) ■ Onset before age 25 years	An 18-year-old male patient is unshaven and dirty. He stares into the mirror, posturing and grimacing, and giggles when he tells the doctor that his stomach is "a monster machine ready to throw me on the train."
Catatonic	■ Stupor or extreme agitation ■ Incoherent speech or muteness ■ Blank facial expression ■ Bizarre posturing (waxy flexibility) ■ Rare since introduction of antipsychotic agents	A 27-year-old patient does not speak and shows extreme psychomotor agitation to the point of physical exhaustion. At times, he holds unusual, uncomfortable-looking body positions.

* Most common to least common.

TABLE 12-5   Differential Diagnosis of Schizophrenia

DISORDER	CHARACTERISTICS
Schizophrenia	■ Psychotic and residual symptoms lasting at least 6 months (see Table 12-2) ■ Normal consciousness and memory function ■ Auditory hallucinations predominate
Psychotic disorder caused by a general medical condition	■ Hallucinations that are visual and changeable rather than auditory and recurrent ■ Occurs in the context of an acute medical illness ■ Symptoms not due to delirium or dementia
Brief psychotic disorder	■ Psychotic and residual symptoms lasting more than 1 day but less than 1 month ■ Obvious precipitating psychosocial factors
Schizophreniform disorder	■ Psychotic and residual symptoms lasting 1–6 months ■ Obvious precipitating psychosocial factors
Schizoaffective disorder	■ Fit criteria for both a mood disorder and schizophrenia ■ Psychotic symptoms present for at least 2 weeks without mood symptoms ■ Mood symptoms present during the psychotic and residual phases ■ Chronic social and occupational impairment
Delusional disorder and shared psychotic disorder (folie à deux)	■ Fixed, non-bizarre delusional system present for at least 1 month ■ Absence of other thought disorders ■ Relatively normal social and occupational functioning
Manic phase of bipolar disorder	■ Psychotic symptoms, elated mood, rapid onset, hyperactivity, rapid speech, and increased sociability ■ Delusions of grandeur ■ Little or no impairment in social or occupational functioning between episodes
Schizoid personality disorder	■ Voluntary social withdrawal ■ No evidence of a thought disorder
Schizotypal personality disorder	■ Negative symptoms ■ Bizarre behavior and odd thought patterns ■ No frank psychosis
Borderline personality disorder	■ Extreme mood swings with uncontrollable anger and episodic suicidal thoughts ■ Mini-psychotic episodes (lasting only minutes)

TABLE 12-5	Differential Diagnosis of Schizophrenia (Continued)
DISORDER	**CHARACTERISTICS**
Substance-induced psychotic disorder	■ Prominent hallucinations (often visual or tactile) or delusions directly related to use or withdrawal of a specific drug (especially amphetamines and hallucinogens) (see Chapter 10) ■ Psychotic symptoms remit when use or withdrawal ends

Adapted from Fadem B., & Simring, S. S. (2003). *High-yield psychiatry (2nd ed.).* Baltimore: Lippincott Williams & Wilkins, Table 11–3.

Treatment

Pharmacological agents are the primary treatments for schizophrenia. These agents include **traditional antipsychotic agents** (dopamine-2 [D_2]-receptor antagonists), such as haloperidol and chlorpromazine, and **atypical antipsychotic agents,** such as clozapine, risperidone, olanzapine, quetiapine, ziprasidone and aripiprazole (see Chapter 19). In part because they cause fewer negative neurological effects like parkinsonism (e.g., resting tremor) or tardive dyskinesia (writhing [choreoathetoid] movements), the atypical agents have recently become first-line pharmacologic treatments for schizophrenia. Significant improvement occurs in approximately 70% of patients on antipsychotic medication. About 25% of this improvement can be attributed to the placebo effect (see Chapter 5).

In part because antipsychotics have unpleasant side effects, the compliance rate with these medications in schizophrenia is low. Treatment of noncompliant patients includes long-acting injectable depot forms of antipsychotic medication, such as **haloperidol decanoate** and **fluphenazine decanoate.** Psychological treatments, including supportive, family, and group psychotherapy (see Chapter 11) are useful adjuncts to pharmacotherapy to provide long-term support for the patient and family and to foster compliance with the drug regimen.

Prognosis

Schizophrenia usually involves repeated psychotic episodes, lifelong impairment, and a chronic, downhill course over years. Although the illness often stabilizes in midlife, suicide is unfortunately common in patients with schizophrenia. More than 50% of persons with schizophrenia attempt suicide, and 10% of those die in the attempt. These attempts often occur when patients are in the characteristic post-psychotic depression or when experiencing "command" hallucinations ordering them to harm themselves. The overall prognosis is better and the suicide risk is lower in patients who have one or more of these characteristics:

■ Are older at the onset of illness
■ Are married

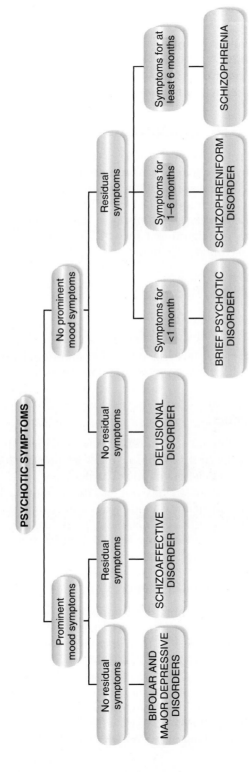

FIGURE 12-1. A diagnostic flowchart for a psychotic patient after medical and pharmacological causes of the symptoms have been ruled out.

- Have social relationships
- Are female
- Have good employment histories
- Have mood symptoms
- Have positive symptoms
- Have experienced relatively few relapses

■OTHER PSYCHOTIC DISORDERS

Psychotic disorders are a group of illnesses characterized at some point during their course by psychosis. Schizophrenia is the most comprehensive model for a psychotic disorder. Other psychotic disorders have similar symptoms but do not include all of the criteria required for the diagnosis of schizophrenia. Unlike schizophrenia, these other disorders often are associated with recent significant stressful life events and abrupt onset of symptoms. These disorders include:

- Brief psychotic disorder
- Schizophreniform disorder
- Schizoaffective disorder
- Delusional (psychotic) disorder
- Shared psychotic disorder (folie à deux)

Psychotic symptoms are also seen in other emotional illnesses (e.g., bipolar disorder; see Chapter 13) and physical illnesses (e.g., delirium; see Chapters 18 and 25).

Duration of the disorders

One DSM-IV-TR requirement for the diagnosis of schizophrenia is that symptoms, both residual and psychotic, must be present for at least 6 months. The diagnosis of **brief psychotic disorder** (see Case 12-2) is made when symptoms last for at least 1 day but less than 1 month. The diagnosis of **schizophreniform disorder** is made when the symptoms last at least 1 month but less than 6 months. Schizoaffective, delusional, and shared delusional disorders can last for more than 6 months, but other criteria distinguish them from schizophrenia (see later text).

Schizoaffective and delusional disorders

If a patient shows significant mood symptoms such as mania or depression along with the diagnostic criteria for schizophrenia, the patient may have **schizoaffective disorder.** For this diagnosis, psychotic symptoms must be present for at least 2 weeks without the mood symptoms, and the mood symptoms must persist during the psychotic and residual phases of the illness. This disorder is usually associated with better premorbid functioning and a better prognosis than schizophrenia.

Patients with **delusional disorder** show highly systematized but non-bizarre (possible in real life) delusions for a period of at least 1 month with

THE PATIENT A 26-year-old medical student is brought to the emergency department by his wife. The wife tells the doctor that her husband, who has been studying for final examinations, has shown odd behavior over the past 2 weeks. In particular, the patient told his wife that his classmates are trying to poison him. The patient has no history of prior substance abuse or psychiatric illness. Physical examination is unremarkable and there is no evidence of current substance use.

COMMENT Because there is no medical explanation for the patient's symptoms, the most appropriate diagnosis for this patient is brief psychotic disorder. This disorder is characterized by psychotic symptoms, like this patient's delusion of being poisoned, lasting more than 1 day but less than 1 month. The stress of final examinations is likely to be a precipitating psychosocial factor for illness in this medical student.

TREATMENT For his own protection, and for assessment and treatment, the patient should be hospitalized. Pharmacologic treatment will involve antipsychotic medications such as haloperidol. Benzodiazepines (antianxiety agents) can also be used to control the agitation caused by the frightening experience of having had psychotic symptoms.

no other symptoms of schizophrenia. In contrast to schizophrenia, delusional disorder commonly starts in middle age and patients are usually socially and occupationally functional. Delusional disorder has subtypes, including::

- **Erotomanic type,** characterized by the conviction that a famous person is in love with the patient
- **Jealous type,** characterized by the belief that one's partner is having sexual relations with someone else
- **Persecutory type,** in which the patient believes that someone is trying to harm her

Shared psychotic disorder (folie à deux) is a related illness characterized by delusional symptoms usually occurring in close relatives of patients with delusional disorder. For example, without any evidence, a married 62-year-old woman with delusional disorder believes that people are putting anthrax dust into her house. When the woman is admitted to the hospital, her husband worries about his ability to remove the dust from the house. If separated for a time from his wife (the inducer), the husband's shared delusion about the anthrax dust is likely to diminish and then disappear.

REVIEW QUESTIONS

1. A 30-year-old woman who has no psychotic, residual, or mood symptoms tells you that sometimes she becomes frightened at night because her desk looks like a seated man lurking in the room. This description is an example of

   (A) an illusion
   (B) a neologism
   (C) a hallucination
   (D) tangentiality
   (E) an idea of reference

2. A 53-year-old hospitalized schizophrenic patient tells her doctor that another patient was talking about her when he said, "A woman won $10,000 in the lottery today." This patient's statement is an example of

   (A) an illusion
   (B) a neologism
   (C) a hallucination
   (D) tangentiality
   (E) an idea of reference

3. A 58-year-old patient tells you that for the last 5 years his coworkers have been trying to get him fired from his job by telling lies about him to the boss. The patient is married and has lived in the same town for 25 years. Physical examination is normal. The most appropriate diagnosis for this patient is

   (A) schizophrenia
   (B) schizoaffective disorder
   (C) schizophreniform disorder
   (D) brief psychotic disorder
   (E) delusional disorder
   (F) shared delusional disorder
   (G) psychosis caused by a general medical condition

4. A 50-year-old man with a history of psychotic symptoms, severe depression, and periods of boundless energy and enthusiasm has held different jobs but none of them for more than 3 months. Physical examination is normal. The patient is successfully treated for his mood symptoms but remains strange and distant. The most appropriate diagnosis for this patient is

   (A) schizophrenia
   (B) schizoaffective disorder
   (C) schizophreniform disorder

(D) brief psychotic disorder

(E) delusional disorder

(F) shared delusional disorder

(G) psychosis due to a general medical condition

5. A 40-year-old lawyer is sure that her husband is stealing money from her and buying gifts for another woman. She threatens him with a knife while angrily accusing him of this behavior and is taken to the emergency room of the local hospital. The husband notes that although she has not been violent before, the patient has been showing increasingly strange behavior over the past 9 months. She is not currently taking any medication. Choreoathetoid movements are observed on physical examination. The history reveals that the patient's father and uncle died in their 50s after deteriorating physically and mentally for many years. The most appropriate diagnosis for this patient is

(A) schizophrenia

(B) schizoaffective disorder

(C) schizophreniform disorder

(D) brief psychotic disorder

(E) delusional disorder

(F) shared delusional disorder

(G) psychosis due to a general medical condition

ANSWERS AND EXPLANATIONS

1-A. This patient is describing an illusion, a misperception of a real external stimulus (the desk as a man). Both normal and psychotic people experience illusions. A neologism is an invented new word; a hallucination is a false perception; and an idea of reference is the false belief of being referred to by others. Tangentiality involves verbally getting further and further from the point one is making as speech continues. The latter four symptoms are characteristically seen in psychotic patients.

2-E. An idea of reference is the false belief of being referred to by others (e.g., another patient talking about this woman) (see also answers to Question 1).

3-E. This patient demonstrates symptoms of delusional disorder. In the persecutory type of the disorder, there is a fixed, nonbizarre delusional system (paranoid in this subtype); few if any other thought disorders; and relatively normal occupational and social functioning (e.g., this patient is employed and has been married for 25 years). In schizophrenia, psychotic and residual symptoms last at least 6 months, and there is lifelong social and occupational impairment. Schizoaffective disorder is characterized by symptoms of a mood disorder, psychotic symptoms, and lifelong social and occupational impairment. Schizophreniform disorder is characterized by psychotic and residual symptoms lasting 1 to 6 months. In shared delusional disorder, a person develops the same delusion as a person with delusional disorder with whom they are in a close relationship.

4-B. This patient has the symptoms of schizoaffective disorder with characteristics of both a mood disorder and schizophrenia (see also answers to Question 3).

5-G. Because of the abnormal physical findings, the most probable diagnosis for this patient is psychosis caused by a general medical condition. The age of the patient and her family history strongly suggest Huntington's chorea, which can present with psychiatric symptoms such as psychosis and depression (see Chapter 25) (see also answers to Questions 3 and 4).

REFERENCES

American Psychiatric Association. (1997). Practice guidelines for the treatment of patients with schizophrenia. *Am J Psychiatry, 154,* (4 Supplement), 1.

American Psychiatric Association. (2001). *Diagnostic and statistical manual of mental disorders* (4th ed.). Text revision. Washington, DC: American Psychiatric Association, pp. 297–343.

Andreasen, N. C., & Flaum, M. (1991). Schizophrenia: The characteristic symptoms. *Schizophenia Bull, 17,* 27.

Fenton, W. S., & McGlashan, T. H. (1991). Natural history of schizophrenia subtypes. *Arch Gen Psychiatry, 48,* 969–977.

Malaspina, D., Harlap, S., Fennig, S., Heiman, D., Nahon, D., Feldman, D., & Susser, E. S. (2001). Advancing paternal age and the risk of schizophrenia. *Arch Gen Psychiatry, 58,* 361–367.

Mortensen, P. B., Pedersen, C. B., Westergaard, T., Wohlfarht, J., Ewald, E., Mors, O., et al. (1999). Effects of family history and place and season of birth on the risk of schizophrenia. *N Engl J Med, 340,* 603–608.

Sawa, A., & Snyder, S. H. (2002). Schizophrenia: Diverse approaches to a complex disease. *Science, 296,* 692–695.

Sørensen, H. J., Mortensen, E. L., Reinisch, J. M., & Mednick, S. A. (2003). Do hypertension and diuretic treatment in pregnancy increase the risk of schizophrenia in offspring? *Am J Psychiatry, 160,* 464–468.

Mood Disorders

13

V ariations in mood are common in everyday life. People normally feel sad when they experience a loss or disappointment and happy when they anticipate or experience a positive event. In contrast, patients with primary mood disorders show discordance between life events and how they feel emotionally. There may be no change in their current social circumstances to account for their emotions, or they may feel increased, decreased, or even contradictory emotional responsiveness to a change. For example, a student who does poorly on an exam remains so sad 9 months later that he has little appetite for food, has lost 10 pounds, and cannot enjoy his favorite activities. Another student who does well on an exam feels elated and believes she can mentally transmit her superior knowledge to others. The first student shows evidence of **depression** and the second shows the elevated mood and psychotic thinking that can characterize **mania.** Two other abnormal mood states, **dysthymia** and **hypomania,** are attenuated versions of depression and mania, respectively.

It can be difficult to distinguish between normal variations in mood and mood disorders. Symptoms such as impaired judgment, problems in physical functioning, and disruption in work or interpersonal relationships help identify the latter. In severe cases, psychotic symptoms such as delusions or hallucinations may help identify a mood disorder patient.

The Diagnostic and Statistical Manual of Mental Disorders, Fourth Edition-Text Revision (DSM-IV-TR) categories of primary mood disorders are **major depressive disorder** and **bipolar disorder (I and II)** and their less severe counterparts, **dysthymic disorder** and **cyclothymic disorder.** The mood states of depression, mania, dysthymia, and hypomania individually or in combination characterize these disorders (Fig. 13-1). If mood symptoms occur because of a medical condition or substance use, (i.e., secondary mood disorders), the correct diagnosis is **mood disorder due to a general medical condition** or **substance-induced mood disorder.**

■ MAJOR DEPRESSIVE DISORDER

Major depressive disorder (MDD) is identified by one episode or recurrent episodes of major depression in an individual's lifetime. The DSM-IV-TR diagnosis for a major depressive episode requires that at least five of nine listed symptoms (Table 13-1) be present most of the time for at least a 2-week period.

Characteristics

An episode of major depression characteristically involves not only unhappiness but also decreased interest and pleasure in one's usual activities and decreased appetite for pleasurable stimuli such as sex and food. Lack of appetite for food often leads to significant (more than 5% of body weight) weight loss. Depressed patients also often have difficulty maintaining sleep (see Chapter 7) and become chronically fatigued. In **atypical depression,** patients are more likely to show weight gain rather than loss, and they are more likely to show excessive somnolence.

Depressed patients may show confused thinking and mild memory problems. In the elderly, these cognitive symptoms may be misdiagnosed as dementia (see Chapters 4 and 18). Depressed patients also typically show diurnal variation in symptoms; they feel more depressed in the morning and better in the evening.

Intense feelings of guilt and suicidal thoughts (ideation) and actions occur in depression. Suicide is a particular danger in depressed patients who feel hopeless, have been hospitalized for depression, or have psychotic symptoms, such as delusions (Bostwick & Pankratz, 2000) (see Chapter 14). If they occur, the delusions of depression commonly are congruent with the negative mood and involve themes of destruction, catastrophe, and fatal illness.

Masked depression and seasonal affective disorder

Physical symptoms, such as headaches and body aches, are common in depressed patients. Up to 50% of depressed patients seem unaware of or deny that they are depressed; instead they report vague physical symptoms. Patients with this **"masked depression"** tend to first seek help from primary care doctors (Green et al., 2000; Whooley & Simon, 2000). The diagnosis of masked depression is considered only when an identifiable

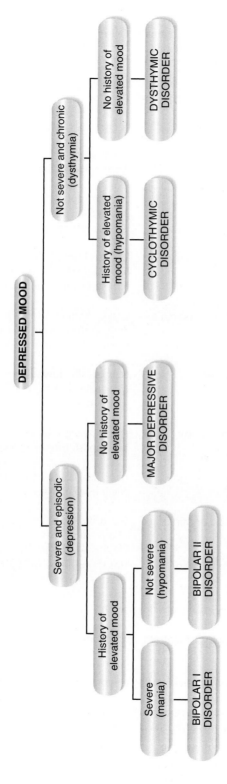

FIGURE 13-1. A diagnostic flowchart for a patient with a depressed mood after medical and pharmacological causes of the symptoms have been ruled out.

TABLE 13-1 DSM-IV-TR Diagnostic Criteria For a Major Depressive Episode

Criterion A. Symptoms: At least 5 of the following present during the same 2-week period. At least one of these must be symptom #1 or #2.

DSM-IV-TR Symptom	Explanation
1. Subjective report or observation by others of depressed mood	Has feelings of sadness, hopelessness, emptiness, and low self-esteem
2. Markedly decreased interest or pleasure in most activities	In severe form, this symptom is called anhedonia, the inability to respond to pleasurable stimuli
3. Change (up or down) in appetite (e.g., change of more than 5% in body weight in a month)	Has less interest than usual in food and loses weight; in atypical depression, patients overeat and gain weight
4. Persistent insomnia or hypersomnia	Wakes frequently at night and too early in the morning; in atypical depression, patients oversleep
5. Psychomotor agitation or retardation	Is physically slowed down (particularly in the elderly) or speeded up
6. Daily fatigue or loss of energy	Has little vigor or desire to accomplish former goals
7. Feelings of worthlessness or guilt	Poor self-image and inappropriate feelings of culpability
8. Problems concentrating or thinking	Has difficulty with attentiveness and memory
9. Recurrent thoughts of death or suicide	Has thoughts of killing himself or tries to take his own life

Criterion B. Symptoms of mania are not present

Criterion C. There is significant distress or impairment in social or occupational functioning

Criterion D. Symptoms are not caused by a substance or medical condition

Criterion E. Symptoms are not caused by bereavement (depression cannot be diagnosed less than 2 months after the loss of a loved one)

organic cause for the physical symptoms is absent and when the patient has other symptoms of depression, such as weight loss and insomnia.

Seasonal affective disorder (SAD), a subtype of major depressive disorder, is associated with the winter season and short days. This disorder can be treated effectively with full-spectrum light exposure.

Etiology and occurrence

The causes of MDD can be biological or social, but MDD is usually caused by a combination of both factors. Biological factors include heredity, altered neurotransmitter activity, and abnormalities of the limbic-hypothalamic-pituitary-adrenal axis (see Chapter 5). The psychosocial etiology of depression includes the loss of a primary attachment figure, such as a parent in childhood, or the catastrophic loss of a loved one, such as a spouse or child, in adulthood. Other psychological factors that have been implicated in depression are low self-esteem and negative interpretations of ordinary life events. Some believe that the symptoms of depression result from feelings of helplessness caused by repeated futile attempts to escape negative life situations (i.e., the "learned helplessness" model of depression) (see Chapter 9). Although there is little association between mood disorders and ethnicity, education, marital status, or income, being female is a significant risk factor for MDD. In the United States, the lifetime prevalence of this disorder, about 5 to 12% for men, is almost twice as high in women. Although the healthy elderly are not more likely to be depressed than younger people, older persons who are chronically ill or those who are widowed are at increased risk for depression.

Treatment

Depression can be treated successfully in most patients. However, only about 25% of depressed patients seek and receive treatment. As with medical illnesses, women are more likely than men to seek professional help.

Patients do not seek treatment for depression for several reasons. They may not realize that their physical symptoms are a result of depression (see masked depression earlier in the chapter). Even if patients know they are depressed, they may not be able to afford treatment. Many health insurance plans do not fully cover the costs of treatment for emotional disorders such as depression. Also, many Americans consider being stoic and uncomplaining about illness a virtue, and illness itself a personal failure or even a moral weakness. These notions are intensified when the patient's illness is emotional rather than physical, and thus less "real."

Without treatment, most episodes of depression are self-limiting and last approximately 6 to 12 months. However, during the episode, the patient is at high risk for accidents, suicide, and social problems, such as job loss and marital difficulties. Most patients have repeated episodes of depression; some, particularly those with comorbid psychiatric disorders such as dysthymic disorder (see later text) or substance abuse (see Chapter 23), remain chronically depressed.

Successfully treated episodes of depression last less than 3 months. The most commonly used and effective treatments are pharmacologic agents, including the **heterocyclic antidepressants, selective serotonin reuptake inhibitors (SSRIs),** and **monoamine oxidase inhibitors (MAOIs)** (see Chapter 19). Because of their more positive side-effect profiles, SSRIs such as fluoxetine (Prozac) and other newer antidepressants are now used as first-line agents (see Chapter 19). Because all antidepressants take at least 3 weeks to work, psychostimulants, which work more quickly, are sometimes used to treat depression. However, in contrast to antidepressants, stimulants can cause tolerance and dependence (see Chapter 23).

Electroconvulsive therapy (ECT), in which a grand mal seizure is induced by passing an electric current through the brain (see Chapter 19), is a much maligned but effective treatment for severe depression that does not respond to antidepressant medications. This therapy is also used when antidepressants are too dangerous or have intolerable side effects, or when rapid resolution of symptoms is necessary because a patient is acutely suicidal.

Psychological treatment for depression, including psychoanalytic, interpersonal, family, behavioral, and cognitive therapies, can be helpful (see Chapter 11). Some evidence indicates that psychological treatment in conjunction with medication is more effective at resolving depressive symptoms than either type of treatment alone.

■ BIPOLAR DISORDER

Bipolar disorder involves discreet episodes of both depression and mania **(bipolar I disorder)** or both depression and hypomania **(bipolar II disorder).** There is no simple manic disorder because depressive symptoms eventually occur. Therefore, one episode of mania or hypomania plus one episode of major depression defines bipolar disorder.

Characteristics

Symptoms of mania include inflated self-image, excessive optimism, increased energy and activity, and rapid thoughts and speech. Patients often have a decreased need for sleep and decreased appetite for food. In contrast, sexual interest is likely to be increased. Manic patients also show an uncharacteristic lack of modesty in dress and behavior and an inability to control aggressive impulses. The DSM-IV-TR criteria for a manic episode require that three to four manic symptoms (Table 13-2) be present for at least a 1-week period (less if hospitalization is required). These symptoms, and the psychotic delusions often seen in mania (see later text), commonly lead to social impairment and legal difficulties.

In a hypomanic episode, mild symptoms of mania such as inflated self-esteem and talkativeness are present for at least a 4-day period. In con-

TABLE 13-2   DSM-IV-TR Diagnostic Criteria For a Manic Episode

Criterion A. A distinct period of abnormally and persistently elevated (happiness and physical well-being), expansive (self-important), or irritable (easily bothered) mood lasting at least 1 week or less if hospitalization is necessary

Criterion B. Symptoms: At least 3 (4 if the mood is only irritable) of the following present

DSM-IV-TR symptom	Explanation
1. Inflated self-esteem or grandiosity	Has feelings of self-importance
2. Decreased need for sleep	Feels rested after little sleep
3. Talkativeness or pressured speech	Seems forced to speak rapidly
4. Flight of ideas	Thoughts move quickly from one to the other
5. Distractibility	Cannot concentrate on relevant stimuli
6. Increased activity or agitation	Engages in nondirected, nonpurposeful movement
7. Engagement in activities that are likely to have negative consequences	Runs up credit card and telephone bills; uncharacteristic involvement in physically dangerous activities

Criterion B. Symptoms of depression are not present

Criterion C. There is significant distress or impairment in social or occupational functioning

Criterion D. Symptoms are not caused by a substance or medical condition

trast to mania, severe social or occupational impairment and psychotic symptoms are absent in hypomania and hospitalization is not required.

Psychotic symptoms can occur in any major mood disorder but are more common in bipolar I disorder than in MDD. These symptoms, primarily delusions, occur mainly during manic episodes. Commonly, the delusions of mania are congruent with a positive mood and often involve themes of power and influence. Despite the occurrence of psychotic symptoms, and in contrast to schizophrenia and schizoaffective disorder in which chronic impairment is seen, the bipolar patient's functioning usually returns to normal between episodes.

THE PATIENT A 22-year-old medical student is taken to the emergency department by police when he attempts to enter a government office building to "have a conference with the President" about conducting a fund drive to "finance my cure for cancer." When police prevent him from entering the building, he becomes irritable and hostile and resists attempts to restrain him. In the emergency room, physical examination is essentially normal. The patient speaks rapidly and his ideas follow each other in rapid succession. Blood tests do not reveal evidence of substance use. The patient's identical twin brother with whom he lives notes that the patient has been showing "strange behavior" for the past few weeks. The brother asks the doctor what is wrong with the patient and whether he himself is at risk for developing the same symptoms.

COMMENT The belief that one is important enough to demand a conference with the President and cure cancer is a grandiose delusion typical of mania. This delusion, combined with the patient's accelerated "pressured" speech and rapid flow "flight" of ideas, indicates that he is having a manic episode. Anger, irritability, and hostility are common in a manic episode. Although bipolar I disorder involves episodes of both mania and major depression, a single episode of mania defines the illness. Although this psychotic patient could be schizophrenic, general withdrawal and apathy and paranoid rather than grandiose delusions are more common in schizophrenic patients. The risk of this patient's twin brother also developing bipolar disorder is high; the concordance rate in monozygotic twins is close to 75% (see Chapter 5).

TREATMENT The emergency room treatment of this psychotic bipolar patient is likely to include benzodiazepines such as clonazepam (Klonopin) and antipsychotics such as olanzapine (Zyprexa). His long-term management will be achieved using lithium or anticonvulsants such as valproic acid (Depakene) or carbamazepine (Tegretol).

Etiology and occurrence

As in MDD, biological factors in bipolar disorder include changes in neurotransmitter availability, endocrine abnormalities, and genetics. The latter is a particularly strong influence in bipolar disorder (see Chapter 5). In contrast to MDD, psychosocial factors are probably not involved in the etiology of mania or hypomania. Bipolar disorder occurs in approximately 1% of the population and, like MDD, shows no sex, cultural, or ethnic differences in its occurrence.

Treatment

Because bipolar disorder usually starts with an episode of depression, bipolar patients may be misdiagnosed with major depression and treated with antidepressants. Unfortunately, antidepressants can provoke a hypomanic or full-blown manic episode in a potentially bipolar patient (see

Chapter 19). To avoid this adverse effect, depressed patients should be questioned about previous hypomanic or manic episodes; for example, "Have you ever felt high or better than normal without mood-altering drugs?" A positive response indicates that the patient may have bipolar disorder rather than MDD.

The treatment of choice for the maintenance of bipolar patients is **lithium** carbonate or citrate. However, lithium has multiple adverse effects, such as renal and thyroid dysfunction; tremor; and weight gain (see Chapter 19). When lithium is contraindicated or when the patient shows rapid-cycling (more than four episodes in a year) bipolar disorder, **anticonvulsants** such as divalproex (Depakote) and carbamazepine (Tegretol) are preferred. Combinations of lithium and anticonvulsants can be used for patients who do not show an adequate response to either. **Sedative agents** such as lorazepam (Ativan) and clonazepam (Klonopin) as well as antipsychotics such as haloperidol (Haldol), olanzapine (Zyprexa), and risperidone (Risperdal) are commonly used to treat acute manic episodes because they resolve symptoms quickly.

While psychological treatments are not useful in the treatment of manic symptoms, as in schizophrenia, supportive, family, and group psychotherapy (see Chapter 11) are helpful adjuncts to pharmacotherapy over the chronic course of bipolar disorder.

■ DYSTHYMIC DISORDER AND CYCLOTHYMIC DISORDER

Dysthymic disorder and **cyclothymic disorder** are less severe forms of MDD and bipolar disorder, respectively. Dysthymic disorder is characterized by the presence of symptoms of dysthymia, such as low self-esteem and decreased productivity, without the extreme symptoms of MDD, such as anhedonia (Table 13-1) and suicidality. Cyclothymic disorder involves the presence of alternating states of dysthymia and hypomania. In contrast to MDD and bipolar disorder, dysthymic disorder and cyclothymic disorder are less severe, are nonepisodic, and are never associated with psychosis. Because people normally have some degree of mood variability, dysthymic disorder and cyclothymic disorder (presence of alternating states of dysthymia and hypomania) can be diagnosed only when the symptoms persist most of the time for at least 2-years. Dysthymic disorder occurs in about 6% of the population, and, like MDD, is at least twice as common in women. Like bipolar disorder, cyclothymic disorder occurs in approximately 1% of the population with no sex difference in its occurrence.

Treatment of dysthymic disorder is similar to that of MDD and involves antidepressant medication and psychotherapy. Mood stabilizing agents similar to those used to treat bipolar disorder are the primary treatments for cyclothymic disorder.

THE PATIENT For the past few months, a 28-year-old woman has seemed full of energy and optimism for no obvious reason. Although she gets only about 6 hours of sleep a night, she has been very productive at work. She is talkative and gregarious and relates that she is having sexual relationships with four different men. A few years previously, friends say she was often pessimistic and seemed tired and "washed out." During that time she continued to work but did not seek out social activities and had little interest in sex. There is no evidence of a thought disorder, and the patient denies suicidality or hopelessness. Physical examination, including body weight, is normal.

COMMENT This patient's symptoms are characteristic of cyclothymic disorder. This disorder involves periods of both hypomania (energy, optimism, talkativeness, and hypersexuality) and periods of dysthymia (pessimism, feeling "washed out," and little interest in socializing or sex). The symptoms persist over at least a 2-year period with no discrete episodes of illness. In contrast to the bipolar patient in Case 13-1, this patient does not show psychotic delusions. Dysthymia is distinguished from depression here by the absence of suicidal ideation and hopelessness, no change in body weight, and the ability to function in the work situation.

TREATMENT The most effective long-term treatment for cyclothymic disorder, as for bipolar disorder, is a mood stabilizer, such as lithium, or an anticonvulsant.

■ DIFFERENTIAL DIAGNOSIS OF MOOD DISORDERS

Mood disorder caused by a general medical condition

Mood symptoms in a medically ill patient may result directly from the illness or its treatment rather than from a primary mood disorder (see Chapter 25). Also, the possibility of a medical etiology should be explored when mood symptoms first appear in the elderly, because primary mood disorders commonly present in early or middle adulthood.

Manic symptoms are associated with endocrine problems such as hyperthyroidism and neurological lesions caused by stroke, neoplasm, or infection (particularly in the orbitofrontal right cortex, a center for the biological control of inhibitions, emotions, and drive states; see Chapter 5), as well as use of medications such as steroids. Medical and psychiatric illnesses that can present with depressive symptoms are listed in Table 13-3 and Table 25-3.

Substance-induced mood disorder

An important consideration in the differential diagnosis of a mood disorder is that the symptoms are caused or exacerbated by use of or withdrawal from drugs of use (see Chapter 25) or abuse (see Chapter 23). Prescription drugs that can cause depressive symptoms include reserpine and other antihypertensives as well as antineoplastic agents and steroids. Steroids can also cause symptoms of elevated mood (see Table 25-4).

TABLE 13-3	Differential Diagnosis of Depression
Medical Conditions	
Cancer, particularly pancreatic and other gastrointestinal tumors	
Viral illness (e.g., pneumonia, influenza, AIDS)	
Endocrinologic abnormalities (e.g., hypothyroidism, Cushing's syndrome)	
Neurologic illness (e.g., Parkinson's disease, multiple sclerosis, Huntington's disease, stroke, dementia)	
Nutritional deficiency	
Renal or cardiopulmonary disease	
Psychiatric and Related Conditions	
Schizophrenia (particularly after an acute psychotic episode)	
Somatoform disorders	
Eating disorders	
Anxiety disorders	
Adjustment disorders	
Substance abuse and withdrawal	

Stimulants such as amphetamines and cocaine are abused drugs likely to elevate mood and cause manic symptoms. Withdrawal of stimulants, opiates, and sedatives commonly results in depression of mood.

Other differential diagnoses

Major depressive episodes sometimes must be distinguished from **adjustment disorder with depressed mood** or normal **bereavement.** The former diagnosis is given when the mood symptoms do not meet the full criteria for a major depressive episode, follow within 2 months of a significant psychosocial stressor, and persist for up to 6 months after the stressor has terminated (see Chapter 15). The latter diagnosis is given within 2 months of the death of a loved one or other significant loss (see Chapter 4), even if the patient meets the DSM-IV-TR criteria for a major depressive episode. Patients whose severe symptoms persist for more than 2 months after the loss can be diagnosed with MDD.

Patients who actually have MDD are sometimes misdiagnosed with another psychiatric illness. For example, a depressed patient who becomes overly worried about imagined dangers may be misdiagnosed with an **anxiety disorder** (see Chapter 15). Likewise, a depressed patient with unexplained physical complaints may be misidentified with hypochondriasis or another **somatoform disorder** (see Chapter 16). In contrast to patients with anxiety or somatoform disorders, the anxiety and physical symptoms in depressed patients dissipate when the depression is treated successfully.

Mood disorder patients who cannot afford health care (see Chapter 27) may delay seeking treatment until they become ill enough to show psychotic symptoms, such as delusions. Because of this and because clinicians tend to underdiagnose mood disorders and overdiagnose schizophrenia in patients from low socioeconomic groups (Roukema et al., 1984), poor bipolar patients are more likely than affluent bipolar patients to be misdiagnosed as schizophrenic.

REVIEW QUESTIONS

1. A 65-year-old man has been diagnosed with advanced prostate cancer. The patient has lost 20 pounds and has decreased energy and difficulty sleeping because of pain. Over the past month he has been expressing fearfulness about dying and strong feelings of guilt about "bad things I've done in my life," which he believes have caused his illness. The sign or symptom most likely to indicate that this patient is experiencing a major depressive episode rather than a normal reaction to serious illness is

   (A) weight loss
   (B) decreased energy
   (C) difficulty sleeping
   (D) excessive guilt
   (E) fear of dying

2. When compared with an American man, the chances that an American woman will develop major depressive disorder (MDD) or bipolar disorder over the course of her lifetime are, respectively:

   (A) higher, lower
   (B) higher, equal
   (C) higher, higher
   (D) lower, higher
   (E) lower, lower
   (F) equal, lower

(G) equal, higher

(H) equal, equal

3. A depressed 25-year-old female patient who is slow moving and shows a flat affect is put on fluoxetine (Prozac). Within 2 weeks, she is showing greatly increased activity level, flight of ideas, and pressured speech. In this patient, the medication has

(A) precipitated a manic episode

(B) had a toxic effect

(C) had a delayed effect

(D) increased anxiety

(E) increased depression

Questions 4 and 5

A 45-year-old man reports a variety of aches, pains, and extreme fatigue that have been present for the past 6 months. Physical examination is unremarkable but the patient has lost 10 pounds without dieting since checkup last year. The patient reports that he wakes 2 hours before his alarm and has significant problems concentrating on his work. The patient denies that he is sad or hopeless. After a 5-week trial of antidepressant medication, the patient's aches and pains are gone, he is sleeping all night, his energy level and concentration are normal, and he has gained 5 pounds.

4. This patient's symptoms before treatment were probably a result of

(A) hypochondriasis

(B) dysthymic disorder

(C) cyclothymic disorder

(D) depression

(E) malingering

5. Analysis of neurotransmitter availability in the brain of this patient before treatment is most likely to reveal which of the following?

(A) Increased dopamine

(B) Decreased histamine

(C) Increased acetylcholine

(D) Decreased acetylcholine

(E) Decreased serotonin

ANSWERS AND EXPLANATIONS

1-D. Feelings of guilt that he has caused his illness are more characteristic of depression than sadness about being very ill. The other symptoms that the patient shows (e.g., weight loss, decreased energy, and sleep problems) are characteristic symptoms of advanced cancer itself. Fear of dying is normal in patients with serious illnesses.

2-B. When compared with a man's risk, the risk that an American woman will develop MDD over the course of her lifetime is higher and the risk that she will develop bipolar disorder is equal.

3-A. In this depressed patient, the antidepressant fluoxetine has precipitated a manic episode (e.g., greatly increased activity level, flight of ideas, and pressured speech). This reaction indicates that the patient has bipolar disorder rather than major depressive disorder. There is no evidence of increased depression, increased anxiety, or a delayed or toxic effect in this patient.

4-D, 5-E. This patient's physical complaints were relieved and weight loss reversed by antidepressant medication. This indicates that these symptoms were manifestations of hidden or masked depression. Bipolar disorder involves episodes of both mania and depression. Cyclothymic disorder involves episodes of hypomania and dysthymia occurring over a 2-year period with no discrete episodes of illness. In hypochondriasis, patients believe that normal body functions or minor illnesses are serious or life threatening (see Chapter 16). There is no evidence in this patient of bipolar disorder, dysthymic disorder, cyclothymic disorder, or malingering (i.e., fabricating symptoms for gain) (see Chapter 16). While not used diagnostically, analysis of neurotransmitter availability in this depressed patient is most likely to reveal decreased serotonin, commonly reflected in decreased plasma levels of its major metabolite 5-HIAA. Increased dopamine is associated with schizophrenia, and decreased acetylcholine is associated with Alzheimer's disease (see Chapter 5).

REFERENCES

American Psychiatric Association. Diagnostic and Statistical Manual of Mental Disorders 4th Edition Text Revision. 2001. Washington, DC, American Psychiatric Association, pp. 345–427.

Bostwick, J. M., & Pankratz, V. S. (2000). Affective disorders and suicide risk. *Am J Psychiatry, 157,* 1925–1932.

Green, A. R., Betancourt, J. R., Carrillo, J. E., Pornnoppadol, C., Simon, G. E., & VonKorff, M. (2000). The relation between somatic symptoms and depression. *N Engl J Med, 342,* 658–659.

Keller, M. B., Lavori, P. W., Mueller, T. I., Endicott, J., Coryell, W., Hirschfield, R. M., & Shea, T. (1992). Time to recovery, chronicity and levels of psychopathology in major depression. A 5-year prospective follow-up of 431 subjects. *Arch Gen Psychiatry, 49,* 809.

Kendler, K. S., Kessler, R. C., Walters, E. E., MacLean, C., Neale, M. C., Heath, A. C., & Eaves, L. J. (1995). Stressful life events, genetics liability and onset of an episode of major depression in women. *Am J Psychiatry, 152,* 883.

Paykel, E. (1993). Workshop in psychopharmacology: Depression in medical illness. *Int Clin Psychopharmacol, 7,* 205.

Rosenberg, D. R., Wright, B., & Gershon, S. (1992). Depression in the elderly. *Dementia, 3,* 157.

Roukema, R., Fadem, B. H., James, B., & Rayford, F. (1984). Bipolar disorder in a low socioeconomic population: Difficulties in diagnosis. *J Nerv Mental Diseases, 172(2),* 76–79.

Seeman, M. V. (1995). *Gender and psychopathology.* Washington, DC: American Psychiatric Press.

Whooley M. A., & Simon, G. E. (2000). Primary care: Managing depression in medical outpatients. *N Engl J Med, 343,* 1942–1950.

Suicide **14**

A patient who wants to take his own life challenges a physician's fundamental purpose. Although the reason for the suicide attempt may not be immediately apparent, people rarely reach this decision easily. In fact, most suicidal patients are ambivalent about their decision to kill themselves; they want to escape an intolerable life situation but at the same time have the often-unconscious desire to be saved from self-destruction. Because this desire leads most suicidal patients to visit a physician with vague physical complaints in the 6 months before the act, a primary care doctor is often in a unique position to save the patient.

People commonly make statements like, "I felt so sick I wanted to die" without suicidal intent. However, whenever such a statement is made to a physician, it must be taken seriously, particularly when the patient is physically ill, depressed, or otherwise emotionally impaired. Although no specific set of characteristics identify a suicidal patient, certain demographic, psychological, social, and physical factors have been associated with increased suicide risk (Table 14-1). No matter what risk factors are present, the physician's good clinical judgment is the most important variable in identifying the patient at risk for suicide.

■ PREVIOUS SUICIDAL BEHAVIOR

A **serious prior suicide attempt,** particularly within the past 3 months, is the most significant risk factor for completed or "successful" suicide. Although there are many more attempts than actual suicides, approximately 30% of people who attempt suicide try it again, and 10% succeed. Characteristics of the previous attempt are important considerations in the assessment of

TABLE 14-1   Risk Factors for Suicide

FACTOR	DECREASED RISK	INCREASED RISK
TOP FIVE RISK FACTORS (IN DESCENDING ORDER)		
1. History	No previous suicidal behavior	Serious prior suicide attempt
2. Age	Younger adults	Older adults
3. Substance use	Little or no substance use	Substance abuse or dependence
4. Behavior	Not impulsive or violent	History of rage and violent behavior
5. Sex	Female	Male
OTHER RISK FACTORS		
Race	African American	White
Social status	Married	Socially isolated
Family history	No family history of suicide	Parent or close relative committed suicide
Religion	Catholic or Muslim	Jewish or Protestant
Psychotic symptoms	No psychotic symptoms	Psychotic symptoms
Health	Good health	Chronic illness
Occupation	Nonprofessional	Professional
Economic conditions	Strong economy	Economic recession or depression
Employment	Job satisfaction	Low job satisfaction

From Fadem, B, & Simring, S. (2003). *High-yield psychiatry* (2nd ed.). Baltimore: Lippincott Williams & Wilkins. Table 13-5.

future suicide risk. Clearly, the more potentially lethal the previous method used, the higher the future suicide risk. Means such as shooting or hanging oneself, jumping from a high place, or crashing one's vehicle are more lethal than ingesting pills or slashing one's wrists. The likelihood of rescue from the previous suicidal act is also important when assessing future risk. A suicide attempt is potentially more lethal if it takes place in a setting where the possibility of rescue is remote. Thus, patients who attempted suicide in an unfamiliar setting where no people were nearby are at higher risk than those who tried suicide in a familiar setting with people nearby (e.g., at home just before a family member was expected to arrive).

DEMOGRAPHIC FACTORS

Suicide is the eighth leading cause of death in the United States, after heart disease, cancer, stroke, chronic obstructive pulmonary disease, accidents, pneumonia, and influenza and diabetes mellitus. The suicide rate in the United States is approximately 12 per 100,000. This rate has been relatively steady for more than 40 years, and it falls in the midrange for developed countries. Scandinavia, Japan, Switzerland, Germany, Austria, and countries in Eastern Europe have suicide rates two times that of the United States. Spain, Italy, Ireland, Egypt, and the Netherlands have lower rates (less than 10 per 100,000) (Sadock & Sadock, 2003).

Age

Suicide is rare in children. However, it is the third leading cause of death in adolescents aged 15 to 19 years, following only accidents (first) and homicide (second). In part because teenagers are inclined to do what other teens do, teen suicide, like teen violence, tends to occur in clusters (Mckeown et al., 1998; Shafii & Shafii, 2002). In adulthood, suicide risk is positively associated with age and increases substantially after age 55. In the elderly, suicide risk decreases as women age but increases as men age (Fig. 14-1); white men 65 years and older are more likely to commit suicide than any other group.

Sex and ethnicity

There are gender and ethnic differences in suicide rates. Although women attempt suicide four times more often than men, men successfully commit suicide three times more often than women. One reason for this difference is that men tend to use more violent and hence lethal means than women. Historically, African Americans have had lower suicide rates than white Americans. However, the race gap is narrowing among males aged 15 to 19 years, particularly for suicide by gun (Joe & Kaplan, 2002). Native-American and Inuit groups have high suicide rates, and immigrants to the United States have higher rates of suicide than the general population in both this and their native countries.

Marital status and religion

People with little social support are at higher risk for suicide than people with strong social support systems, such as marriage and religion (Van Ness, 2002). Separated, divorced, or widowed people are more likely to

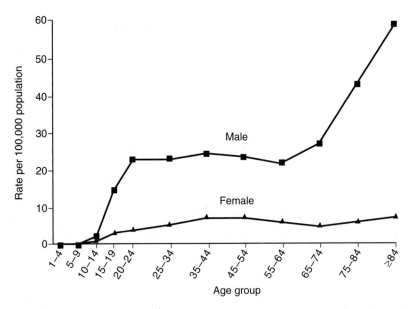

FIGURE 14-1. Suicide rates in men and women by age in the United States in 1998.

(Reprinted with permission from Vastag, B. (2001). Suicide prevention plan calls for physicians' help. JAMA, 285, 2701).

kill themselves than married people, particularly if the loss of the partner occurred in the recent past. Suicide is proscribed in all religions; however, perhaps because the Catholic and Muslim religions specifically and strongly prohibit suicide, rates are lower in these groups than in Jewish groups. Protestants have the highest suicide rates (Van Ness & Larson, 2002; Roy, 2000; Cross & Hirschfield, 1989).

Occupation

Professional people are at higher risk for suicide than nonprofessionals (Sadock & Sadock, 2003). Access to a means for suicide is an important differentiating factor for this risk. For example, physicians (particularly females) and dentists may be at increased risk for suicide because they have access to prescription drugs. Professionals with access to guns (such as police officers) are also at higher risk (Violanti & Paton, 1996). Although the reasons are less obvious, musicians and attorneys also seem to be at higher risk for suicide than the general population.

■ OTHER RISK FACTORS

Other factors to consider when assessing the risk of suicide include substance abuse, previous behavior, genetics, family history, and mental and physical health.

Substance abuse and history of aggressive behavior

Chronic and acute use of substances, including alcohol, greatly increases suicide risk. Alcoholics are at particularly high risk for suicide if they have recently lost a significant other, such as a spouse or close friend. Aggressive, impulsive, and violent people are at increased risk for suicide and, because drug and alcohol use tend to decrease inhibitions against risk-taking behavior, such people are at even greater risk for suicide when intoxicated.

Genetic factors

Genetic factors are associated with both depression (see Chapter 13) and increased suicide risk. Suicide rates of adults adopted as children are more similar to those of their natural parents than of their adoptive parents, and concordance rates for suicide are higher in monozygotic twins than in dizygotic twins.

Family history

Family history of suicide is associated with increased suicide risk. Specifically, death of a parent by suicide, death of a parent in a child younger than age 11, or loss of a parent by divorce in adolescence are risk factors for both depression and suicide.

Mental health and physical health

Although many seriously depressed patients are at risk for suicide, some are at higher risk than others. Of the characteristics of major depression, the one most closely linked to suicide risk is hopelessness, the feeling that one's circumstances will never improve. In patients with major depressive disorder, psychotic symptoms, a history of hospitalization for depression, and a short length of time since the last hospitalization are specific risk factors for suicide (Bostwick & Pankratz, 2000) (see Chapter 13).

Severely depressed patients rarely have the clarity of thought or energy needed to plan and commit suicide. However, suicide risk increases when the patient is in the initial stages of recovery from depression. One explanation for this is that the patient's energy and clear thinking return before the depressed mood lifts, facilitating execution of the suicidal plan. Schizophrenic patients are also at high suicide risk; at least half attempt suicide at some time in their lives (see Chapter 12).

Loss of physical health or even the perception of serious illness is associated with increased suicide risk. When seriously or terminally ill patients express their suicidal thoughts, it is important to distinguish between a normal desire to avoid pain and suffering and an abnormal mental state of major depression. In the latter instance, successful treatment of the depression can reduce the risk of suicide, allowing patients to use and even to enjoy the remainder of their lives.

■ HOSPITALIZING A SUICIDAL PATIENT

If a physician determines that a patient is at high risk for suicide, hospitalization is indicated. If a patient refuses to comply, the patient can be detained against his will for 1 to 2 days, depending on state law (Case 14-1). More prolonged detention can be imposed by the state court system when patients who pose a threat to themselves refuse to be detained. Physicians can be held legally responsible if they fail to identify or detain a suicidal patient or if they give a patient medication that is used later in a suicide attempt. Although all suicidal patients are at risk, Table 14-2 contains specific indications for hospitalization.

CASE 14-1

THE PATIENT When a hospitalized 65-year-old man is told that the lesion just removed from his colon is malignant, he becomes very agitated and upset. He states that "life is just too hard to go on any longer." The patient is clearly mentally competent, but he has been despondent since his wife's recent death. The doctor is concerned and asks the patient to stay in the hospital overnight. The next day, the patient seems much calmer. He tells the doctor that he does not want any further treatment and would like to be released immediately. He also asks the doctor not to tell his adult children that he is leaving the hospital.

COMMENT This patient is at high risk for suicide. He is mentally depressed, physically ill, and has lost an important family member. Although he could be showing a normal grief reaction to the losses he has experienced, the patient's refusal to be treated for a treatable condition and his wish to hide his whereabouts from relatives are evidence of the distorted reasoning that can characterize clinical depression. The sudden appearance of peacefulness in this previously agitated patient is further evidence that he has reached an internal decision to kill himself and is now calm.

TREATMENT Competent patients have the right to refuse treatment, even if death will result (see Chapter 26). However, this patient's decision to refuse treatment is more likely to be the result of clinical depression than of a measured decision to end his life. When the depression lifts, this patient is likely to change his mind and accept treatment. Therefore, the doctor should suggest that the patient remain in the hospital until he can be evaluated for suicide risk and treated for depression. If it is determined that he is at risk to himself, the patient can be held against his will for his own protection for a period of 1 to 2 days. A court order must be obtained to hold the patient longer. The patient's family should be told of the doctor's concerns about suicide. Confidentiality is secondary to safety and does not need to be maintained when a patient like this one is clearly suicidal (see Chapter 26).

TABLE 14-2	Indications for Hospitalizing a Suicidal Patient
INDICATION	**COMMENT**
Possession of a means for suicide	Has access to a gun or to medication
Presence of a plan for suicide	Has chosen the time, place, or circumstances
Acute intoxication	Shows evidence of reduced impulse control
Expresses feeling out of control	Cannot restrain the urge to kill himself
Psychotic symptoms	Has "command" hallucinations
Lack of social support	There is no responsible, caring adult in the home
History of repeated suicide attempts	There were a number of attempts in the recent past
Patient is unreliable	The physician is uncertain about the risk

REVIEW QUESTIONS

1. A hospitalized, depressed 20-year-old woman tells her physician that she will kill herself with her brother's gun when she is released from the hospital. When the doctor suggests that she remain in the hospital, she refuses. Her brother, with whom she lives, says that he will get rid of the gun and insists that his sister be allowed to come home. The doctor should next do which of the following?

(A) Release the woman into the care of her brother

(B) Hold the woman involuntarily for 24 to 48 hours for evaluation

(C) Ask the brother to provide proof that the gun was removed and then release the woman

(D) Commit the woman to a mental health facility for 30 days

(E) Make an appointment for the woman to receive outpatient counseling

Questions 2–4

A 40-year-old Muslim woman has been abusing alcohol for the past 5 years. Her history reveals that she has been married for the past 15 years.

2. Which of the following characteristics is this patient's greatest risk factor for suicide?

(A) Alcoholism

(B) Sex

(C) Marital status

(D) Religion

(E) Age

3. This woman is at the highest risk for suicide if she works as a

   (A) messenger

   (B) secretary

   (C) teacher

   (D) nurse

   (E) physician

4. If this patient tries to commit suicide, the method most likely to fail is

   (A) shooting herself with a gun

   (B) crashing her car

   (C) slashing her wrists

   (D) jumping from a high place

   (E) hanging herself

5. After a doctor tells a patient that he needs additional medical tests, the patient says, "Doc, maybe my time is up." The most appropriate next statement by the physician is

   (A) "Please tell me what you mean by that."

   (B) "It's not so bad, the tests are not painful."

   (C) "Don't worry, you will be fine."

   (D) "How long have you felt suicidal?"

   (E) "Have you ever tried to kill yourself?"

ANSWERS AND EXPLANATIONS

1-B. Because she poses an immediate threat to her own life, the patient can be held involuntarily for 24 to 48 hours (depending on state law) until a court hearing can be conducted. At the hearing it will be determined whether the patient will be held for a longer period (i.e., "committed" for her own protection). Simply removing access to the gun will not prevent suicide in this patient. She will simply find another means of accomplishing this goal. Outpatient counseling alone is not appropriate for this suicidal patient.

2-A, 3-E, 4-C. This woman's highest risk factor for suicide is alcohol abuse. Her sex, age, marital status, and religion are not risk factors for suicide. Professionals are at higher suicide risk than nonprofessionals; among the professions listed, physicians are at highest risk. The method of suicide most likely to fail is slashing her wrists. Shooting, crashing a car, jumping from a high place, and hanging are more lethal methods of committing suicide.

5-A. Statements like "maybe my time is up" may or may not indicate suicidal intent. However, when made to a physician by a physically ill patient, a statement like this must be taken seriously. "Please tell me what you mean by that" can help to clarify the patient's intent. The statements "it's not so bad" and "don't worry" are patronizing and do not address the issue of suicidality. Specific questions like "How long have you felt suicidal?" and "Have you ever tried to kill yourself?" can be asked if the doctor determines that the patient's statement indicated suicidal intent.

REFERENCES

Bostwick, J. M., & Pankratz, V. S. (2000). Affective disorders and suicide risk. *Am J Psychiatry, 157,* 1925–1932.

Cross, C. K., & Hirschfeld, R. M. A. (1989). Epidemiology of disorders in adulthood: Suicide. In R. Michels (Ed.), *Psychiatry* (2nd ed.) (Vol. 3, pp. 1–15). Philadelphia: Lippincott, Williams & Wilkins. 1–15.

Goleman, D. (1991, December 4). Missing in talk of right to die: Depression's grip on a patient. *The New York Times.*

Joe, S. & Kaplan, M. (2002). Firearm-related suicide among young African-American males. *Psych Services, 53,* 332–334.

Mckeown, R. E., Garrison, C. Z., Cuffe, S. P., Waller, J. L., Jackson, K. L., & Addy, C. L. (1998). Incidence and predictors of suicidal behaviors in a longitudinal sample of young adolescents. *J Am Acad Child Adolesc Psychiatry*, 37, 612–619.

Robins, L. N., & Kulbok, P. A. (1988). Epidemiological studies in suicide. *Psychiatr Ann, 18,* 619–627.

Roy, A. (2000). Suicide. In B. J. Sadock & V. A. Sadock (Eds.), *Comprehensive Textbook of Psychiatry* (7th ed.). Baltimore: Lippincott Williams & Wilkins.

Sadock, B. J., & Sadock, V. A. (2003). *Synopsis of psychiatry* (9th ed., pp. 913–914). Baltimore: Lippincott Williams & Wilkins.

Shafii, M., & Shafii, S. L. (2002). School violence: Assessment, management, prevention. *Psychiatr Serv, 53,* 354–355.

Van Ness, P. H., & Larson, D. B. (2002). Religion, senescence and mental health. *Am J Geriatric Psychiatry, 10,* 386–397.

Violanti, J. M., & Paton, D. (1996). *Traumatic stress in critical occupations: Recognition, consequences, & treatment* (pp. 260). Springfield, Illinois: Charles C. Thomas.

Anxiety Disorders and Related Disorders   **15**

A woman is approached by a strange man on a dark street. Her body responds rapidly. Her heart rate increases, she starts shaking and sweating, and she has an intense desire to run to safety. Another woman experiences the same sympathetic nervous system responses whenever she leaves her home, despite the fact that there is no one approaching her.

Although the terms **fear** and **anxiety** are often used interchangeably, their meanings are actually quite different. The first woman is responding with fear, a normal reaction to a real external threat. The second woman is responding with anxiety; she feels threatened, but the source of the threat is not known, not recognized, or inadequate to account for her symptoms. The first woman quickly calms down when she finds refuge and the source of her fear is removed. Because the source of the second woman's anxiety is obscure, her symptoms are likely to persist and may even intensify over time.

■ OVERVIEW OF ANXIETY DISORDERS

All anxiety disorders are characterized by symptoms of fear without adequate cause. Because most people experience anxiety at some time in their lives, normal anxiety must often be distinguished from an anxiety disorder. To diagnose an anxiety disorder, the symptoms must be present for an extended period (often at least 6 months), interfere with a person's normal functioning, and cause significant distress.

General characteristics

The physiologic manifestations of anxiety include sympathetic nervous system symptoms such as shakiness, sweating, **mydriasis** (pupil dilation), and the subjective experience of **tachycardia,** which patients may refer to as "palpitations." Anxious patients also commonly report gastrointestinal symptoms (e.g., diarrhea) and urinary disturbances (e.g., increased frequency). The **hyperventilation** that can accompany these sympathetic responses can lead to dizziness and syncope (fainting) as well as tingling sensations in the extremities and loss of sensation or numbness around the mouth. Symptoms of anxiety can be situational or free-floating. **Situational anxiety** is caused by an overreaction to an identifiable, external, environmental stressor, whereas **free-floating anxiety** has no particular external trigger.

DSM-IV-TR classification of anxiety disorders

The Diagnostic and Statistical Manual of Mental Disorders, Fourth Edition-Text Revision (DSM-IV-TR) classification of anxiety disorders includes:

- **Generalized anxiety disorder (GAD)**
- **Panic disorder (with or without agoraphobia)**
- **Specific and social phobias**
- **Obsessive-compulsive disorder (OCD)**
- **Post-traumatic stress disorder (PTSD)**
- **Acute stress disorder (ASD)**

The diagnoses **anxiety disorder caused by a general medical condition** and **substance-induced anxiety disorder** are given if a medical illness or substance use or withdrawal is the main cause of the anxiety symptoms.

The anxiety disorders are distinguished from each other by the presence or absence of an obvious environmental stressor (present in the phobias, PTSD, and ASD; absent in panic disorder, OCD, and GAD) as well as the pattern of symptom appearance and disappearance (e.g., acute in panic disorder; chronic in GAD). Descriptions of the anxiety disorders follow; specific examples of patients with each disorder are given in Table 15-1.

TABLE 15-1 Patient examples of DSM-IV-TR Anxiety Disorders

CLASSIFICATION	CHARACTERISTIC PATIENT
Generalized anxiety disorder	A 40-year-old woman complains of "palpitations," shortness of breath, and chronic indigestion. She tells you that for as long as she can remember she has been "a high-strung person."
Panic disorder	A 22-year-old female medical student comes to the emergency room after a sudden onset of tachycardia, sweating, and dyspnea. She is certain that she is having a heart attack. Aside from the elevated pulse rate, physical examination is normal. The patient had two other episodes of these symptoms, each lasting about 30 minutes, during the past week.
Agoraphobia	A 25-year-old woman reports that she has not left her home in 6 months because she becomes very "nervous" when she goes anywhere. She has therefore had little direct contact with family and friends. She reports that her sleep, appetite, and energy are normal.
Specific phobia	A 32-year-old woman who is afraid of dogs refuses to leave her house to go to work because she may see a dog on the street.
Social phobia (social anxiety disorder)	He tries to avoid it, but a 29-year-old man must take a client to dinner in a restaurant. Although he knows the client well, he is so afraid that he will make a mess while eating and embarrass himself that he says he is not hungry and sips from a glass of water instead.
Obsessive compulsive disorder	Before she can go to sleep at night, a 25-year-old woman must count the tiles on the ceiling a minimum of 5 times. She has had a few minor car accidents because she is distracted by counting all the traffic lights as she drives through them.
Post-traumatic stress disorder	A 35-year-old woman who was raped 5 years ago reports that vivid memories of the rape accompanied by intense anxiety frequently intrude during her daily activities, and nightmares about the event often wake her. The symptoms intensified when a coworker was raped 2 months ago.

Etiology

The anxiety disorders are among the most commonly treated mental health problems. Both psychosocial and biological factors are involved in their etiology. Psychosocial factors include maladaptive learning that results in fear of a harmless thing or situation (see Chapter 9) and exposure to an extreme stressor. Biological factors include genetics and gender. Anxiety disorders are more common in the family members of patients than in the general population, and their concordance rates are higher in monozygotic than in dizygotic twins. Compared with men, women are two to three times more likely to have panic disorder, twice as likely to develop PTSD when exposed to an extreme stressor, and slightly more likely to have GAD (55 to 60% versus 40 to 45%).

Neurobiological associations

Altered neurotransmitter activity is associated with symptoms of anxiety; specifically, decreased activity of serotonin and γ-aminobutyric acid (GABA); decreased GABA-benzodiazepine receptor binding (Malizia et al., 1998); and increased activity of norepinephrine (see Chapter 5). Neuroanatomically, the locus ceruleus, the site of noradrenergic neurons; the raphe nuclei, the site of serotonergic neurons; the temporal cortex; the frontal cortex; and the caudate nucleus (particularly in OCD) are implicated in the development of anxiety disorders (see Chapter 5, Figures 5-4 and 5-5).

Differential diagnosis

Organic causes of the symptoms of anxiety include excessive caffeine intake, substance abuse and withdrawal, hyperthyroidism, vitamin B_{12} deficiency, hypo- or hyperglycemia, anemia, and **pheochromocytoma,** an epinephrine-secreting adrenal medullary tumor. Because symptoms of anxiety (e.g., shortness of breath, chest discomfort, tachycardia, and sweating) also occur in cardiovascular disorders such as arrhythmias and respiratory disorders such as chronic obstructive pulmonary disease (COPD), these disorders must also be ruled out.

Anxiety is marked in many depressed patients, and patients with anxiety disorders are often comorbid for major depressive disorder and dysthymic disorder (see Chapter 13). It can therefore be difficult to distinguish between anxiety and depressive disorders. The close biological association between these groups of disorders is supported by research showing that neuroendocrine abnormalities and electroencephalographic (EEG) changes during sleep (see Chapter 7) are similar in patients with OCD and major depressive disorder.

Anxiety disorders must also be distinguished from the prodrome and psychotic phases of schizophrenia where anxiety is often prominent (see Chapter 12) and hypochondriasis, in which there is unfounded but significant distress about having a serious illness (see Chapter 16).

■ GENERALIZED ANXIETY DISORDER

Characteristics

Patients with GAD have persistent symptoms of anxiety, including hyperarousal and excessive worrying over at least a 6-month period. Their "free-floating" symptoms cause them significant distress but cannot be related to a specific person or situation.

Occurrence and prognosis

Generalized anxiety disorder is present in about 3 to 5% of the population and is commonly comorbid with major depression. In about 50% of patients, onset of GAD occurs in childhood or adolescence. Symptoms are chronic and tend to worsen during stressful times. Treatment is often needed indefinitely, although some GAD patients become relatively asymptomatic within a few years.

CASE 15-1

THE PATIENT A 45-year-old woman says that she frequently feels "nervous" and often has an "upset stomach," which includes heartburn, indigestion, and diarrhea. Physical examination (including blood pressure) and laboratory values (including thyroid function tests) are unremarkable. She notes that she often finds herself worrying about whether she will lose her job and whether her elderly parents will become ill. She says that she has been "a worrier" since she was a teenager and notes that other family members also tend to worry excessively.

COMMENT This patient is showing the symptoms of generalized anxiety disorder (GAD). She has a chronic, subjective sense of fear with no obvious precipitant, unexplained gastrointestinal problems, and a family history of anxiety. She does not have panic disorder because, although her anxiety symptoms have lasted at least 6 months, there have been no distinct attacks. Normal thyroid function and blood pressure indicate that physiological causes of her anxiety symptoms, such as hyperthyroidism and pheochromocytoma, are unlikely.

TREATMENT Antianxiety agents such as buspirone (BuSpar) and antidepressant agents such as paroxetine (Paxil), venlafaxine (Effexor), and doxepin (Adapin, Sinequan) are effective for the long-term treatment of patients with GAD. Unlike benzodiazepines, these agents do not cause dependence or tolerance. If benzodiazepines are used to treat this patient, the most effective ones are those that have an intermediate length of action like lorazepam (Ativan), because they have less addiction potential than short-acting agents yet work quickly enough to relieve the patient's symptoms.

PANIC DISORDER (WITH OR WITHOUT AGORAPHOBIA)

Characteristics

Panic disorder is characterized by episodic **panic attacks,** periods of intense anxiety that have a sudden onset and increase in intensity over an approximately 10-minute period. Panic attacks commonly occur about twice weekly and last about 30 minutes each, although they rarely follow a fixed pattern. During an attack, the patient has striking cardiac and respiratory symptoms that lead her to believe that she is about to die. Although mitral valve prolapse is often found in patients with panic disorder, no causal relationship between the two conditions has been demonstrated. Between attacks, the patient often develops **anticipatory anxiety,** an intense fear of having another attack, which further limits her functioning.

In panic disorder with **agoraphobia,** panic attacks are associated with fear and avoidance of public places or situations where escape is impossible or help is unavailable. For example, a patient with panic disorder with agoraphobia may have a panic attack whenever he goes outside alone but not when he goes out with his wife. Patients may avoid shopping malls, theaters (unless they sit at the end of the row), and driving in heavy traffic.

For experimental diagnostic purposes, a panic attack can be induced in a panic disorder patient by intravenous administration of sodium lactate or by hyperventilation or inhalation of CO_2 (see Chapter 6).

Occurrence and prognosis

Panic disorder has a lifetime prevalence of 1.5 to 3.5%, and the mean age of onset is 25 years. Genetic factors and social factors, such as divorce or marital separation in the patient's recent past, are involved in the etiology of panic disorder. When compared with the general population, adults who have panic disorder with agoraphobia are more likely to have experienced separation anxiety disorder in childhood (see Chapter 2). The course of panic disorder is chronic, with many recurrent episodes and an increased risk of depression and suicide.

PHOBIAS

Characteristics

Phobias are characterized by unfounded, irrational fears of certain things or situations. **Specific phobia** is an irrational fear of things such as snakes, elevators, or closed-in areas (claustrophobia). The nature of the stimulus (e.g., natural phenomenon or animal) that precipitates the symptoms divides specific phobias into subtypes (Table 15-2). **Social phobia,** also called **social anxiety disorder,** is an exaggerated fear of embarrassing oneself in a social or performance setting such as while giving a speech, eating in public, or using a public restroom.

TABLE 15-2   Subtypes of Specific Phobia

SUBTYPE (IN DESCENDING ORDER OF FREQUENCY FOUND IN ADULT CLINICAL SITUATIONS)	FEAR OF
Situational	Tunnels, bridges, public transportation, flying, closed places
Natural environment	Lightening, thunder, heights, deep water (often onset in childhood)
Blood-injection-injury	Receiving an injection or treatment requiring invasion of the body
Animal	Animals including insects
Other type	Loud sounds, costumed characters (in children), falling, contracting an illness, choking

Occurrence and prognosis

Phobias are among the most common mental health problems. Specific phobia is present in up to 5% of men and 10% of women. Social phobia is reported in about 3% of the population with no sex difference in its occurrence. Ninety-five percent of patients who are diagnosed with agoraphobia also have a diagnosis of panic disorder (see above). The differential diagnosis of phobias includes normal shyness. It also includes disorders such as delusional disorder, in which irrational fears are caused by psychotic thinking processes (see Chapter 12), and personality disorders (PDs) involving pathological suspiciousness of others (paranoid PD), avoidance of other people due to fear of rejection (avoidant PD), and preference for social isolation (schizoid PD) (see Chapter 24).

A phobia may not be problematic if the person is not exposed to the phobic stimulus. For example, a person who has a snake phobia and lives in a large city may never see a snake. However, if the phobic stimulus is encountered in everyday life (e.g., eating in a public place), its avoidance often leads to occupational and social difficulties, including employment problems, school dropout, and failure to establish social relationships.

■ OBSESSIVE-COMPULSIVE DISORDER

Characteristics

Patients with OCD experience recurrent, unwanted, intrusive feelings, thoughts, and images (obsessions) and anxiety. This anxiety is relieved to some extent by performing repetitive actions (compulsions) and sometimes by the obsessive thinking itself. A common symptom in OCD is avoidance of hand contamination and a compulsive, ritualistic need to wash the hands repeatedly after touching things. Repeated checking of door locks and gas jets and counting of objects are other common compulsions. Such behaviors can consume hours of time and lead to medical consequences (e.g., skin damage from vigorous hand washing). Patients with OCD usually have insight; they realize that these thoughts and behaviors are irrational and want to eliminate them.

Because Tourette's disorder and temporal lobe epilepsy also involve repetitive motor movements, OCD must be distinguished from these disorders. Although they are different illnesses, OCD and Tourette's disorder are genetically related; there is a higher rate of OCD in first-degree relatives of patients with Tourette's disorder than in the general population. Patients with OCD must also be distinguished from those with obsessive-compulsive PD, a condition in which a conscious need for perfection may manifest in repetitive behavior, but in which rituals like hand washing are not prominent (see Chapter 24).

Occurrence and prognosis

Although it can begin in childhood, OCD usually starts in early adulthood. It is present in 2 to 3% of the population, with no sex differences. One third of patients with OCD improve significantly with treatment and one half improve moderately; the remainder fails to improve or shows progressive deterioration in functioning over time.

■ THE STRESS DISORDERS AND ADJUSTMENT DISORDER

Characteristics

Approximately one half of all people are exposed to a significant psychological trauma during their lives. Most of these people recover completely; others have continuing symptoms and may be diagnosed with the stress disorders—post-traumatic stress disorder (PTSD) and acute stress disorder (ASD). For these diagnoses, there must be exposure to a life-threatening or potentially fatal event affecting the patient or the patient's close friend or relative. Examples of such events include sexual assault, war, earthquake, fire, and serious accident. Symptoms must last for more than 1 month to fulfill the DSM-IV-TR diagnostic criteria for PTSD that in chronic form can last for years. Symptoms lasting 2 days to 4 weeks are diagnosed as acute stress disorder (ASD) rather than PTSD.

The symptoms of the stress disorders can be divided into four types: re-experiencing, hyperarousal, emotional numbing, and avoidance.

■ **Re-experiencing** includes intrusive thoughts or memories of the event that occur unexpectedly **(flashbacks)** as well as recurrent nightmares of the event.

- **Hyperarousal** includes anxiety, increased startle response, impaired sleep, and increased or hypervigilance (e.g., jumping at every sound).
- **Emotional numbing** includes decreased emotionality, an inability to experience happiness, and difficulty connecting emotionally with others.
- **Avoidance** includes guilt about having escaped while others died or were seriously injured (**survivor's guilt**); dissociation and social withdrawal; and feelings of helplessness and being overwhelmed.

Differential diagnosis of the stress disorders

Post-traumatic stress disorder and ASD may have to be distinguished from the behavioral sequelae of brain injury caused by the traumatic event. Stress disorders must also be distinguished from **adjustment disorders.** The latter are common and generally milder conditions not fitting the criteria for PTSD or ASD. Adjustment disorders are characterized by emotional symptoms (e.g., anxiety, depression, conduct problems, or mixed emotional symptoms) that cause social, school, or work impairment occurring within 3 months and lasting less than 6 months after termination of a serious but usually not life-threatening stressor (e.g., divorce, bankruptcy, or changing residence). For example, if a previously normal 10-year-old boy is jittery and upset 4 months after a move to a new home, has little interest in playing with his friends, and begins to do poorly at school, he may be diagnosed with **adjustment disorder with anxiety.** With chronic or enduring stressors, the symptoms of adjustment disorder can persist for longer than 6 months.

Occurrence and prognosis

The lifetime prevalence of PTSD is 1 to 14% in the general population and 3 to 58% in people at particular risk, such as survivors of sexual assault, earthquake, or combat. Risk factors for the stress disorders include female gender and prior personal or family psychiatric history. About one third of patients with PTSD are comorbid for major depressive disorder.

Complete recovery occurs within 3 months in about one third of patients with PTSD. Another third of patients have persistent symptoms after 10 years. Alcohol abuse and childhood trauma, such as sexual abuse, appear to increase the duration of PTSD.

TREATMENT OF THE ANXIETY DISORDERS

Pharmacological agents and psychological therapies are used in the treatment of anxiety disorders (Table 15-3).

Pharmacologic treatment

Antianxiety agents, including **benzodiazepines, buspirone,** and **beta-blockers,** relieve symptoms of anxiety (see Chapter 19). Among the benzodiazepines, fast-acting agents such as clonazepam (Klonopin), alprazo-

THE PATIENT On September 25, 2001, a 43-year-old stockbroker who escaped from World Trade Center Tower One describes continuing intense feelings of fear, anxiety, and helplessness. She also expresses feelings of guilt because none of her coworkers made it out of the building. Although she is unable to recall specific details of her escape from the tower, thoughts about that day often intrude during her daily activities, and vivid nightmares about it awaken her each night.

COMMENT This woman is showing evidence of ASD, a common occurrence in survivors in the month after September 11th. This disorder is characterized by anxiety and intrusive memories, as well as nightmares and guilt about having survived while others died. This woman's diagnosis may change to PTSD if her significant symptoms persist beyond 1 month.

TREATMENT A support group consisting of other victims of the World Trade Center attack will be helpful for this patient. Medication such as selective serotonin reuptake inhibitors (SSRIs) and propranolol (Inderal) can also be useful if her symptoms persist (Table 15-3).

lam (Xanax), and diazepam (Valium), and intermediate-acting agents like lorazepam (Ativan), are most commonly used for acute symptoms, particularly for panic attacks. Because benzodiazepines carry a risk of dependence and addiction, they are often used for only a limited amount of time (e.g., 8 to 12 months), to treat acute exacerbations of anxiety symptoms and then are gradually withdrawn. However, some patients benefit from long-term monotherapy with an intermediate-acting (e.g., lorazepam) or long-acting (e.g., clonazepam) agent. Benzodiazepines are also used in conjunction with antidepressants (see later text) with gradual weaning from the agent when the patient's symptoms improve (Goddard et al., 2001).

Buspirone (BuSpar) is a relatively new antianxiety agent. Because it takes up to 2 weeks to work, buspirone is less useful for acute symptoms of anxiety than benzodiazepines. However, because of its low abuse potential, buspirone is useful as long-term maintenance therapy for patients with chronic anxiety such as those with GAD, particularly for patients who have never been treated with benzodiazepines.

Beta-adrenergic antagonists (i.e., **beta-blockers**) such as propranolol (Inderal) and atenolol (Tenormin) are used to control autonomic symptoms such as tachycardia in anxiety disorders. These agents are particularly useful for anxiety associated with performing in public or taking an examination because they are less likely than benzodiazepines to cause sedation and impaired thinking.

Antidepressants, including monoamine oxidase inhibitors (MAOIs), heterocyclics such as clomipramine (Anafranil), and especially selective serotonin reuptake inhibitors (SSRIs) such as paroxetine (Paxil), fluoxetine (Prozac), fluvoxamine (Luvox), and sertraline (Zoloft) (Pohl et al., 1998), in

TABLE 15-3   Treatment of the Anxiety Disorders

TREATMENTS
(IN DESCENDING ORDER OF UTILITY FOR EACH CLASSIFICATION)

CLASSIFICATION	PHARMACOLOGIC	PSYCHOLOGIC
Panic disorder with or without agoraphobia	■ Emergency treatment: fast-acting BZ ■ Long-term treatment: SSRI ■ Combination of an SSRI and a BZ ■ Intermediate- or long-acting BZ ■ Beta-adrenergic antagonist (e.g., propranolol [Inderal]) for autonomic symptoms	■ Systematic desensitization and cognitive-behavioral therapy are useful adjuncts to pharmacotherapy
Specific phobia	■ There is no good pharmacologic treatment ■ Beta-adrenergic antagonist	■ Cognitive-behavioral therapy ■ Systematic desensitization ■ Other behavioral therapy (e.g., flooding and implosion; see Chapter 27) ■ Hypnosis, family therapy, and psychotherapy
Social phobia	■ SSRI (e.g., paroxetine [Paxil]) or venlafaxine (Effexor) ■ MAOI (e.g., phenelzine [Nardil]) ■ Beta-adrenergic antagonist	■ Assertiveness training ■ Group therapy
Obsessive-compulsive disorder	■ SSRI (e.g., fluvoxamine [Luvox]) ■ Clomipramine (Anafranil)	■ Behavior therapy ■ Supportive psychotherapy (see Chapter 28)
Generalized anxiety disorder	■ Buspirone (BuSpar) ■ Venlafaxine ■ Doxepin (Adapin) ■ Intermediate-acting BZ (e.g., lorazepam [Ativan]) ■ Beta-adrenergic antagonist	■ Cognitive-behavioral therapy and other behavioral therapy are useful for chronic symptoms

TABLE 15-3	Treatment of the Anxiety Disorders (Continued)

	TREATMENTS (IN DESCENDING ORDER OF UTILITY FOR EACH CLASSIFICATION)	
CLASSIFICATION	PHARMACOLOGIC	PSYCHOLOGIC
Post-traumatic stress disorder	■ SSRI (e.g., sertraline [Zoloft]) ■ Anticonvulsant (e.g., carbamazepine [Tegretol)) ■ Antipsychotic (e.g., olanzapine [Zyprexa]) ■ Beta-adrenergic antagonist	■ Support groups, such as survivor groups ■ Psychotherapy

BZ, benzodiazepine; MAOI, monoamine oxidase inhibitor; SSRI, selective serotonin reuptake inhibitor.

doses similar to those used to treat depression, are the most effective long-term (maintenance) therapy for panic disorder and OCD. The antidepressants doxepin (Adapin, Sinequan) and venlafaxine (Effexor and Effexor ER) have Food and Drug Administration (FDA) indications for the treatment of GAD (Gelenberg et al., 2000), but other antidepressants can also be effective. Paroxetine, sertraline, and venlafaxine have FDA indications for social phobia, and extended treatment (at least 8 weeks) may be needed for the full therapeutic effect (Katzelnick, 1995; Stein et al., 1998).

Pharmacotherapy has limited effectiveness in PTSD. Sertraline and paroxetine are FDA indicated for PTSD but are not helpful for the sleep disturbances often associated with this disorder (Marshall et al., 2001). In patients who are SSRI resistant, antipsychotics like olanzapine (Zyprexa) may be helpful alone or in combination with SSRI s (Stern et al., 2002) to treat the hyperarousal of PTSD. Anticonvulsants such as carbamazepine or valproic acid are also useful, particularly for flashbacks and nightmares.

Psychological treatment

Cognitive-behavioral therapy and systematic desensitization with reciprocal inhibition are the most effective treatments for phobias and are useful adjuncts to pharmacotherapy in other anxiety disorders. Behavioral therapies such as flooding and implosion can also be helpful for treating phobias. Group therapy and leaderless group therapy (e.g., victim survivor groups; see Chapter 11) are particularly effective for patients with ASD and PTSD.

Some studies show that the efficacy of cognitive therapy in treating anxiety disorders is about equal to that of pharmacotherapy. Patients who do not respond to either may be helped by a combination of both (Barlow et al., 2000).

REVIEW QUESTIONS

Questions 1 and 2

A 22-year-old medical student relates that she has recently begun to experience sudden bouts of dizziness and shortness of breath that last about 20 minutes and then subside. Because of these attacks, she must sit near the door of the lecture hall so that she can leave in a hurry. This student has no history of asthma. Other than an increased pulse rate, physical findings are normal.

1. Of the following, the most effective immediate treatment for this patient when she develops these symptoms is

    (A) an antidepressant

    (B) psychotherapy

    (C) a benzodiazepine

    (D) buspirone

    (E) a beta-blocker

2. Of the following, the most effective long-term treatment for this patient is

    (A) an antidepressant

    (B) psychotherapy

    (C) a benzodiazepine

    (D) buspirone

    (E) a beta-blocker

3. A 26-year-old, fourth-year medical student with no previous psychiatric history reports that he has had a recurring thought over the past year that he will kill a patient before he graduates. The student has never harmed a patient and has no intention of doing so. When he snaps his fingers repeatedly, he feels somewhat calmer. This student is most likely to be experiencing

    (A) panic disorder

    (B) obsessive-compulsive disorder (OCD)

    (C) generalized anxiety disorder (GAD)

    (D) social phobia

    (E) adjustment disorder

4. A 45-year-old diabetic man is admitted to the hospital with a serious foot infection. During the last year, his wife divorced him and he declared personal bankruptcy. After this, he moved to a new apartment. On his first day in the apartment he was robbed at knife point in the elevator. Which of the events experienced by this man is most likely to result in PTSD?

(A) Divorce

(B) Bankruptcy

(C) Serious illness

(D) Changing residence

(E) Robbery

5. A 23-year-old student reports that he becomes very "uptight" when he must use a public restroom but otherwise does not report episodes of anxiety. Because he becomes so uncomfortable about using public restrooms, he refuses when his classmates ask him to join them when they go out. Of the following, the pharmacologic agent which has FDA approval for the long-term treatment of this student's symptoms is

(A) imipramine (Tofranil)

(B) chlordiazepoxide (Librium)

(C) clomipramine (Anafranil)

(D) venlafaxine (Effexor)

(E) clonazepam (Klonopin)

ANSWERS AND EXPLANATIONS

1-C, 2-A. This student is showing the symptoms of panic disorder. This condition is characterized by panic attacks, which consist of increased heart rate, dizziness, sweating, shortness of breath, fainting, and the conviction that one is about to die. Attacks commonly occur twice weekly and last about 30 minutes and are most common in young women. Although the most effective immediate treatment for this patient is a benzodiazepine because it works quickly, the most effective long-term (maintenance) treatment for this patient is an antidepressant, particularly a selective serotonin-reuptake inhibitor (SSRI) such as paroxetine (Paxil).

3-B. This student's symptoms suggest obsessive-compulsive disorder (OCD). Recurrent, unwanted thoughts like killing a patient are typical obsessions of OCD. The finger snapping is a compulsion that relieves his anxiety. The most effective long-term treatment for OCD is an antidepressant, particularly a selective serotonin reuptake inhibitor (SSRI), such as fluvoxamine.

4-E. Robbery, a life-threatening event, is most likely to result in posttraumatic stress disorder (PTSD). Although life events such as divorce, bankruptcy, illness, and changing residence are stressful, they are rarely life threatening. Psychological symptoms occurring after events such as these are more likely to be evidence of adjustment disorder, not PTSD or acute stress disorder.

5-D. This student's symptoms of anxiety in a public situation (such as using public restrooms) but not in other situations suggest social phobia (social anxiety disorder). This phobia has limited the patient's ability to socialize freely. Of the listed agents, venlafaxine (Effexor) is FDA approved to treat social phobia (see Table 15-3). Heterocyclic antidepressants such as imipramine and clomipramine, benzodiazepines such as chlordiazepoxide, and clonazepam may be helpful. However, they are less likely to be used for the long-term treatment of this disorder.

REFERENCES

American Psychiatric Association: Diagnostic and Statistical Manual of Mental Disorders, Fourth Edition-Text Revision. (2001). Washington, DC: American Psychiatric Association, pp. 429–484.

Barlow, D. H., Gorman, J. M., Shear, M. K., & Woods, S. W. (2000). Cognitive-behavioral therapy, imipramine, or their combination for panic disorder: A randomized controlled trial. *JAMA, 283,* 2529–2536.

Gelenberg, A. J., Lydiard, R. B., Rudolph, R. L., Aguiar, G., Haskins, J. T., & Salinas, E. (2000). Efficacy of venlafaxine extended-release capsules in nondepressed outpatients with generalized anxiety disorder: A 6-month randomized controlled trial. *JAMA, 283,* 3082–3088.

Hollander, E. (ed.). (1993). *Obsessive-compulsive related disorders.* Washington, DC: American Psychiatric Press.

Katzelnick, D. J., Kobak, K. A., Greist, J. H., Jefferson, J. W., CMantle, J. M., & Serlin, R. C. (1995). Sertraline for social phobia: A double-blind, placebo-controlled crossover study. *Am J Psychiatry, 152,* 1368–1371.

Kessler, R. C., Stang, P. E., Wittchen, H. U., Ustun, T. B., Roy-burne, P. P., & Walters, E. E. (1998). Lifetime panic-depression comorbidity in the National Comorbidity Survey. *Arch Gen Psychiatry, 55,* 801.

Magee, W. J., Eaton, W. W., Wittchen, H. U., McGonagle, K. A., & Kessler, R. C. (1996). Agoraphobia, simple phobia and social phobia in the National Comorbidity Survey. *Arch Gen Psychiatry, 53,* 159.

Malizia, A. L., Cunningham, V. J., Bell, C. J., Liddle, P. F., Jones, T., & Nutt, D. J. (1998). Decreased brain $GABA_A$-benzodiazepine receptor binding in panic disorder: Preliminary results from a quantitative PET study. *Arch Gen Psychiatry, 55,* 715–720.

Marshall, R. D., Beebe, K. L., Oldham , M., & Zaninelli, R. (2001). Efficacy and safety of paroxetine treatment for chronic PTSD: A fixed-dose, placebo-controlled study. *Am J Psychiatry, 158,* 1982–1988.

Pohl, R. B., Wolkow, R. M., & Clary, C. M. (1998). Sertraline in the treatment of panic disorder: A double-blind multicenter trial. *Am J Psychiatry, 155,* 1189–1195.

Stein, M. B., Liebowitz, M. R., Lydiard, R. B., Pitts, C. D., Bushnell W., & Gergel, I. (1998). Paroxetine treatment of generalized social phobia (social anxiety disorder): A randomized controlled trial. *JAMA, 280,* 708–713.

Stein, M. B., Kline, N. A., & Matloff, J. L. (2002). Adjunctive olanzapine for SSRI-resistant combat-related PTSD: A double-blind, placebo-controlled study. *Am J Psychiatry, 159,* 1777–1779.

Wolf, M. E., Mosnaim, A. D. (eds.). (1990). *Post-traumatic stress disorder: Etiology, phenomenology and treatment.* Washington, DC: American Psychiatric Press.

Somatoform **16**
Disorders,
Factitious
Disorders, and
Malingering

A t least 30% of the physical complaints of primary care patients cannot be explained by organic illness (Kroenke et al., 1994). Although understanding the social and psychiatric influences on these complaints is essential for appropriate management, patients with unexplained symptoms present a diagnostic and treatment challenge for even the most empathic and dedicated doctor (Hartz et al., 2000).

Patients with unexplained physical symptoms fall into two general categories (Fig. 16-1). In the first category, symptom formation is unconscious. These patients come to the doctor believing that they are medically ill. This category includes patients with **somatoform disorders,** a group of emotional disorders characterized by physical symptoms that suggest organic pathology (see later text); and patients with depressive illnesses, because **"masked depression"** (see Chapter 13) commonly presents with physical symptoms. In the second general category symptom, formation is conscious. Individuals with these conditions, which include **factitious disorders** and **malingering,** feign mental or physical illness or actually induce physical illness in themselves or in others. In factitious disorders, the symptoms are feigned for psychological reasons (e.g., to gain attention and

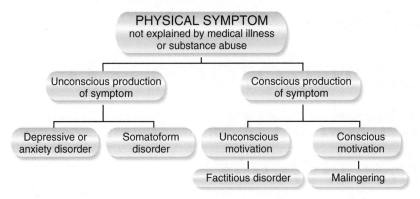

```
                    PHYSICAL SYMPTOM
                  not explained by medical illness
                        or substance abuse

          ┌─────────────────────┴──────────────────────┐
   Unconscious production                        Conscious production
       of symptom                                    of symptom

   ┌──────────┴──────────┐                  ┌──────────┴──────────┐
Depressive or       Somatoform         Unconscious            Conscious
anxiety disorder      disorder         motivation            motivation

                                            │                      │
                                    Factitious disorder        Malingering
```

FIGURE 16-1. The differential diagnosis of a patient with medically unexplained physical symptoms.

care from medical personnel). In malingering, the symptoms are invented for tangible gain, such as money in a lawsuit or release from legal, work, or school responsibilities.

■ SOMATOFORM DISORDERS

Persons who have somatoform disorders are not lying; they truly believe that they have physical problems. They tend to seek medical attention, typically visiting many different doctors searching for help (**"doctor shopping"**). Their symptoms commonly lead to impairment in social or occupational functioning. Approximately 50% of patients with a somatoform disorder also have another mental symptom, most commonly depression or anxiety (Simon et al., 1999; Green et al., 2000; Otto et al., 2001).

Classification

The five major Diagnostic and Statistical Manual of Mental Disorders, Fourth Edition-Text Revision (DSM-IV-TR) classifications of somatoform disorders are **somatization disorder, conversion disorder, hypochondriasis, body dysmorphic disorder,** and **pain disorder.** Selected DSM-IV-TR criteria for and specific examples of patients with each disorder are listed in Table 16-1. **Undifferentiated somatoform disorder** is diagnosed when the unexplained symptoms, such as fatigue, loss of appetite, and gastrointestinal or genitourinary complaints, do not fit the diagnostic criteria for any of these disorders.

Etiology

Social factors are involved in the etiology of the somatoform disorders. Although the patient is not consciously aware of it, primary or secondary gain may result from the symptoms. **Primary gain** involves using the defense mechanism of somatization (see Chapter 8) to unconsciously express an

TABLE 16-1	Somatoform Disorders

SELECTED DSM-IV-TR DIAGNOSTIC CRITERIA	PATIENT EXAMPLE
Somatization Disorder	
■ History over years of at least 4 pain symptoms, 2 GI symptoms, 1 sexual symptom, and 1 pseudoneurological symptom ■ Symptoms begin before age 30 years	A 39-year-old woman has a 20-year history of somatic complaints such as headache (pain symptom), nausea (GI symptom), menstrual irregularities (sexual symptom), and temporary loss of sensation in her hands (pseudoneurological symptom). She tells the doctor that she is always sick but that her previous doctors never seem to identify the problem and were unable to help her.
Conversion Disorder	
■ One or more symptoms affecting voluntary motor or sensory function and suggesting a neurologic etiology ■ The symptom is produced or preceded by psychological stress or conflict	A 28-year-old woman experiences a sudden loss of vision but appears unconcerned. Medical tests are essentially normal. The patient reports that just before the onset of her blindness, she saw her child dart out into the street.
Hypochondriasis	
■ Preoccupation over at least 6 months with fear or idea of having a serious disease based on misinterpretation of bodily symptoms ■ Fear persists despite negative medical findings and physician's reassurance	A 41-year-old man reports that he has seen many doctors for his persistent illnesses but is frustrated because they have ultimately referred him to mental health clinicians. He now fears that he has stomach cancer because his stomach makes noises after he eats. Medical tests are negative and his doctor has repeatedly told him that nothing is wrong with him.
Body Dysmorphic Disorder	
■ Preoccupation with an imagined problem with one's appearance or an insignificant physical abnormality ■ The preoccupation is not accounted for by anorexia nervosa (see Chapter 17)	A 28-year-old woman seeks rhinoplasty for her "huge" nose. She rarely goes out in the daytime because she believes that this characteristic makes her look "like a hag." On physical examination, her nose appears completely normal.

TABLE 16-1	Somatoform Disorders (Continued)

SELECTED DSM-IV-TR DIAGNOSTIC CRITERIA	PATIENT EXAMPLE
Pain Disorder	
▪ Pain severe enough to seek medical attention ▪ Psychological factors are involved in the onset or other aspect of the pain	A 40-year-old man who suffered a minor knee injury playing ball 11 months ago continues to complain of severe knee pain although there is no evidence of pathology.

GI, gastrointestinal.
Adapted from Fadem, B. & Simring, S. (2003). *High-yield psychiatry.* Baltimore: Lippincott Williams & Wilkins.

unacceptable emotion as a physical symptom to avoid dealing with the emotion. **Secondary gain** means that the symptom, once established, serves a useful purpose, such as getting attention from others or avoiding responsibility (e.g., "I cannot take care of myself, so you will have to take care of me").

Genetic and familial factors have also been associated with the somatoform disorders. Somatization disorder, pain disorder, and hypochondriasis tend to run in families and have a higher concordance rate in monozygotic than in dizygotic twins. A family history of mood disorder and obsessive-compulsive disorder is more common in patients with hypochondriasis and pain disorder, and a family history of antisocial personality disorder and alcoholism is more common in patients with somatization disorder than in people without these disorders.

The somatoform disorders tend to start in early adulthood and have chronic symptoms that worsen during times of stress and that improve when life conditions are more favorable. Most of these disorders are more common in women, although hypochondriasis occurs equally in men and women.

Somatization disorder (formerly "Briquet syndrome")

Somatization disorder is a specific somatoform disorder characterized by a history of at least eight physical symptoms, including pain and gastrointestinal, sexual, and neurological symptoms, for which no cause or inadequate cause is found. The symptoms tend to be chronic and total remission is rare. Because the physical symptoms of somatization disorder vary by culture, social factors and learning may be involved in its etiology.

Hypochondriasis

In contrast to somatization disorder, in which the symptoms of illness predominate, fear of having a serious illness is the focus of **hypochondriasis.** Because of the persistent and repetitive nature of these concerns, hypochondriasis may have a similar etiology to other disorders characterized by recurrent unwanted thoughts and behaviors, such as obsessive-compulsive disorder (OCD) (see Chapter 15) and impulse control disorders (e.g., trichotillomania [compulsive hair pulling]) (see Chapter 22). As evidence for an etiologic similarity, selective serotonin reuptake inhibitors, such as fluoxetine (Prozac), that improve symptoms in patients with OCD and impulse control disorders also improve symptoms in nondepressed hypochondriacal patients (O'Malley et al., 1999).

Conversion disorder

Conversion disorder involves the sudden, dramatic loss of motor function (e.g., paralysis) or sensory function (e.g., hearing or vision). In describing this disorder, Freud noted that the symptoms had obvious and symbolic significance associated with a particular stressful life event. For example, a woman getting married in the near future finds that she is suddenly unable to move her legs. Perhaps because conversion symptoms decrease the individual's anxiety about the life stressor that provokes them, patients with conversion disorder typically appear relatively unworried about their serious symptoms, a phenomenon known as **"la belle indifference."**

The most common conversion motor symptoms include paralysis that shifts to different areas of the body, bizarre seizures (**pseudoseizures**), and

---

CASE 16-1

THE PATIENT Three months ago, a 25-year-old woman's 65-year-old father had a stroke that paralyzed the right side of his body. The woman tells her physician that she has recently begun to experience numbness and tingling on the right side of her body. She relates this alarming symptom in a calm and thoughtful way. Physical examination, laboratory testing, and neuroimaging reveal no evidence of pathology.

COMMENT This case illustrates several aspects of conversion disorder. First, the patient has a dramatic neurological symptom (numbness and tingling) without adequate physical cause. Second, the symptom appeared suddenly after a stressful life event (her father's illness). Typically, patients with conversion disorder unconsciously model their symptoms on those of a person close to them (use of identification as a defense mechanism). Finally, the woman shows "la belle indifference"—she appears relatively unconcerned about the symptom. Factitious disorder and malingering are unlikely in this patient because there is no history of attention-seeking from doctors, nor is there obvious benefit to be gained by producing this symptom.

TREATMENT Symptoms of conversion disorder commonly remit without treatment after a brief period. Because this patient is not particularly distressed, the best approach is to reassure her that the symptoms will disappear in time and to train her in relaxation techniques. If the symptoms persist, further medical investigation is indicated. If this testing is negative, hypnosis or drug-assisted interviewing may speed remission of symptoms.

---

globus hystericus (i.e., lump in the throat). The most common sensory presentations are paresthesias (abnormal sensations), anesthesias (loss of sensation often inconsistent with anatomic innervation), and visual problems (e.g., blindness or tunnel vision). Although evoked potentials and other measures of neurological function (see Chapter 6) are typically normal in patients with conversion disorder, these tests have low sensitivity and may be normal also in patients with "real" neurological illnesses.

Conversion disorder is more common in psychiatrically unsophisticated patients, such as adolescents, young adults, and people from rural areas. It is often comorbid with histrionic personality disorder (see Chapter 24) and depression. Symptoms are commonly self-limited and remission usually takes place in less than 1 month. While the reasons are not clear, hypnosis or drug-assisted interviewing (see Chapter 6) is often quickly followed by remission of symptoms.

Body dysmorphic disorder

In **body dysmorphic disorder,** a patient who appears normal is focused on a minor or imagined physical defect in appearance, usually of the face or head (Phillips et al., 1993; Otto, et al., 2002). The excessive concern over the offending physical feature varies over time. Plastic surgery or other medical treatments to correct the perceived defect must be used with great caution because it rarely relieves symptoms.

Pain disorder

Pain disorder involves protracted, intense pain not adequately explained by physical causes. The age of onset is usually in the 30s and 40s, and the disorder can be acute (lasting less than 6 months) or chronic (lasting more than 6 months). The pain, which is often present along with a real but minor medical condition, can be disabling, and the patient may become dependent on pain medication.

Differential diagnosis of the somatoform disorders

The most important differential diagnosis of the somatoform disorders is the possibility that the patient really has an unidentified organic ailment. Diagnosis must therefore be approached carefully because misdiagnosis can delay treatment for an underlying medical problem. For example, globus hystericus, thought to be almost pathognomonic for conversion disorder, may also be caused by unusual organic conditions, such as cranial nerve disorders. Similarly, severe neurological pain may be caused by disorders such as spinal arachnoiditis (progressive, often iatrogenic, intradural scarring; Faure et al., 2002) and spinal whiplash injuries, which may be difficult to identify with commonly used imaging or nerve-testing techniques.

Other physical illnesses likely to be misdiagnosed as somatoform disorders are early-stage connective tissue disorders, such as systemic lupus erythematosus and rheumatoid arthritis; central nervous system disorders, such as brain tumor, multiple sclerosis, epilepsy, dementia, stroke (small intracranial hemorrhage, ischemic stroke, or spinal infarct), and myasthenia gravis; and endocrine disorders, such as hypoglycemia, thyroid dysfunction, and porphyria. Medically unexplained illnesses that have no consistent pathognomonic features or laboratory findings, such as **chronic fatigue syndrome** (unexplained fatigue lasting more than 6 months) and **fibromyalgia** (unexplained widespread musculoskeletal pain and multiple sites of hyperalgesia [tenderpoints]), must also be considered. Unexplained physical complaints are also seen in many depressed (see Chapter 13) and anxious (see Chapter 15) patients. Factitious disorder and malingering (see later text), in which symptoms are feigned, must also be ruled out in the differential diagnosis of somatoform disorders. Finally, presence of a somatoform disorder does not preclude the presence of comorbid organic pathology, a possibility that must be explored when evaluating patients with somatoform disorders.

Treatment

The most useful strategy for treating the somatoform disorders and their associated conditions, such as chronic fatigue syndrome and fibromyalgia, involves the establishment of a strong and supportive doctor-patient relationship. The physician can best do this by scheduling regular appointments and by providing reassurance to the patient (see Chapter 24). Formation of liaisons with other medical professionals, including mental health professionals, provides a **multidisciplinary approach** that is essential to treating these patients successfully. Another important treatment strategy is to identify and decrease social difficulties in the patient's life that may aggravate the symptoms. Also, it is helpful to identify the secondary gain that the physical symptoms provide for the patient, such as increased attention and avoidance of responsibility. These and other goals for the medical management of patients with somatoform disorders are listed in Table 16-2.

Pharmacotherapy has limited usefulness in somatoform disorders unless there is a comorbid psychiatric illness, such as depression or anxiety. However, antidepressants with **serotonergic action** (e.g., selective serotonin reuptake inhibitors) may be useful, particularly in hypochondriasis, body dysmorphic disorder, and pain disorder (O'Malley et al., 1999). Individual and group psychotherapy, hypnosis, behavioral relaxation therapy, and cognitive-behavioral therapy (Kroenke & Swindle, 2001) can be helpful in all somatoform disorders. Unfortunately, although pharmacological and psychological treatment may help to control the manifestations of these disorders, there is no "cure," and the symptoms often return in time.

■ FACTITIOUS DISORDERS AND MALINGERING

While individuals with somatoform disorders truly believe that they are ill, patients with factitious disorders and malingering feign mental or

TABLE 16-2	Goals of Medical Management in Patients With Somatoform Disorders
To increase the patient's	▪ Trust in the physician ▪ Physical functioning ▪ Activity level (if inactive) ▪ Use of conservative medical management ▪ Appropriate lifestyle modification ▪ Ability to deal with medical uncertainty ▪ Understanding of the underlying causes of the symptoms
To decrease the patient's	▪ Use of invasive or risky procedures with low probability of success ▪ Secondary gain ▪ "Doctor shopping" ▪ Social difficulties

physical illness or actually induce physical illness in themselves or others for psychological gain (factitious disorder) or tangible gain (malingering).

Factitious disorders

Factitious disorder (formerly Munchausen Syndrome) is a rare disorder in which patients fake or induce medical or emotional symptoms for attention and care from medical personnel. However, they typically do not consciously understand why they need to do this. The most commonly feigned symptoms are abdominal pain, fever (by heating the thermometer), blood in the urine (by adding blood from a needle stick), and seizures. The most commonly induced symptoms include causing skin lesions by injuring easily reached body areas and inducing tachycardia by drug administration. Multiple cross-hatched abdominal scars giving the appearance of a **"grid abdomen"** are evidence of previous but usually unnecessary surgical procedures that the factitious disorder patient has provoked. Typically, patients with factitious disorder have worked in the medical field and have specific knowledge of how to imitate medical illness realistically.

In **factitious disorder by proxy,** an adult, usually a parent, feigns or induces illness in a child to gain attention for him or herself. Factitious disorder by proxy is considered a form of child abuse and must be reported to child welfare authorities.

Individuals with factitious disorder and factitious disorder by proxy often have a history of serious childhood illness that resulted in medical treatment or hospitalization in which the patient felt cared for and protected. There also may be a history of childhood abuse or neglect. Preoccupation with illness and medical care negatively affects the individual's work, school, and social relationships. Patients also may be put at risk by unnecessary surgery, medical procedures, or medications.

THE PATIENT A 39-year-old woman takes her 6-year-old son to a physician's office. She says that the child often experiences episodes of breathing problems and abdominal pain. The child's medical record since birth shows many office visits and four abdominal surgical procedures that have resulted in crosshatched abdominal scarring, although no abnormalities were ever found. When the doctor confronts the mother with the suspicion that she is fabricating the illness in the child, the mother angrily grabs the child and leaves the office immediately.

COMMENT This clinical presentation is an example of factitious disorder by proxy. The mother has faked the child's illness for attention from medical personnel. This faking has resulted in multiple surgical procedures in which no abnormalities were identified, resulting in a "grid abdomen." Because she knows she is lying, the mother becomes angry and quickly leaves the office when she is confronted with the truth.

TREATMENT Factitious disorder by proxy is a form of child abuse. Therefore, the first thing the physician should do is notify the appropriate state social service agency to report this suspicion. Delaying action could result in further injury or even death to the child. The child probably has no knowledge of his mother's behavior.

Malingering

Malingering is the conscious simulation or exaggeration of physical or mental illness for financial or other obvious gain, such as avoiding school, work, or a prison term. In contrast to somatoform disorders and factitious disorders, malingering is not a psychiatric illness and is listed under "other conditions that may be a focus of clinical attention" in the DSM-IV-TR (see Chapter 12). Incarcerated individuals or people involved in lawsuits are more likely to malinger than those in the general population. In contrast to patients with factitious disorder who actively seek medical attention and treatment for attention, people who are malingering tend to avoid doctors and treatment (unless they must provide evidence for a lawsuit or are substance abusers seeking prescription drugs). The malingerer's symptoms improve dramatically as soon as the desired gain is obtained.

REVIEW QUESTIONS

Questions 1 and 2

A 15-year-old girl is admitted to the hospital with a diagnosis of "abdominal pain of unknown origin." Her parents state that she is interested in going into nursing. After extensive testing has failed to identify a cause for the pain, the teenager is seen reading a medical textbook by flashlight under the blanket at night.

1. This clinical presentation is most consistent with

    (A) factitious disorder

    (B) conversion disorder

    (C) factitious disorder by proxy

    (D) somatization disorder

    (E) malingering

    (F) hypochondriasis

    (G) somatoform pain disorder

2. Which of the following best describes symptom production and motivation in this teenager?

    (A) Symptom production conscious, motivation primarily conscious

    (B) Symptom production unconscious, motivation primarily conscious

    (C) Symptom production conscious, motivation primarily unconscious

    (D) Symptom production unconscious, motivation primarily unconscious

3. A 40-year-old woman comes to the emergency room on a Sunday afternoon complaining of intolerable, unremitting foot pain. She is sweating profusely and seems agitated. Radiographic and laboratory studies fail to reveal any pathology. After the patient receives an injection of meperidine hydrochloride (Demerol) and instructions to visit her family physician for further evaluation, her agitation and sweating improve and she quickly leaves the hospital. Later, a check of her medical records reveals that she has visited the emergency room on at least three other occasions with complaints of severe headache, toothache, and stomach pain for which she also received meperidine injections. This clinical presentation is most consistent with

    (A) factitious disorder

    (B) conversion disorder

    (C) factitious disorder by proxy

    (D) somatization disorder

    (E) malingering

    (F) hypochondriasis

    (G) somatoform pain disorder

4. A second-year medical student complains of a "tight" feeling in his abdomen after eating which has been present over the past eight months. He believes that the pain indicates that he has hepatitis because of eating at the school cafeteria salad bar. Physical examination is normal

and all tests are negative but he continues to believe that he is ill. His preoccupation with his symptom has negatively affected his school-work and social life. Which disorder best fits this clinical picture?

(A) Factitious disorder

(B) Conversion disorder

(C) Factitious disorder by proxy

(D) Somatization disorder

(E) Malingering

(F) Hypochondriasis

(G) Somatoform pain disorder

5. A 48-year-old man from Ohio is found in Alaska working as a night watchman. He states that he cannot remember who is he or where he previously lived. The police discover that the man is wanted in Ohio for armed robbery. This clinical presentation is an example of

(A) factitious disorder

(B) conversion disorder

(C) factitious disorder by proxy

(D) somatization disorder

(E) malingering

(F) hypochondriasis

(G) somatoform pain disorder

6. A 48-year-old woman reports persistent muscle pain for which no medical cause can be found. There is no reason to believe that the patient is malingering. Which of the following is the most effective strategy for the primary care doctor to take in dealing with this patient?

(A) Refer her to a mental health clinician

(B) Prescribe antidepressant medication

(C) Prescribe an analgesic

(D) Establish a multidisciplinary treatment approach

(E) Explain to the patient that her symptoms are not real

(F) Terminate her care as soon as possible

ANSWERS AND EXPLANATIONS

1-A, 2-C. This clinical presentation is an example of factitious disorder. In contrast to patients with somatoform disorders such as conversion, somatization, and hypochondriasis who really believe that they are ill, patients with factitious disorder are conscious of the fact that they are faking their illness. Abdominal pain is one of the most commonly feigned symptoms, and this patient's nighttime reading is providing her with specific knowledge of how to fake the illness realistically. Like this patient, factitious disorder patients commonly have an interest in or have worked in the medical field. Although she is consciously producing her abdominal symptoms, she is not receiving tangible benefit for her behavior. Thus, in contrast to individuals who are consciously faking illness for obvious gain (i.e., malingering, see Question 3), the motivation for this patient's faking behavior is primarily unconscious.

3-E. The sweating and agitation that this woman shows are symptoms of opiate withdrawal. She is feigning pain symptoms to obtain opiates (obvious gain for this addicted woman), and thus is malingering. In conversion disorder, somatization disorder, factious disorder, and factitious disorder by proxy, there is no obvious gain related to physical or mental symptoms.

4-F. This student, who continues to believe that he is ill despite reassurance from medical personnel, is demonstrating hypochondriasis—exaggerated concern over normal physical sensations (e.g., a tight feeling in the abdomen after eating) and minor ailments (see also response to question 1) which affect his ability to function socially and at school.

5-E. This presentation is an example of malingering—feigning illness (mental illness in this case) for obvious gain. The obvious gain here is avoiding a prison sentence for robbery.

6-D. Antidepressants, analgesics, and counseling all may be beneficial to this patient with unexplained physical symptoms. Therefore, the primary care doctor's most effective recommendation is to establish a multidisciplinary approach to her treatment, including mental health and medical professionals. Explaining that her symptoms are not real will not help, and terminating treatment is not appropriate, even though this patient's symptoms are probably not caused by physical illness.

REFERENCES

American Psychiatric Association: Diagnostic and Statistical Manual of Mental Disorders, Fourth Edition-Text Revision. (2001) (pp. 485–517). Washington, DC: American Psychiatric Association.

Cloninger, C. R. (1993). Somatoform and dissociative disorders. In: Winokur, G., Clayton, P. J. , *Medical basis of psychiatry* (2nd ed.) (pp. 169–192). Philadelphia: WB Saunders.

Faure, A., Khalfallah, M., Perrouin-Verbe, B., Caillon, F., Deschamps, C., Bord, E., Mathe, J.-F., & Robert, R. (2002). Arachnoiditis ossificans of the cauda equina. Case report and review of the literature. *J Neurosurg, 97,* 239–243.

Green, A. R., Betancourt, J. R., Carrillo, J. E., Pornnoppadol, C., Simon, G. E., & VonKorff, M. (2000). The relation between somatic symptoms and depression. *N Engl J Med, 342,* 658–659.

Hartz, A. J., Noyes, R., & Bentler, S. E. (2000). Unexplained symptoms in primary care: Perspectives of the doctors and the patients. *Gen Hosp Psychiatry, 22,* 144–152.

Hollender, E. (1993). Obsessive-compulsive spectrum disorders: An overview. *Psychiatr Ann, 23,* 355–358.

Kellner, R. (1990). Somatization: theories and research. *J Nerv Ment Dis, 178,* 150–160.

Kroenke, K., & Swindle, R. (2000). Cognitive-behavioral therapy for somatization and symptom syndromes: A critical review of clinical trials. *Psychother Psychosom, 69,* 205–215.

Kroenke, K., Sptizer, R. L., Williams, J. B. W., Lenzer, M., Hahn, S. R., deGruy, F. V., & Brody, D. (1994). Physical symptoms in primary care: Predictors of psychiatric disorders and functional impairment. *Arch Fam Med, 3,* 774–779.

O'Malley, P. G., Jackson, J. L., Tomkins, G., Santory, J., Balden, E., & Kroenke, K. (1999). Antidepressant therapy for unexplained symptoms and symptom syndromes: A critical review. *J Fam Pract, 46,* 980–993.

Otto, M. W., Wilhelm, S., Cohen, L. S., & Harlow, B. L. (2001). Prevalence of body dysmorphic disorder in a community sample of women. *Am J Psychiatry, 158,* 2061–2063.

Phillips, K. A., McElroy, S. I., & Keck, P. E., Jr. (1993). Body dysmorphic disorder: 30 cases of imagined ugliness. *Am J Psychiatry, 150,* 302–308.

Simon, G. E., VonKorff, M., Piccinelli, M., Fullerton, C., & Ormel, J. (1999). An international study of the relation between somatic symptoms and depression. *N Engl J Med, 341,* 1329–1335.

Obesity and the Eating Disorders

17

" **Y**ou cannot be too rich or too thin." This tongue-in-cheek quote, attributed to Wallace Simpson, the reed-thin American wife of the late Duke of Windsor, reflects the attitude of many Americans toward body weight. That is, they equate being thin with being successful, while being obese reflects laziness and lack of self-control. This idealized view of thin people and the negative view of overweight people are significant contributing factors to the financial success of the American weight control industry and, unfortunately, to the high prevalence of eating disorders such as anorexia nervosa and bulimia nervosa in the U.S. population.

OBESITY

Obesity is a common health concern in the United States. Between 25 and 50% of American adults are obese, and their numbers are increasing.

Characteristics

Obesity is defined as more than 20% over ideal weight based on insurance company standard height and weight. **Body mass index (BMI),** the ratio of body weight in kg to height in m^2, may be a more accurate indicator of obesity than body weight. Normal BMI is in the range of 20 to 25 (Fig. 17-1).

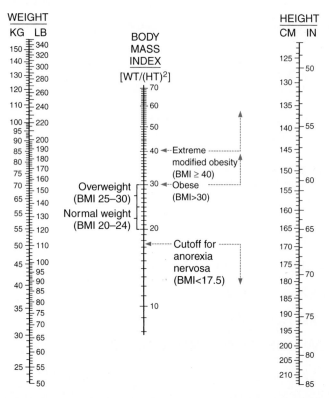

FIGURE 17-1. Body mass index (BMI). BMI is calculated by placing a straight edge between the body-weight column (left) and the height column (right) and reading the BMI from the point at which the straight edge crosses the BMI column.

(Adapted from Bray, G. A. (1978). Definitions, measurements and classification of the syndromes of obesity. Int J Obes, 2, 99.)

A BMI higher than 25 usually indicates that an individual is overweight, and a person with a BMI of greater than 30 is considered obese.

The formula for calculating BMI from body weight in pounds is body weight (lb) × 705/height (inches)/height (inches). For example, for a man weighing 170 lb who is 70 inches tall, BMI = 170 × 705 = 119,850; 119,850/70 = 1712.14; 1712.14/70 = 24.46 (normal).

The prevalence of obesity in the United States varies by ethnic group in women but not in men (Flegal et al., 2002). In most groups, it is more common in women than in men (Table 17-1). In children, the term **overweight** is used to describe excess body weight and is defined as at or above the 95th percentile of the sex-specific BMI for age growth charts. The prevalence of overweight children, which is increasing among children aged 2 through 19 years, is currently highest among Mexican-American and non-Hispanic African-American adolescents ages 12 to 19 years (Ogden et al., 2002).

TABLE 17-1 Obesity Prevalence Data for Selected U.S. Adults, by Sex

GROUP	PERCENT MALES	FEMALES	FEMALE:MALE
Non-Hispanic whites, 1988–94, age ≥20[a]	20	23	1.2
Non-Hispanic whites, 1988–91, age ≥25, <grade 12 education[b]	39	39	1.0
Non-Hispanic whites, 1988–91, age ≥25, grade 12 education[b]	36	38	1.1
Non-Hispanic whites, 1988–91, age ≥25, >grade 12 education[b]	30	30	1.0
Non-Hispanic African Americans, 1988–94, age ≥20[a]	21	37	1.8
Non-Hispanic African Americans, 1988–91, age ≥25, <grade 12 education[b]	29	55	1.8
Non-Hispanic African Americans, 1988–91, age ≥25, grade 12 education[b]	29	51	1.8
Non-Hispanic African Americans, 1988–91, age ≥ 25, >grade 12 education[b]	36	49	1.4
Mexican Americans, 1988–94, age ≥20[b]	21	33	1.6
Mexican Americans, 1988–91, age ≥ 25, <grade 12 education[b]	39	53	1.4
Mexican Americans, 1988–91, age ≥25, grade 12 education[b]	43	40	0.9
Mexican Americans, 1988–91, age ≥25, >grade 12 education[b]	40	47	1.2
Puerto Ricans, 1982–84, age 20–74[b]	25	37	1.5
Cuban Americans 1982–84, age 20–74[b]	29	34	1.2
American Indians in OK, 1994–96[b] (questionnaire)	38	36	0.9
American Indians in NM and AZ, 1994–96[b] (questionnaire)	33	34	1.0

GROUP	PERCENT		
	MALES	FEMALES	FEMALE:MALE
American Indians in WA and OR, 1994–96[b] (questionnaire)	33	43	1.3
American Indians in ND and SD, 1994–96[b] (questionnaire)	46	47	1.0
Alaska Natives, 1996[b] (questionnaire)	41	30	1.0
Asian Americans, ages 18–59[c] (questionnaire)	57	38	0.7
Samoans in Manu'a[b]	56	77	1.4
Samoans in Oahu[b]	75	80	1.1

[a]Obesity was defined as a body mass index of ≥30 kilograms per square meter.
[b]Obesity was defined as a body mass index of ≥27.8 kilograms per square meter for males and a body mass index of ≥27.3 kilograms per square meter for females.
[c]Obesity was defined as a body mass index of ≥25 kilograms per square meter.
Reproduced with permission from Wizemann, T. M., & Pardue, M-. L. (Eds.). (2001). Exploring the biological contributions to human health: Does sex matter? Washington, DC: National Academy Press, p. 134.

Health problems associated with obesity include cardiorespiratory problems (e.g., hypertension) and increased risk for hypercholesteremia, cancer, diabetes, orthopedic problems, and early death (Calle et al., 2003). A specific disorder of obesity, **Pickwickian syndrome,** is characterized by a body weight more than twice that of normal, as well as respiratory (e.g., alveolar hypoventilation), cardiovascular, and sleep problems (see Chapter 7).

Etiology

Obesity is not an eating disorder. Many elements, including biological, social, and psychological factors, are involved in its etiology. There is a strong genetic component; adult body weight is closer to that of biologic rather than of adoptive parents. Also, many obese patients have a family history of obesity. Mutations in at least two genes, the leptin receptor (LEPR) gene and melanocortin 4 receptor (MC4R) gene, have been implicated in obesity (List & Habener, 2003; Farooqui et al., 2003; Branson et al., 2003). Endocrine disorders such as Cushing's disease, hypothyroidism, and use of psychoactive agents such as antipsychotics and antidepressants also are associated with obesity.

Because physical activity is important in the maintenance of body weight, the sedentary lifestyle and reliance on automobiles of the mechanized American society are significant factors in the rising obesity rates. As evidence for this association, obesity and its associated complications are increasing in Asia as more of that population moves to large cities and becomes more sedentary (Mydans, 2003). No specific psychological component has been associated with the development of obesity. In fact, the type and degree of psychopathology of overweight and obese people are quite similar to those of the normal-weight population.

Treatment

Although many commercial dieting and weight loss programs are effective initially, most weight lost is regained within a 5-year period. Surgical techniques such as **gastric bypass,** in which food is rerouted past part of the stomach and small intestine, and **gastric banding,** in which the size of the stomach is effectively reduced, result in initial weight loss. A variety of serious sequelae, including vomiting, diarrhea, intestinal obstructions, electrolyte disturbances, and the well-documented problems associated with exposing obese patients to major surgery, limit the usefulness of these procedures. Whether such procedures are effective for lasting maintenance of body weight is not yet known, and they are currently used only when less invasive strategies have failed.

    Amphetamines such as dextroamphetamine decrease appetite (see Chapter 23) and were once commonly used in weight loss programs. However, the abuse potential of these agents has limited their utility, and they are now rarely prescribed for weight loss. The amphetamine-like agent **phentermine** (Ionamin), a sympathomimetic amine, is still used for some patients; however, the related agents **dexfenfluramine** (Redux) and **fenfluramine** (Pondimin) were taken off the market because they were associated with heart valve abnormalities. Two newer, FDA-approved weight-loss agents, **orlistat** (Xenical) and **sibutramine hydrochloride** (Meridia), are not appetite suppressants. Orlistat is a pancreatic lipase inhibitor that limits the breakdown of dietary fats, thereby decreasing their absorption by about 33%. Sibutramine blocks monoamine reuptake, which increases feelings of satiety. Although these agents are indicated for weight loss in patients with BMIs greater than 30 kg/m^2 (or greater than 27 kg/m^2 in the presence of other risk factors, such as hypertension or diabetes), they may have negative effects such as gastrointestinal problems (orlistat) and elevated blood pressure (sibutramine). Two anticonvulsants, topiramate (Topamax) and zonisamide (Zonegran), appear to have weight-loss potential but do not yet have FDA approval for this use (Grady, 2003).

    For most people, maintenance of weight loss is best achieved by a combination of sensible dieting and exercise tailored to the person's capabilities. Typically, sensible dieting involves a low-calorie, high-carbohydrate, low-fat regimen (conventional diet). Recent preliminary studies indicate that when compared with a conventional diet, the low-carbohydrate, high protein, high-fat (Atkins) diet may produce greater weight loss and more improvement in some risk factors for heart disease (Foster et al., 2003;

Samaha et al., 2003). **Twelve-step peer-support programs** based on the Alcoholics Anonymous (AA) model (see Chapter 23) also can be helpful in long-term maintenance of weight loss.

▪ OVERVIEW OF THE EATING DISORDERS

Characteristics

Patients with the eating disorders **anorexia nervosa** and **bulimia nervosa** typically have normal appetites but show abnormal behavior associated with food. Such patients also often use compensatory mechanisms to avoid weight gain, such as vomiting and abuse of diuretics, enemas, and laxatives. This **purging** behavior can lead to malnutrition and electrolyte disturbances which can lead to serious cardiovascular problems, such as life-threatening arrhythmias. Laxative abuse may result in **melanosis coli,** a blackened area of mucosa identified during examination of the colon. Patients with eating disorders may also use drugs or thyroid hormones to lose weight, or they may seek surgical procedures like **liposuction** to remove body fat.

Patients with eating disorders tend to engage excessively in sports and strenuous exercise aimed at weight loss, behavior that has been called **hypergymnasia.** Gymnastics and ballet dancing in particular are seen in patients with these disorders, probably because they require that participants have low body weight. Characteristically, and despite normal or below normal body weight, eating disorder patients show disturbances of body image and often feel that they look fat.

Occurrence

Anorexia nervosa and bulimia nervosa are more common in women; each occurs in about 1 to 3% of women and 0.1 to 0.2% of men. These disorders are more common in late adolescence and young adulthood and are more likely to be seen in high academic achievers and in higher socioeconomic groups. Table 17-2 compares the physical and psychological characteristics of anorexia nervosa and bulimia nervosa.

Differential diagnosis

The eating disorders, particularly anorexia nervosa, must be distinguished from medical conditions that cause weight loss, such as occult malignancy, regional enteritis, and chronic infection.. Major depressive disorder resulting in lack of appetite and weight loss is also an important differential diagnosis, and many patients with eating disorders are comorbid for major depression. **Kleine-Levin syndrome** (episodic eating binges and hypersomnia [see Chapter 7] must also be considered in the diagnosis of an eating disorder. However, in contrast to the eating disorders, this syndrome is not associated with over-concern about weight gain. Personality disorders such as borderline personality disorder, which is characterized by

TABLE 17-2	Comparison of the Physical and Psychological Characteristics of Anorexia Nervosa and Bulimia Nervosa	
CATEGORY	ANOREXIA NERVOSA	BULIMIA NERVOSA
PHYSICAL CHARACTERISTICS		
Body weight	■ Significantly below normal	■ Relatively normal
Menstrual cycle	■ Amenorrhea	■ Menstrual irregularities
Laboratory tests	■ Hypokalemia ■ Metabolic acidosis: Hypercholesteremia Abnormal serum electrolytes Increased liver enzymes Increased serum urea nitrogen Decreased thyroid hormone Decreased serum glucose Mild anemia and leukopenia	■ Hypokalemia ■ Other metabolic abnormalities (not as severe as in anorexia nervosa)
Other characteristics	■ Lanugo (downy body hair on the shoulders and trunk) ■ Decreased bone density (due to prolonged starvation) ■ Cold intolerance ■ Cyanotic hands and feet ■ Syncope or near-syncope	If purging type: ■ Esophageal varices (caused by repeated vomiting) ■ Enamel erosion resulting in dental caries caused by presence of gastric acid in the mouth ■ Swelling or infection of parotid glands ■ Metacarpal-phalangeal calluses (Russell's sign) from the teeth because the hand is used to induce gagging
PSYCHOLOGICAL CHARACTERISTICS		
Major concern	■ Intense fear of obesity	■ Worry about gaining weight
Self-image	■ Not congruent with actual appearance	■ Poor self-image
Insight	■ Denial of the disorder	■ Distress about having the disorder
Sexuality	■ Lack of interest in sex	■ Relatively normal sexuality

TABLE 17-2	Comparison of the Physical and Psychological Characteristics of Anorexia Nervosa and Bulimia Nervosa (Continued)	
CATEGORY	ANOREXIA NERVOSA	BULIMIA NERVOSA
Depression	■ Denies depression	■ Reports depression
Treatment	■ Antidepressants less helpful	■ Antidepressants helpful

poor impulse control (including impulsive eating; see Chapter 18), are also included in the differential diagnosis of eating disorders.

■ ANOREXIA NERVOSA

Anorexia nervosa is one of the few life-threatening psychiatric disorders. Mortality rates for patients with anorexia nervosa range up to approximately 18%. Causes of death in anorexic patients include cardiac arrhythmias due to metabolic abnormalities such as **hypokalemia** (serum potassium level below 3.5 mEq/L) and malnutrition. The Diagnostic and Statistical Manual of Mental Disorders, Fourth Edition-Text Revision (DSM-IV-TR) diagnostic criteria for anorexia nervosa require that the patient have a body weight less than 85% of the normal expected weight (equal to or below a BMI of 17.5 kg/m^2) or fails to gain weight during a period of expected growth. Patients must also have a strong fear of gaining weight and a disturbed body image. Finally, post-menarcheal women must have missed three consecutive menstrual periods. Eating disorder not otherwise specified (NOS) is diagnosed when a patient does not meet all of these diagnostic criteria (e.g., she continues to menstruate).

Treatment and prognosis

Treatment of anorexia nervosa has two stages. The first stage aims to restore body weight and save the patient's life. The second, a long-term phase, involves strategies to prevent relapse. Because prolonged starvation can result in death, initial treatment is directed at reinstating the patient's nutritional condition. If body weight is not too low, nutritional reinstatement can be accomplished on an outpatient basis using frequent regular office visits and weigh-ins. If body weight falls to 20% or more below normal, the patient should be admitted to the hospital and retained until near-normal body weight is achieved.

Anorexic patients often resist hospitalization. Patients under 18 can be hospitalized and treated against their will. Patients 18 and older who are at imminent risk for death from malnutrition can sometimes be hospitalized involuntarily (see Chapter 26 and Case 17-1 in later text), but such decisions are made on an individual basis.

Antidepressants such as amitriptyline (Elavil) and the SSRIs like fluoxetine (Prozac) can be effective in some anorexic patients. However, these agents are more effective in treating bulimia. Although lack of appetite is not the cause of anorexia nervosa, cyproheptadine [Periactin] may help increase appetite and eating in patients whose body weight is not yet dangerously low.

CASE 17-1

THE PATIENT A 23-year-old ballet student is brought to the emergency room complaining of severe pain in her right foot. The pain began that afternoon during rehearsal for a performance. Physical examination reveals a very thin young woman with a growth of fine, soft body hair on her shoulders and arms. The patient reports that she has not menstruated in more than 1 year. When asked if she could be pregnant, she states that she has not desired nor had a romantic or sexual relationship in more than 2 years. When offered a snack during her wait for a radiograph, the patient tells the doctor that she is on a diet and really needs to lose at least 10 pounds for her career in dance. The patient weighs 90 pounds (42 kg) and is 5 feet 5 inches tall (1.65 m). Her body mass index (BMI: wt/ht^2) is $42/1.65^2 = 42/2.72 = 15.4$. Radiologic studies indicate a fracture of the right metatarsal and evidence of prior healed fractures of the foot. Blood work and an electrocardiogram (EKG) are ordered. Serum potassium level is 2.2, hemoglobin is 10 g/100mL, and hematocrit is 34%. The patient reports her mood as "good."

COMMENT This case illustrates several characteristics of a patient with an eating disorder. First, the patient's BMI is below the cutoff for anorexia nervosa (<17.5) (Fig 17-1). In spite of this, the patient feels that she needs to diet and lose more weight. She also does not menstruate and expresses no interest in sexuality. Hypokalemia (serum potassium level <3.5 mEq/L) and mild anemia (hemoglobin <12 g/100 mL; hematocrit <37) give further evidence of starvation. Osteoporosis may have contributed to this patient's foot fractures, which, along with lanugo (fine body hair), are caused by the chronic starvation seen in anorexic patients.

TREATMENT After treating the fracture, the physician should assess whether this patient's eating disorder is life-threatening. EKG changes associated with hypokalemia (e.g., prominent U wave, prolonged P-R interval, S-T depression, and decreased T-wave elevation) can presage life-threatening arrhythmias. If the patient is in imminent danger, the doctor should explain to her the risk of foregoing treatment and suggest that she be treated in the hospital until she is out of danger. In most jurisdictions the doctor can hold such a patient for 24 to 48 hours if she resists hospitalization. During that time, if warranted, the case can be brought before a judge who will determine whether the patient understands the risk to her life if she refuses treatment. The judge will then decide whether to issue a court order holding and treating the patient against her will (see Chapter 26).

In the hospital, the patient will receive a normalized diet and constant supervision to ensure that she eats. She may also receive calcium supplements and bisphosphonates, such as alendronate (Fosamax) or salmon calcitonin (Miacalcin), to help prevent further progression of osteoporosis. During and after hospitalization, ongoing group and family therapy and antidepressant medication will be useful in her treatment.

Typically, the anorexic patient was obedient and a good student, in fact a "perfect child," prior to the onset of the disorder. However, the patient's insistence on dieting despite obvious evidence of starvation ultimately leads to conflict with parents. Because of this and because interfamily difficulties such as marital problems or an overcontrolling mother are believed to be involved in the etiology of the disorder, the most effective form of psychotherapy is family therapy (see Chapter 11).

Early age of onset and treatment and few or no previous hospitalizations predict a positive outcome for patients with anorexia nervosa. However, even when patients recover from the most severe symptoms, chronically low body weight and over-concern about food and eating typically continue throughout life.

■ BULIMIA NERVOSA

The DSM-IV-TR criteria for bulimia nervosa require recurrent episodes of eating large amounts of food (binge-eating) coupled with feeling out of control over the binge-eating during the episode. There is usually also some type of inappropriate compensatory mechanism or purging behavior such as laxative or diuretic abuse or, more commonly, self-induced vomiting. Medical consequences of the repeated vomiting include parotid gland swelling and infection, as well as tooth enamel erosion (Fig. 17-2), which leads to dental caries. This binge-eating and purging behavior must occur at least twice a week for at least 3 months for the diagnosis of **bulimia nervosa, binge-eating/purging type.** Patients who binge eat but use other inappropriate compensatory mechanisms, such as hypergymnasia rather than purging to avoid gaining weight, have the **non-purging type of bulimia.** If a patient has the essential features of anorexia but binges and

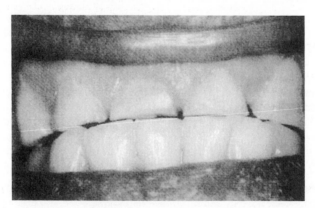

FIGURE 17-2. Erosion of the upper front teeth of a patient with long-term bulimia nervosa; binge-eating/purging type.

(Reproduced with permission from Walsh, B. T. (1997). Eating disorders. In A. Tasman, J. Kay, J. A. Lieberman (Eds.), Psychiatry (Vol. 2). Philadelphia: WB Saunders.)

TABLE 17-3 DSM-IV-TR Subtypes of Bulimia Nervosa and Anorexia Nervosa

EATING DISORDER	TYPE	BEHAVIOR
Bulimia nervosa	Purging type	■ Binge-eating (consuming large quantities of high calorie food all at one time and in secret) ■ Purging (vomiting, or misuse of laxatives, diuretics or enemas to avoid weight gain)
	Nonpurging type	■ Binge-eating ■ Excessive fasting or exercising (to lose weight or avoid weight gain) ■ No purging
Anorexia nervosa	Restricting type	■ Excessive fasting, dieting or exercising ■ No purging or binge-eating
	Binge-eating/ purging type	■ Excessive fasting, dieting, or exercising ■ Purging or binge-eating

DSM-IV-TR, Diagnostic and Statistical Manual of Mental Disorders, Fourth Edition-Text Revision.

purges, the diagnosis is **anorexia nervosa, binge-eating/purging type,** not bulimia nervosa. The subtypes of bulimia nervosa and anorexia nervosa are described in Table 17-3.

Treatment and prognosis

Psychological treatment of bulimia nervosa includes cognitive and behavioral therapies. Pharmacologic treatment includes antidepressants, such as heterocyclics, monoamine oxidase inhibitors, and, particularly, selective serotonin reuptake inhibitors such as fluoxetine (Prozac). Combinations of psychotherapy and antidepressants are more effective than either modality alone. At 10-year follow-up, 50% of bulimic patients are free of symptoms; most others are improved.

REVIEW QUESTIONS

1. The mother of a 10-year-old child who is in the 99th percentile for body weight reports that "he is not eating well." The most appropriate thing for the doctor to say at this time is

   (A) "There are many treatments for obesity; let's discuss them."

   (B) "Please tell me what you mean by 'he is not eating well'."

(C) "Many overweight children slim down at puberty."

(D) "The nurse will discuss with you an appropriate diet for the child."

(E) "The best treatment for obesity is diet and exercise."

2. A 22-year-old medical student comes to the physician complaining of facial swelling and pain. The student is 5 feet, 7 inches tall and weighs 128 pounds. Physical examination reveals a parotid gland abscess. Aside from the abscess and metacarpal-phalangeal calluses on her right hand, physical findings are unremarkable. The patient seems distressed when the physician questions her about her eating habits and tells him that she feels like she is "out of control." This clinical picture most closely suggests

(A) anorexia nervosa restricting type

(B) anorexia nervosa binge-eating/purging type

(C) bulimia nervosa binge-eating/purging type

(D) hypochondriasis

(E) acute stress disorder

3. A 16-year-old gymnast who is 5 feet, 2 inches tall (1.58 m) and weighs 80 pounds (36.5 kg) visits a physician for a school physical. Findings on physical examination are normal; however, laboratory tests reveal evidence of hypokalemia and hypercholesteremia. Which of the following is most likely to characterize this teenager?

(A) Lack of appetite

(B) Belief that she is significantly underweight

(C) High sexual interest

(D) Conflict with her mother

(E) Poor school performance

Questions 4 and 5

A 20-year-old college student who is 5 feet, 9 inches tall and weighs 320 pounds tells the physician that he has been overweight ever since he can remember. He reports that he peaked at 380 pounds 2 years ago, lost 100 pounds over the next year, and gained back 40 pounds during the last few months. He asks the physician for help losing weight and keeping it off. Physical examination and laboratory tests are essentially normal.

4. Of the following, the physician's best recommendation for non-pharmacologic treatment is

(A) gastric stapling

(B) gastric bypass surgery

(C) a low-fat, high-carbohydrate diet

(D) a high-fat, low-carbohydrate diet

(E) a sensible diet and exercise program

5. Of the following, the physician's best recommendation for pharmacologic treatment is

(A) dexfenfluramine (Redux)

(B) fenfluramine (Pondimin)

(C) cyproheptadine (Periactin)

(D) sibutramine (Meridia)

(E) alendronate (Fosamax)

ANSWERS AND EXPLANATIONS

1-B. Before proceeding, the doctor must clarify what the mother means by the statement "is not eating well." An obese child such as this one may be overeating, may be eating high-calorie foods exclusively, or may be showing some other abnormal eating behavior. A metabolic or endocrine disorder such as hypothyroidism is another possibility. After identifying possible contributors to the child's obesity, the doctor can discuss treatment options with the mother.

2-C. The correct diagnosis for this patient is bulimia nervosa, binge-eating/purging type. Calluses on the knuckles (Russell's sign) and the parotid gland abscess are evidence of self-induced vomiting. Because her body weight is normal and she expresses feeling out of control, it is unlikely that this patient has anorexia nervosa, binge-eating/purging type. This patient is not worrying excessively about her health, as would a person with hypochondriasis, nor does she report exposure to a life-threatening stressor, as would someone with acute stress disorder.

3-D. This patient has a BMI ($36.5/1.58^2 = 14.6$) and electrolyte abnormalities characteristics of anorexia nervosa. Because gymnasts must be slim, gymnastics is closely associated with the development of this disorder. Anorexia is also characterized by family conflicts (particularly with the mother), normal appetite, perception of being of normal weight or overweight, low sexual interest, and good school performance.

4-E, 5-D. The safest and most effective nonpharmacologic recommendation for long-term maintenance of weight loss in this obese patient is a combination of sensible dieting and exercise tailored to his abilities. Although helpful for some patients, the efficacy for maintenance of long-term weight loss of high-fat, low-carbohydrate or low-fat, high-carbohydrate diets have not been proven. Surgical procedures are generally used only as a last resort in obese patients. Of the listed pharmacologic agents, sibutramine is indicated for weight loss in obese patients; dexfenfluramine and fenfluramine have been taken off the market. Alendronate is a bisphosphonate used to treat osteoporosis, and cyproheptadine is used to increase, not decrease, appetite.

REFERENCES

American Psychiatric Association (2001). *Diagnostic and statistical manual of mental disorders* (4th ed., text revision, pp. 583–595). Washington, DC: American Psychiatric Association.

Branson, R., Potoczna, N., Kral, J. G., Lentes, K. -U., Hoehe, M. R., & Horber, F. F. (2002). Binge-eating as a major phenotype of melanocortin 4 receptor gene mutations. *N Engl J Med, 348,* 1096–1103.

Farooqi, I. S., Keogh, J. M., Yeo, G. S. H., Lank, E. J., Cheetham, T., & O'Rahilly, S. (2003). Clinical spectrum of obesity and mutations in the melanocortin 4 receptor gene. *N Engl J Med, 348,* 1085–1095.

Flegal, K. M., Carroll, M. D., Ogden, C. L., & Johnson, C. L. (2002). Prevalence and trends in obesity among US adults, 1999–2000. *JAMA, 288,* 1723–1727.

Foster, G. D, Wyatt, H. R., Hill, J. O., McGuckin, B. G., Brill, C., Mohammed, B. S., et al. (2003). A randomized trial of a low-carbohydrate diet for obesity. *N Engl J Med, 348,* 2082–2090.

Gordon, R. A. (1990). *Anorexia and bulimia: Anatomy of a social epidemic.* Cambridge: Basil Blackwell.

Grady, D. (2003, April 15). Quest for weight-loss drug takes an unusual turn. *The New York Times.*

Institute of Medicine. (2001). In T. M. Wizemann & L. Pardue (Eds.), *Exploring the biological contributions to human health: Does sex matter?* Washington, DC: National Academy Press.

List, J. F., & Habener, J. F. (2003). Defective melanocortin 4 receptors in hyperphagia and morbid obesity. *N Engl J Med, 348,* 1160–1163.

Mydans, S. (2003, March 13). Clustering in cities, Asians are becoming obese. *The New York Times.*

Ogden, C. L., Flegal, K. M., Carroll, M. D., & Johnson, L. (2002). Prevalence and trends in overweight among US children and adolescents, 1999–2000. *JAMA, 28,* 1728–1732.

Pi-Sunyen, F. X. (1994). In M. E. Shils, J. A. Olson, M. Shike (Eds.), *Obesity in modern nutrition.* Malvern, PA: Lea and Febiger.

Samaha, F. F., Iqbal, N., Seshadri, P., Chicano, K. L., Daily, D. A., McGrory, J., et al. (2003). A low-carbohydrate as compared with a low-fat diet in severe obesity. *N Engl J Med, 348,* 2074–2081.

Walsh, B. T., & Devlin, M. J. (1995). Eating disorders. *Child Adolescent Psychiatry Clin North Am, 4,* 343.

Wardlaw, G. M. (2001). *Contemporary nutrition: Issues and insights* (4th ed.). St. Louis: McGraw-Hill.

Cognitive and Dissociative Disorders 18

A person who forgets his identity and turns out to be the long-lost heir to a fortune is the stuff of novels and movies. In the real world, **amnesia** (loss of memory) rarely has a romantic or exciting outcome. Two groups of disorders, the cognitive disorders and the dissociative disorders, are characterized by deficits in memory function as well as personality changes and unusual behavior. Although they may have similar presentations, the etiology of these two groups of disorders is quite different. In the cognitive disorders, symptoms result from anatomic or metabolic abnormalities in the brain itself. In the dissociative disorders, symptoms are psychological, often associated with emotional stress that has occurred in the individual's recent or remote past.

COGNITIVE DISORDERS

Cognitive disorders involve problems with memory, as well as difficulty with orientation to person, place, and time (**orientation times three**), level of consciousness, and other cognitive or "thinking" functions. These symptoms are caused by abnormalities in neural chemistry, structure, or physiology originating in the brain or secondary to systemic illness. Patients with cognitive disorders may have psychiatric symptoms, such as mood changes, anxiety, irritability, paranoia, and psychosis. These symptoms, while secondary to the cognitive losses, can lead to misdiagnosis. The famous folk singer Woody Guthrie, who died of Huntington's disease in 1967, was diagnosed early in the illness with "schizophrenia, paranoid type."

Because all psychiatric symptoms are mediated by the brain, it is theoretically difficult to separate organic from nonorganic disorders. Therefore, cognitive disorders are no longer termed **organic mental disorders.** The major cognitive disorders are delirium, dementia, and amnestic disorder.

Differential diagnosis of the cognitive disorders

Many patients with cognitive disorders are elderly. Because normal aging is associated with minor cognitive changes, such as reduction in the ability to learn new things quickly and a general slowing of mental processes, it may be necessary for a physician to make the distinction between normal aging and a cognitive disorder in an individual patient. One important distinction between these two entities is that, in contrast to patients with cognitive disorders whose functioning is quite impaired, normally aging patients are able to care for themselves and carry on a normal life.

Depressed patients, particularly when elderly, often show difficulties in concentration and decreased speed of mental process. This presentation of depression is called **pseudodementia** because it mimics cognitive impairment (see Chapter 3) (Table 18-1).

Delirium

Delirium is a syndrome of cognitive impairment that results from central nervous system dysfunction; it is characterized by clouding of consciousness. Commonly, delirious patients are oriented to person but are not fully attentive, and they are not oriented to time or place. The patient also often appears to be hyperactive or hypoactive and seems anxious and confused. Sleep disturbances and autonomic dysfunction are common in delirium.

Delirium usually presents in the course of an acute medical illness. It is the most common psychiatric syndrome seen in hospitalized patients, particularly those in surgical and coronary intensive care units, and in elderly nursing home patients with illnesses such as systemic infections (e.g., urosepsis). The disorder is more common also, in children, and in patients with preexisting brain damage or a history of psychiatric illness.

Some of the most common causes of delirium are diseases of the central nervous system, such as meningitis and encephalitis; systemic illnesses originating in the liver, kidney, heart, or lungs; and substance abuse and withdrawal, particularly involving the sedative drugs, such as alcohol. Other causes of delirium include acute electrolyte changes, fever, postoperative states, and medications such as anticholinergics (see Table 25-4).

Delirium can progress to dementia or death if left untreated. However, if a delirious patient is identified (using an instrument such as the Folstein Mini-Mental State Examination; see Table 6-5) and the underlying medical cause treated effectively, the prognosis is good. Psychological management includes providing patients with ongoing orienting information

TABLE 18-1	Comparison of Depression, Delirium, and Dementia	
DEPRESSION	**DELIRIUM**	**DEMENTIA**
Hallmark: sad mood	Hallmark: impaired consciousness	Hallmark: loss of intellectual ability
Patient example: A 67-year-old retired former banker cannot remember to pay his bills. He has also lost more than 10 pounds and wakes 2 hours before his alarm. His symptoms started after he gave up his driver's license.	Patient example: One week after an acute myocardial infarction, a 67-year-old former policeman with no prior history of psychiatric illness seems confused and agitated and reports seeing strange animals in his room.	Patient example: A 67-year-old retired legal secretary is alert but has shown marked memory disturbance for the past year. She does not know what day it is, nor can she precisely identify her daughter who is sitting next to her.
Consciousness not impaired	Consciousness impaired or clouded	Consciousness not impaired
Mood fluctuates	Fluctuations and lucid intervals	Steady course
Develops slowly	Develops quickly	Develops slowly
Normal level of arousal	Stupor or agitation	Normal level of arousal
Illusions, delusions, and hallucinations uncommon	Illusions, delusions, and hallucinations (often visual) present	Illusions, delusions, and hallucinations uncommon
Little autonomic dysfunction	Severe autonomic dysfunction	Little autonomic dysfunction
EEG usually normal	EEG fast wave activity or generalized slowing	EEG usually normal
Diurnal variability, worse in the morning	Diurnal variability, worse at night (i.e., "sun downers")	Little diurnal variability
Usually reversible with antidepressant treatment	Usually reversible if the underlying medical cause is removed	Rarely reversible

EEG, electroencephalogram.

about where they are and who their caregivers are as well as the current location, date, and time of day.

Dementia

Dementia is characterized by gradual loss of memory and intellectual abilities without impairment of consciousness. It most commonly occurs in the elderly; more than 20% of individuals 80 years of age and older exhibit some form of this disorder. **Dementia of the Alzheimer's type** (hereinafter **Alzheimer's disease**), makes up one-half to two-thirds of cases of dementia. Other causes of dementia include **vascular dementia** and **Lewy body dementia,** as well as dementias caused by HIV and other infectious agents (e.g., Creutzfeldt-Jakob disease).

Alzheimer's disease

Alzheimer's disease is diagnosed when other obvious causes for a patient's symptoms have been eliminated. Its etiology is unknown; however, factors that have been implicated include micro- and macroscopic neuroanatomical changes (e.g., accumulation of β-amyloid plaques at the ends of degenerating neurons [Helmuth, 2002]) and genetic components (e.g., possession of at least one copy of the apolipoprotein E_4 gene [Bartrez-Faz, 2002]). Other factors include neurotransmitter alterations, such as reduction in brain levels of choline acetyltransferase that is needed to synthesize acetylcholine, and overstimulation of the N-methyl-D-aspartate (NMDA) receptor by glutamate (Reisberg et al., 2003) (Table 18-2).

Alzheimer's disease has a slow, insidious onset and a progressive, irreversible, downhill course. Cognitive function deteriorates; however, patients usually have a normal level of consciousness and retain motor ability until the later stage of the illness. Neuroanatomically, the illness typically progresses from temporal to frontal and parietal lobes (Fig. 18-1), sparing the occipital lobes and primary motor and sensory strips. A patient with Alzheimer's disease typically first shows memory loss; then has difficulty finding the right words; then becomes unable to copy a simple drawing.

Frontal involvement is associated with the development of emotional symptoms such as anger, depression, and anxiety, difficulty controlling impulses, and lack of judgment. Late-stage symptoms include confusion, psychosis, apathy, and agitation that progress to coma and death, usually within 8 to 10 years of diagnosis.

Management of patients with Alzheimer's disease

The most effective initial interventions in Alzheimer's disease involve providing a structured environment for the patient, including visual orienting cues. Such cues include labels over the doors of rooms identifying their function; daily posting of the day of the week, date, and year; and daily written activity schedules. Practical safety measures, such as disconnect-

| TABLE 18-2 | Pathophysiology of Alzheimer's Dementia |

GROSS NEUROANATOMY

Enlarged ventricles
Diffuse atrophy
Flattened cortical sulci

MICROSCOPIC NEUROANATOMY

Senile/amyloid plaques
Neurofibrillary tangles (seen also in Down's syndrome and, to a lesser extent, in normal aging) in cortex, hippocampus, locus ceruleus, and substantia nigra
Loss of cholinergic neurons in the basal forebrain
Neuronal loss and degeneration in the hippocampus and cortex

NEUROPHYSIOLOGY

Reduction in brain levels of choline acetyltransferase which is needed to synthesize acetylcholine
Abnormal processing of amyloid precursor protein
Decreased membrane fluidity caused by abnormal regulation of membrane phospholipid metabolism

GENETIC ASSOCIATIONS

Abnormalities of chromosome 21, site of gene for amyloid precursor protein (most patients with Down's syndrome ultimately develop Alzheimer's disease)
Abnormalities of chromosome 1 and 14 (particularly in the type occurring before age 65 years)
Possession of at least one copy of the apolipoprotein E_4 gene (apoE$_4$) on chromosome 19 (particularly in women)
Having a close relative with Alzheimer's disease
Female gender

NEUROTRANSMITTER RELATIONSHIPS

Hypoactivity of acetylcholine and norepinephrine
Overstimulation of the NMDA receptor by glutamate
Hypoactivity of somatostatin, vasoactive intestinal peptide, and corticotropin

NMDA, N-methyl-D-aspartate.

ing the stove, are also advisable. Providing a nutritious diet, exercise, and recreational therapy for the patient, as well as psychotherapy and support groups for family caretakers, is crucial in managing the Alzheimer's patient. Despite such interventions, increasing levels of dementia and disability ultimately lead to nursing home placement for most patients.

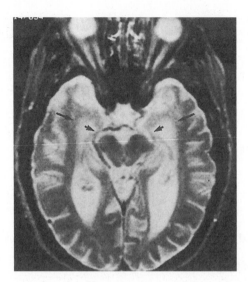

FIGURE 18-1. MRI of a 76-year-old man with Alzheimer's disease. This image shows atrophy within the temporal lobe (short and long arrows).

(From Sirven, J. I., & Malamut, B. L. (Eds.). (2002). Clinical neurology of the older adult. Baltimore: Lippincott Williams & Wilkins, p. 9.)

Although there is currently no agent that can restore cognitive function, pharmacotherapy has a role in the treatment of patients with Alzheimer's disease. **Cholinesterase inhibitors** (see Chapter 19) prevent the breakdown of acetylcholine, improve cognitive function transiently, and slow the progression of disease in about 25% of patients. Donepezil (Aricept) and newer cholinesterase inhibitors such as rivastigmine (Exelon) and galantamine (Reminyl) have fewer adverse hepatic and gastrointestinal effects than an older agent, tacrine (Cognex). Recently, a NMDA antagonist, memantine (Namanda), was shown to be effective in slowing clinical deterioration in patients with moderate to severe Alzheimer's disease (Reisberg et al., 2003). Agents are currently in development that decrease the amount of β-amyloid in brain by promoting immune system attack on β-amyloid plaques and decreasing cholesterol that fosters β-amyloid production (Helmuth, 2002; Vega et al., 2003). Antianxiety agents, antidepressants, and antipsychotics (see Chapter 19) can be helpful for treating the associated emotional symptoms of Alzheimer's.

Vascular dementia

Vascular dementia (formerly multi-infarct dementia) makes up about 15 to 30% of dementias. Vascular dementia is caused by multiple, small cerebral infarctions resulting from atherosclerosis, valvular heart disease, or

THE PATIENT A 75-year-old man is brought to the emergency department after being burned in a house fire. This is the patient's third emergency visit in 2 months. His other visits occurred after he inhaled natural gas when he left the stove on without a flame and when he fell down the porch stairs after wandering out of the house during the night. The patient's wife tells the physician that the patient is very withdrawn and tends to sleep excessively. There is no evidence of physical illness and no history of substance abuse. His wife is distressed and begs the doctor to let her husband come home.

COMMENT This case illustrates a number of aspects of Alzheimer's disease. The patient is getting injured because he is forgetful (e.g., forgetting to turn off the gas jet) and wanders out of the house because he cannot distinguish between the closet or bathroom door and the outside door. There is no evidence of a medical cause for his symptoms as there would be in delirium. There is no evidence of a negative life event precipitating depression or of a history of alcohol abuse as in amnestic disorder. The patient's withdrawal and excessive sleeping could be evidence of depression, a common and treatable occurrence that may occur along with the cognitive losses in Alzheimer's patients.

TREATMENT Because there is a caretaker willing to look after the patient, the most effective initial intervention for this patient is provision of a structured environment. Giving the patient visual cues for orientation (labeling doors for function) and taking practical measures to protect him from household dangers are recommended. Although antidepressant medications can help to improve this patient's concurrent symptoms of depression, neither these agents nor cholinesterase inhibitors will reverse the patient's cognitive losses.

arrhythmias. Between 30 and 40% of patients with Alzheimer's disease have a vascular component to their symptoms. In contrast to Alzheimer's dementia, vascular dementias are characterized by the following:

- Sudden rather than gradual onset of cognitive dysfunction
- Stepwise, abrupt loss of some function with each infarct rather than steady deterioration (e.g., an elderly patient whose mental functioning has been normal suddenly cannot remember what to do with the phone when it rings or how to turn on the microwave)
- Better preservation of the patient's personality characteristics
- Higher risk for men than women
- Increased likelihood of focal neurologic signs

To treat vascular dementias, it is important to reduce the likelihood of new infarcts by treating medical risk factors associated with cerebrovascular disease, such as hypertension and cardiac arrhythmias. In addition, behavioral risk factors need to decrease, such as excessive body weight, smoking, and alcohol abuse.

Other dementias

Lewy body dementia has been viewed as both a variant of Alzheimer's disease and a distinct clinical disorder. It is characterized by a gradually progressive dementia, including fluctuations in cognitive abilities, visual hallucinations, and Parkinsonism. Neuroanatomical findings include Lewy inclusion bodies in the brainstem and cerebral cortex. As in Alzheimer's disease, there are multiple neuritic plaques in Lewy body dementia, although relatively few neurofibrillary tangles are seen. The incidence of Lewy body dementia is not known; however, two characteristics make it important in psychiatry. First, patients often present with positive psychotic symptoms (see Chapter 12); second, patients typically have adverse responses to the antipsychotic medications used to treat these symptoms (Ballard et al., 1999).

Dementia due to HIV infection can result from a direct infection of the brain that causes cortical atrophy, inflammation, and demyelination. Alternatively, dementia in patients infected with HIV can result from cerebral lymphomas or opportunistic brain infections. Death occurs in 50 to 75% of patients with HIV dementia within 6 months.

Other causes of dementia include brain tumor or metastasis to brain, Parkinson's disease, head trauma, multiple sclerosis, Pick's disease (frontotemporal dementia), and Huntington's disease.

Amnestic disorders

Amnestic disorders are characterized specifically by memory loss. Unlike the cognitive disorders, amnestic disorder is associated with little or no other cognitive impairment. In contrast to delirium, there is a normal level of consciousness. Both **retrograde amnesia** (i.e., memory for past events, particularly the recent past) and **anterograde amnesia** (i.e., inability to establish new memories) occur in amnestic disorder. Commonly, the patient fabricates forgotten information to cover up memory loss, a phenomenon known as **confabulation.** For example, when an alert middle-aged man with a history of alcoholism tells the physician that he got his first job in 1999, amnestic disorder should be suspected.

The primary cause of amnestic disorder is thiamine deficiency as a result of long-term alcohol abuse, which leads to destruction of mediotemporal lobe structures, such as the mammillary bodies, hippocampus, and fornix (**Korsakoff's syndrome**). Head injury or cerebrovascular disease involving the temporal lobes, such as **herpes simplex encephalitis,** as well as prolonged substance use, particularly of benzodiazepines and exposure to neurotoxins, are other conditions that may contribute to amnestic disorder. The treatment and prognosis of amnestic disorder depend on the underlying cause.

■ DISSOCIATIVE DISORDERS

Dissociative disorders are characterized by a sudden but temporary loss of memory or identity or feelings of detachment from oneself or the environment in the presence of a normal level of consciousness. In contrast to the cognitive disorders, which are caused by problems in the biological function of the brain, memory loss in the dissociative disorders is a result of emotional factors. The four major Diagnostic and Statistical Manual of Mental Disorders, Fourth Edition-Text Revision (DSM-IV-TR) classifications are dissociative amnesia, dissociative fugue, dissociative identity disorder (multiple personality disorder), and depersonalization disorder (derealization is a variant of this disorder) (Table 18–3). The first three disorders are quite rare; depersonalization disorder in mild form is relatively common.

Differential diagnosis of the dissociative disorders

In addition to the cognitive disorders, medical differential diagnoses for the dissociative disorders include substance abuse, sequelae of electroconvulsive therapy or anesthesia, seizure disorders, and head injury (see Case 18-2). A major psychological differential diagnosis for the dissociative disorders is **posttraumatic stress disorder (PTSD)**, in which memory problems and psychological symptoms (such as anxiety and depression) are caused by exposure to a potentially life-threatening event (see Chapter 15). When the patient presents in a legal or forensic setting, malingering (see Chapter 16) and alcohol abuse must be ruled out, particularly when there are symptoms of dissociative identity disorder.

Dissociation is not necessarily abnormal. In certain religions or cultures, altered states of perception, identity, or consciousness are seen in the framework of particular life experiences.

CASE 18-2

THE PATIENT   A 65-year-old man is brought by the police to the hospital emergency room in Eugene, Oregon after he is found wandering around a mall after closing hours. The patient is alert but has no memory of who he is or where he lives. Medical examination is essentially normal, except for a large resolving hematoma on the right temple. A check of the patient's identity reveals that he is a resident of New Jersey who disappeared from his home 2 weeks ago. There is no evidence that the patient had legal or social difficulties prior to his disappearance.

COMMENT   This clinical picture looks like dissociative fugue, a psychiatric disorder characterized by memory loss and wandering from home. However, because this patient has evidence of a head injury, it is much more likely that his amnesia is caused by physical injury to his brain. Malingering must be considered in the differential diagnosis but is unlikely because there is no obvious reason for the patient to have "faked" his memory problems.

TREATMENT   Treatment of this patient depends on the cause of his memory loss. A cognitive disorder caused by head injury must be ruled out by neurological examination and imaging studies before a diagnosis like dissociative fugue can be considered.

Etiology of the dissociative disorders

The etiology of the dissociative disorders can involve use of the defense mechanisms of dissociation, denial, and repression (see Chapter 8), particularly in response to an emotionally stressful event in the recent past. Early life stressors, especially incest or sexual abuse in childhood or adolescence, are also implicated in the etiology of these disorders. Dissociative disorders commonly start in early adulthood, occur episodically, and may continue for years.

Specific dissociative disorders

Patients with **dissociative amnesia** and **dissociative fugue** experience a sudden inability to remember pertinent and important information about themselves. The amnesia usually resolves in minutes or days but may last for years. In dissociative fugue, which can be associated specifically with a history of excessive alcohol use, memory problems are coupled with leaving home and taking on a different identity.

Dissociative identity disorder was formerly called multiple personality disorder. This dramatic disorder involves many different personalities, or **alters,** sometimes of different genders, in one individual. Typically, one personality rules the others. The disorder is uncommon in severe form and is far more common in women, particularly those sexually abused in childhood. Mild forms of dissociative identity disorder may resemble borderline personality disorder or schizophrenia. The disorder is often chronic and is associated with other psychiatric symptoms, such as depression and anxiety.

Depersonalization disorder is characterized by repeated, chronic feelings of detachment. This disorder occurs in many people in transient form, often following exposure to an acute stressor. Symptoms of depersonalization and **derealization** are often present in other psychiatric disorders such as schizophrenia, depression, anxiety, and histrionic personality disorder. However, in contrast to some of the other dissociative disorders and psychotic disorders (see Chapter 11), patients with depersonalization have insight and know that their unusual perceptions are, in fact, only feelings.

Treatment of the dissociative disorders

Treatment of the dissociative disorders includes hypnosis, drug-assisted interviews (see Chapter 5), and long-term psychoanalytically oriented psychotherapy (see Chapter 16). These treatments help the patient with dissociative identity disorder to integrate their many personalities into one. They also help the dissociative amnesia and fugue patient to recover repressed, or "lost," memories of disturbing emotional experiences and to consciously address this recovered material. Controversy exists, however,

TABLE 18-3 Dissociative Disorders

DSM-IV-TR CHARACTERISTICS	PATIENT EXAMPLES
Dissociative Amnesia	
■ Failure to remember important information about oneself ■ More common in young adults and in women	A 20-year-old soldier cannot recall any of the events of a battle in which half of his platoon was killed.
Dissociative Fugue	
■ Failure to remember pertinent personal information ■ Wandering from home and adopting a new identity	A 32-year-old woman has been living in a town in Texas for more than 3 years and working for the post office. She has no memory of how she got to Texas or of her life in New York as a waitress prior to 3 years ago.
Dissociative Identity Disorder (Multiple Personality Disorder)	
■ At least two distinct personalities in one individual ■ Commonly there are 5–10 personalities	A 28-year-old physician who is married and has three children usually dresses conservatively. A colleague shows her a recent photograph of herself in a skimpy swimsuit. She does not remember the man who took the picture or posing for the photograph.
Depersonalization Disorder	
■ Recurrent, persistent feelings of detachment and unreality about one's own body, the social situation, or the environment (derealization) ■ Normal reality testing	A 40-year-old man tells his physician that when he is under stress he often perceives objects in the environment as much smaller than they really are (micropsia). The patient states that he knows that this is only a feeling and that the objects are really of normal size.

over the value of these techniques, because an interviewer may unknowingly shape the form and content of the memories, which results in the phenomenon of **false recovered memories** (Sheflin & Brown, 1997; van der Kolk et al., 2001). Antidepressants, antianxiety agents, and anticonvulsant agents may also be helpful for associated symptoms in dissociative disorder patients.

REVIEW QUESTIONS

Questions 1–2

A 78-year-old retired pediatrician reports that she has been confused and forgetful over the past 10 months. She also has difficulty sleeping, her appetite is poor, and she has lost 12 pounds. Questioning reveals that her 18-year-old cat died 10 months ago.

1. This clinical picture is most suggestive of

(A) delirium

(B) pseudodementia

(C) dementia of the Alzheimer's type

(D) dissociative fugue

(E) amnestic disorder

(F) depersonalization disorder

2. Of the following, the most effective intervention for this patient is

(A) antipsychotic medication

(B) provision of a structured environment

(C) antidepressant medication

(D) tacrine

(E) reassurance

3. A 45-year-old, mildly mentally retarded patient has recently started to experience memory loss. The patient has odd facial features. The chromosomal abnormality most likely to be responsible for this clinical picture is chromosome

(A) 1

(B) 14

(C) 19

(D) 21

4. An 84-year-old woman is brought to the emergency room by a neighbor who found her wandering down the street in her nightclothes. The patient seems confused and mistakes the emergency room physician for her nephew. Further examination of this patient and details of her history reveal evidence of pneumonia and presence of a high fever. The neighbor notes that before today, the patient always appeared oriented and alert. This clinical picture is most suggestive of

(A) delirium

(B) pseudodementia

(C) dementia of the Alzheimer's type

(D) dissociative fugue

(E) amnestic disorder

(F) depersonalization disorder

5. A 35-year-old female patient tells the physician that she often feels as though she is living her life in a dream and is watching herself perform as though she were in a stage play. Although the patient states, "I know this is not real," the feeling of distance from the world gets even stronger when she is under stress. Physical examination is normal. This clinical picture is most suggestive of

(A) delirium

(B) pseudodementia

(C) dementia of the Alzheimer's type

(D) dissociative fugue

(E) amnestic disorder

(F) depersonalization disorder

6. An 80-year-old patient with Alzheimer's disease can no longer live alone. Which of the following factors is most important in determining if the patient can live with an adult child or should be cared for in a nursing home setting?

(A) The sex of the adult child

(B) The responsibilities of the adult child outside the home

(C) The level of the patient's dementia

(D) The age of the grandchildren in the home

(E) The proximity of the nursing home

ANSWERS AND EXPLANATIONS

1-B, 2-C. This woman is showing evidence of pseudodementia, depression that mimics dementia. Although common in the elderly, depression is an illness (see Chapter 13), not a natural consequence of aging. In the elderly, depression is often associated with cognitive problems as well as sleep and eating problems. Evidence of depression is provided by the fact that this patient's symptoms began with the loss of an important relationship (i.e., the death of her pet). Delirium and dementia are caused by physiological abnormalities. Dissociative fugue involves wandering from home, and amnestic disorder is usually associated with a history of alcoholism. Depersonalization disorder is associated with feelings of detachment from the social situation. The most effective intervention for this depressed patient is antidepressant medication. When the medication relieves the depressive symptoms, her memory will improve. Antipsychotic medication, provision of a structured environment, tacrine, and simple reassurance are not appropriate for this depressed patient.

3-D. This patient with mild mental retardation and unusual facial features has Down's syndrome. If they live to middle age, Down's syndrome patients commonly develop Alzheimer's disease. Chromosome 21 is associated with both Down's syndrome and Alzheimer's disease.

4-A. This clinical presentation, including sudden onset of impaired consciousness and illusions (believing the doctor is her nephew; see Table 18-1) in the presence of serious physical illness, is most suggestive of delirium (see answers to Questions 1 and 2).

5-F. This clinical picture of feelings of being in a dream or performance that worsens during stress is most suggestive of depersonalization disorder. Typically, the patient with this disorder has insight and knows these perceptions are not real (see answers to Questions 1 and 2).

6-C. Of the choices, the most important factor in determining whether this patient will live with an adult child or enter a nursing home is the level of her dementia. As she becomes more debilitated, she increases the danger of self-injury, making nursing home placement more likely. The sex of the adult child, responsibilities of the adult child outside the home, the age of the grandchildren in the home, and the proximity of the nursing home are all less important than the patient's cognitive condition.

REFERENCES

American Psychiatric Association. (2001). *Diagnostic and statistical manual of mental disorders* (4th ed., text revision) (pp. 135–180; 519–533). Washington, DC: American Psychiatric Association.

American Psychiatric Association. (1997). Practice guidelines for the treatment of patients with Alzheimer's disease and other dementias of late life. *Am J Psychiatr, 154,* (Suppl. 5), 1.

Ballard, C., Holmes, C., McKeith, I., Neill, D., O'Brien, J., Cairns, N., et al. (1999). Psychiatric morbidity in dementia with Lewy bodies: A prospective clinical and neuropathological comparative study with Alzheimer's disease. *Am J Psychiatry, 156,* 1039–1045.

Bartres-Faz, D., Junque, C., Moral, P., Lopez-Alomar, A., Sanchez-Aldeguer, J., & Clemente, I. C. (2002). Apolipoprotein E gender effects on cognitive performance in age-associated memory impairment. *J Neuropsychiatry Clin Neurosci, 14,* 80–83.

Ellason, J. W., & Ross, C. A. (1997). Two-year follow-up of inpatients with dissociative identity disorder. *Am J Psychiatry, 154,* 832.

Helmuth, L. (2002). New Alzheimer's treatments that may ease the mind. *Science, 297,* 1260–1263.

Pompei, P. (1995). Delirium in hospitalized elderly patients. *Hosp Pract, 28,* 69.

Reisberg, B., Doody, R., Stööffler, A., Schmitt, F., Ferris, S., & Mööbius, H. J. (2003). Memantine in moderate-to-severe Alzheimer's disease *N Engl J Med, 348,* 1333–1341.

Scheflin, A. W., & Brown, D. (1996). Repressed memory or dissociative amnesia: What the science says. *J Psychiatry Law, 24,* 143–188.

Steinberg, M. (1995). *Handbook for the assessment of dissociation: A clinical guide.* Washington, DC: American Psychiatric Press.

van der Kolk, B. A., Hopper, J. W., & Osterman, J. E. (2001). Exploring the nature of traumatic memory: Combining clinical knowledge with laboratory methods. *J Aggression Maltreatment Trauma, 4,* 9–31.

Vega, G. L., Weiner, M. F., Lipton, A. M., von Bergmann, K., Lütjohann, D., Moore, C., & Svetlik, D. (2003). Reduction in levels of 24S-hydroxycholesterol by statin treatment in patients with Alzheimer disease. *Arch Neurol, 60,* 510–515.

Yessauge, J. (1993). Differential diagnosis between depression and dementia. *Am J Med, 94,* (Suppl. 5), 235.

Biological Therapies **19**

U ntil the late 1940s, patients with serious psychiatric illnesses had few treatment options. They might have received insulin shock therapy, electroconvulsive therapy (without anesthesia), or barbiturate or narcotic sedation. They almost certainly were confined for the tenure of their illness to a secure institution where they may have been kept in physical restraints.

In the 1950s, the treatment of psychiatric patients changed dramatically. With the discovery of medications to treat specific symptoms of psychiatric illness, the most florid and debilitating symptoms of psychotic and mood disorders could now be controlled. For this reason, as well as for economic and humanitarian concerns, attitudes toward the treatment of the mentally ill also changed at that time. The focus of therapeutic intervention shifted from long-term institutionalization to outpatient treatment and support in the form of day-care programs and partial-care centers.

The mechanisms by which biological therapies such as psychopharmacologic agents and electroconvulsive therapy (ECT) work is not completely clear. Studies suggest that these treatments work primarily by regulating abnormal concentrations of synaptic neurotransmitters that are believed to play a role in the production of psychiatric symptoms

TABLE 19-1 Putative Mode of Action of Psychopharmacologic Agents on Psychiatric Symptoms

MAJOR TARGET SYMPTOM	CATEGORY OF AGENT	MAJOR PUTATIVE MODES OF ACTION
Psychosis	Antipsychotics	Block postsynaptic dopamine-2 (D_2) and serotonin 2A ($5\text{-}HT_{2A}$) receptors inhibiting the hyperactivity of dopamine and serotonin
Depression	Antidepressants	Downregulate postsynaptic β-noradrenergic and serotonin receptors over a 3–6 week period by increasing synaptic norepinephrine and serotonin concentrations via inhibition of reuptake mechanisms or blockade of monoamine oxidase activity
Mania	Lithium	Modifies second messenger signal transduction, stabilizes neuronal membranes, augments the function of serotonin, and corrects desynchronization in circadian rhythms
Anxiety	Benzodiazepines	Activate binding sites on the $GABA_A$ receptor, causing an influx of chloride leading to hyperpolarization of the neuronal membrane and decreased neuronal firing

(Table 19-1). However, although they can improve and even relieve symptoms, biological therapies cannot cure psychiatric disorders.

■ ANTIPSYCHOTIC AGENTS

Antipsychotic agents (formerly called neuroleptics or major tranquilizers) are used to treat psychotic symptoms associated with schizophrenia and other psychiatric and physical disorders. They can also relieve symptoms such as anxiety and agitation resulting from medical and psychiatric conditions. Although antipsychotics are commonly taken daily by mouth, fast-acting injectable forms can be used for agitated psychotic patients. In addition, long-acting injectable **"depot"** forms, such as haloperidol decanoate or fluphenazine decanoate, administered intramuscularly every 2 to 4 weeks, can be used to treat noncompliant patients. Whatever the mode of administration, all antipsychotic agents must be used carefully. Drug interactions can occur between antipsychotics and commonly used medications such as antihypertensives, anticholinergics, antidepressants, central nervous system depressants, antacids, nicotine, epinephrine, propranolol, and warfarin. Antipsychotic agents are classified as "traditional" or "atypical" depending on their neurological action and side effect profiles.

Traditional antipsychotics

Hyperactivity of dopamine in the mesolimbic tract is associated with production of positive psychotic symptoms (see Chapter 5). Traditional antipsychotic agents (Table 19-2) act primarily by blocking central dopamine-2 (D_2) receptors on postsynaptic neurons, an action that is believed to inhibit the activity of dopamine along this tract. Thus, although negative symptoms of schizophrenia, such as withdrawal, may improve with continued treatment, traditional antipsychotic agents are most effective against positive symptoms such as hallucinations and delusions (see Chapter 12).

TABLE 19-2	Traditional Antipsychotic Agents	
AGENT	ORAL DOSE (MG/DAY)	CLINICAL USES IN ADDITION TO PSYCHOTIC DISORDERS
Traditional Low-Potency Agents		
Chlorpromazine (Thorazine)	100–800	■ Nausea and vomiting ■ Hiccups
Thioridazine (Mellaril)	200–600	■ Depression with intense anxiety or agitation
Traditional High-Potency Agents		
Haloperidol (Haldol)	2–20	■ Psychosis secondary to organic syndromes, Tourette's disorder, and Huntington's disease ■ Available in long-acting decanoate form
Fluphenazine (Prolixin)	2–15	■ Available in long-acting decanoate form
Trifluoperazine (Stelazine)	4–20	■ Nonpsychotic anxiety (may be used for up to 12 weeks)
Perphenazine (Trilafon)	8–64	■ Nausea and vomiting
Pimozide (Orap)	1–10	■ Tourette's disorder ■ Body dysmorphic disorder ■ Adjuvant to SSRIs in obsessive compulsive disorder

SSRIs, selective serotonin reuptake inhibitors.

Traditional antipsychotic drugs are classified according to their potency. Low-potency agents such as chlorpromazine (Thorazine) and thioridazine (Mellaril) are primarily associated with non-neurologic adverse effects. Their coincidental blockade of muscarinic acetylcholine receptors leads to adverse effects, such as dry mouth, blurred vision, urine retention, and constipation. These agents also block histamine receptors, resulting in weight gain and sedation. Low-potency antipsychotic agents also have negative effects on the circulatory, endocrine, hematologic, hepatic, dermatologic, and ophthalmologic systems (Table 19-3). High-

TABLE 19-3	Non-Neurological Adverse Effects of Antipsychotic Agents (More Common with Traditional, Low-Potency Agents)
SYSTEM	ADVERSE EFFECTS
Circulatory	■ Orthostatic (postural) hypotension (most common with chlorpromazine) ■ Electrocardiogram abnormalities (prolongation of QT and PR intervals) ■ Thioridazine is most cardiotoxic in overdose
Endocrine	■ Increase in prolactin level results in gynecomastia (breast enlargement), galactorrhea, erectile dysfunction, amenorrhea, and decreased libido
Hematologic	■ Leukopenia; agranulocytosis (decreased number of certain white blood cells, particularly polymorphonuclear leukocytes) ■ Usually occur in the first 3 months of treatment
Hepatic	■ Jaundice; elevated liver enzyme levels ■ Usually occur in the first month of treatment ■ More common with chlorpromazine
Dermatologic	■ Skin eruptions, photosensitivity, and blue-gray skin discoloration ■ More common with chlorpromazine
Ophthalmologic	■ Irreversible retinal pigmentation with thioridazine ■ Deposits in lens and cornea with chlorpromazine
Anticholinergic	■ Peripheral effects: dry mouth, constipation, urinary retention, and blurred vision ■ Central effects: agitation and disorientation
Antihistaminergic	■ Weight gain and sedation ■ Chlorpromazine is most sedating

potency agents such as haloperidol (Haldol), fluphenazine (Prolixin), pimozide (Orap), trifluoperazine (Stelazine), and perphenazine (Trilafon) are primarily associated with neurological adverse effects. These effects, which include extrapyramidal effects (e.g., acute dystonia, akathisia, and pseudoparkinsonism), neuroleptic malignant syndrome, tardive dyskinesia, and decreased seizure threshold, can be life-threatening (Table 19-4).

Atypical antipsychotics

Atypical antipsychotic agents include clozapine (Clozaril), risperidone (Risperdal), olanzapine (Zyprexa), quetiapine (Seroquel), ziprasidone (Geodon), and aripiprazole (Abilify) (Kane et al., 2002). In contrast to traditional agents, atypical agents also work on serotonergic systems, particularly as antagonists of serotonin type 2A (5-HT_{2A}) receptors. They also act on other dopaminergic receptors and on noradrenergic systems (Table 19-5).

Like traditional agents, atypical antipsychotics are effective against the positive symptoms of schizophrenia. However, they may be more effective than traditional agents against the negative, chronic, and refractory symptoms of this disorder (see Chapter 12). Improvement in both positive and negative symptoms results from the ability of these agents to not only block dopaminergic activity in the mesolimbic tract like traditional agents, but to increase dopaminergic activity in the mesocortical tract (see Chapter 5) (Stahl, 2001).

Compared with traditional agents, atypical agents are less likely to cause extrapyramidal symptoms (e.g., acute dystonia, akathisia and pseudo parkinsonism), tardive dyskinesia, and neuroleptic malignant syndrome. Atypical agents can also decrease the risk of relapse in clinically stable patients with schizophrenia or schizoaffective disorder (Csernansky et al., 2002). Because of these advantages, atypical agents such as risperidone and olanzapine are being used more frequently as first-line agents in treating psychotic symptoms. Clozapine is also the first pharmacologic agent to receive U.S. Food and Drug Administration (FDA) approval for treating psychotic patients who show suicidal behavior (Meltzer et al., 2003).

Disadvantages of atypical agents (clozapine in particular) include increased likelihood of hematologic problems such as **agranulocytosis.** This disorder, characterized by white blood count under 2,000 or granulocyte count less than 1,000, can lead to life-threatening infections that typically present with pharyngitis and high fever. To identify the disorder early, patients who take clozapine must be monitored with weekly blood tests for the first 6 months of treatment, and every other week after that. Atypical agents also increase the risk of seizures, anticholinergic effects and pancreatitis. Weight gain is also problematic—clozapine and olanzapine cause the most weight gain, and ziprasidone causes the least. The tendency to cause weight gain may be linked to the propensity of some atypical agents to induce or exacerbate type 2 diabetes (Gianfrancesco et al., 2002).

	TABLE 19-4	Neurological Adverse Effects of Antipsychotic Agents (More Common With Traditional, High-Potency Agents)		

EFFECT	ADVERSE DESCRIPTION	OCCURRENCE	TREATMENT (IN ORDER OF HIGH TO LOW UTILITY)
Pseudo parkinsonism	■ Muscle rigidity ■ Slowed movement (bradykinesia) ■ Shuffling gait ■ Resting tremor ■ Mask-like facial expression ■ Cogwheel rigidity ■ Drooling	■ Develops within a few weeks of treatment ■ More common in women over age 40 years	■ Anticholinergic agent [e.g., benztropine (Cogentin)] ■ Propranolol Amantadine (Symmetrel) ■ Benzodiazepine ■ Reduce dose of medication
Akathisia	■ Subjective feeling of motor restlessness ■ Inability to remain still ■ Pacing ■ Rocking	■ Develops within 1–6 weeks of treatment	■ Antihistaminergic agent (e.g., diphenhydramine [Benadryl]) ■ Propranolol ■ Benzodiazepine ■ Anticholinergic agent ■ Reduce dose of medication
Acute dystonia	■ Prolonged muscular spasms of the neck (torticollis), eyelids (blepharospasm), pharynx (glossopharyngeal dystonia), eyes (oculogyric crisis), jaw, tongue or whole body (opisthotonus)	■ Develops within a few hours of treatment ■ More common in men under age 40 years	■ Benzodiazepine administered intramuscularly ■ Anticholinergic or antihistamine
Neuroleptic malignant syndrome	■ High fever (hyperpyrexia) ■ Sweating (diaphoresis) ■ Increased pulse and blood pressure ■ Dystonia ■ Apathy	■ Develops early in treatment ■ More common in men ■ Lasts up to 2 weeks ■ Mortality rate about 20%	■ Stop agent ■ Provide medical support ■ Dantrolene (Dantrium) ■ Bromocriptine (Parlodel)

TABLE 19-4	Neurological Adverse Effects of Antipsychotic Agents (More Common With Traditional, High-Potency Agents) (Continued)		
ADVERSE EFFECT	DESCRIPTION	OCCURRENCE	TREATMENT (IN ORDER OF HIGH TO LOW UTILITY)
	■ Decreased gesturing (akinesia) ■ Agitation		
Tardive dyskinesia (TD)	■ Abnormal writhing movements of the tongue, face, and body	■ Develops after at least 6 months of treatment ■ More common in women	■ Substitute low-potency or atypical antipsychotic agent ■ Tetrabenzene (a central amine depleting agent which is not yet approved for TD)

TABLE 19-5	Atypical Antipsychotic Agents			
AGENT (BRAND NAME)	ORAL DOSE (MG/DAY)	SEROTONIN (5-HT), DOPAMINE (D) AND ADRENERGIC (α) RECEPTOR ANTAGONIST ACTIVITY		SIDE EFFECTS
Clozapine (Clozaril)	300–900	5-HT_2, D_1, D_3,D_4, α_1		■ Agranulocytosis ■ Weight gain ■ Diabetes
Risperidone (Risperdal)	4–6	5-HT_2, D_2,α_1,α_2		■ Extrapyramidal symptoms at high doses ■ Increased prolactin
Olanzapine (Zyprexa)	10–20	5-HT_2, D_1, D_2, D_3,D_4, α1		■ Sedation ■ Weight gain ■ Diabetes
Quetiapine (Seroquel)	200–800	5-HT_2, 5-HT_6,α_1,α_2		■ Sedation ■ Cataracts
Ziprasidone (Geodon)	40–160	5-HT_2, D_1, D_3,D_4,α_1		■ Prolongation of QT interval
Aripiprazole (Abilify)	10–30	5-HT_{2A}, α_1; partial agonist at D_2, 5-HT_{1A}		■ Similar to risperidone ■ Dopamine system stabilizer

THE PATIENT A 25-year-old male patient with schizophrenia who has taken haloperidol for the past 2 months is brought to the hospital with a temperature of 104.1°F, blood pressure of 190/110, and muscular rigidity.

COMMENT The elevated body temperature, elevated blood pressure, and muscular rigidity indicate that this patient has a serious and potentially fatal antipsychotic medication adverse effect known as neuroleptic malignant syndrome (NMS). NMS, characterized by extrapyramidal rigidity causing hyperthermia, is seen more commonly in young male patients in the first few weeks of taking a high potency antipsychotic.

TREATMENT This patient's symptoms are best relieved by stopping the antipsychotic medication and providing medical support. The patient can also be given dantrolene (Dantrium) to relieve muscle rigidity. Agents such as bromocriptine (Parlodel), a dopamine-receptor agonist, may also be used to reverse the dopamine receptor blockade induced by the antipsychotic. After recovering from this life-threatening condition, the patient will be maintained on an atypical or low-potency antipsychotic agent.

ANTIDEPRESSANT AGENTS

At the beginning of the 21st century, more than 7 million Americans were taking **antidepressant agents,** making this group the second largest selling class (with cardiovascular agents first) of prescription drug in the United States. The antidepressants include heterocyclic antidepressants (HCAs), monoamine oxidase inhibitors (MAOIs), selective serotonin reuptake inhibitors (SSRIs), selective serotonin and norepinephrine reuptake inhibitors (SSNRIs), and atypical agents. All antidepressants are believed to increase the availability of neurotransmitters in the synapse via inhibition of reuptake mechanisms (HCAs, SSRIs, SSNRIs) or blockade of MAO (MAOIs), which ultimately leads to down-regulation of post-synaptic receptors (see Table 19-1 and Chapter 5) and improvement in mood. Besides treating depression, antidepressants have other clinical uses in medicine and psychiatry (Table 19-6).

All antidepressants take approximately 3 to 6 weeks to work and all have about equal efficacy in relieving depression. In part because they do not elevate mood in nondepressed people, antidepressants have no abuse potential. However, these agents can be dangerous in overdose (particularly HCAs and MAOIs) and can precipitate manic episodes (particularly tricyclic HCAs) in 15–20% of potentially bipolar patients. Although HCAs were once the mainstay of treatment for depression, SSRIs such as fluoxetine (Prozac), SSNRIs such as venlafaxine (Effexor), and atypical agents such as bupropion (Wellbutrin) are now used as first-line agents because of their more positive side-effect profiles. Psychoactive stimulants such as

| TABLE 19-6 | Antidepressant Agents | | |

AGENT (CURRENT OR FORMER BRAND NAME)	ORAL DOSE (MG/DAY)	EFFECTS	CLINICAL USES IN ADDITION TO DEPRESSION
HETEROCYCLIC AGENTS (HCAS)			
Desipramine (Norpramin, Pertofrane)	75–300	■ 2^0 tricyclic ■ Least sedating ■ Least anticholinergic ■ Most potent norepinephrine reuptake inhibitor ■ Stimulates appetite	■ Depression in the elderly ■ Eating disorders
Nortriptyline (Aventyl, Pamelor)	50–150	■ 2^0 tricyclic ■ Unlikely to cause orthostatic hypotension ■ Anticholinergic	■ Depression in the elderly ■ Depression in patients with cardiac disease ■ Pruritus (itching)
Amitriptyline (Elavil)	75–300	■ 3^0 tricyclic ■ Most sedating and anticholinergic of HCAs	■ Depression with insomnia ■ Chronic pain ■ Migraine prophylaxis ■ Enuresis
Clomipramine (Anafranil)	100–250	■ 3^0 tricyclic ■ Most serotonin-specific of the HCAs	■ OCD ■ Panic disorder
Doxepin (Adapin, Sinequan)	150–300	■ 3^0 tricyclic ■ Sedating ■ Antihistaminergic ■ Anticholinergic	■ GAD ■ Peptic ulcer disease ■ Pruritus
Imipramine (Tofranil)	150–300	■ 3^0 tricyclic ■ Likely to cause orthostatic hypotension	■ Panic disorder with agoraphobia ■ Enuresis ■ Eating disorders
Maprotiline (Ludiomil)	150–225	■ Tetracyclic ■ Low cardiotoxicity ■ May cause seizures	■ Anxiety with depressive features

TABLE 19-6   Antidepressant Agents (Continued)

AGENT (CURRENT OR FORMER BRAND NAME)	ORAL DOSE (MG/DAY)	EFFECTS	CLINICAL USES IN ADDITION TO DEPRESSION
SELECTIVE SEROTONIN REUPTAKE INHIBITORS (SSRIS)			
Citalopram (Celexa)	20–60	■ May be more dangerous in overdose than other SSRIs (cardiac conduction problems) ■ Low cytochrome P450 effects	■ OCD (all SSRIs) ■ Premenstrual dysphoric disorder (fluoxetine [Sarafem], sertraline) ■ Premature ejaculation (fluoxetine)
Escitalopram (Lexapro)	10–20	■ Isomer of citalopram ■ Most serotonin-specific of the SSRIs ■ Low cytochrome P450 effects ■ Fewer side effects than citalopram	■ Hypochondriasis (fluoxetine) ■ Social phobia (paroxetine) ■ Chronic pain (paroxetine) ■ PTSD (sertraline) ■ Panic disorder (all SSRIs except citalopram)
Fluoxetine (Prozac, Sarafem, Prozac Weekly)	20–80 (Prozac) 20–60 (Sarafem) 90 (Prozac Weekly)	■ Initial agitation and insomnia ■ Sexual dysfunction	■ Paraphilias (all SSRIs except citalopram) ■ Depression in children (fluoxetine, sertraline)
Paroxetine (Paxil, Paxil CR [long-acting form])	20–60	■ Most sedating SSRI ■ Potent serotonin reuptake inhibition ■ Most anticholinergic SSRI ■ Shorter half-life than other SSRIs (must be tapered off more slowly) ■ Sexual dysfunction	
Sertraline (Zoloft)	50–200	■ Most likely of the SSRIs to cause gastrointestinal disturbances (e.g., diarrhea) ■ Sexual dysfunction	
Fluvoxamine (Luvox)	100–300	■ Currently indicated only for OCD	

TABLE 19-6	Antidepressant Agents (Continued)

AGENT (CURRENT OR FORMER BRAND NAME)	ORAL DOSE (MG/DAY)	EFFECTS	CLINICAL USES IN ADDITION TO DEPRESSION
SELECTIVE SEROTONIN AND NOREPINEPHRINE REUPTAKE INHIBITORS (SSNRIS)			
Duloxetine (Cymbalta)	60	■ Rapid symptom relief ■ Few sexual side effects	■ Refractory depression ■ Urinary stress incontinence
Venlafaxine (Effexor, Effexor XR [extended-release form])	75–375 (75–225 for XR form)	■ Rapid symptom relief ■ Few sexual side effects ■ Low cytochrome P450 effects ■ Increased diastolic blood pressure at higher doses (less common with XR form) ■ High remission rate	■ Refractory depression ■ Generalized anxiety disorder
MONOAMINE OXIDASE INHIBITORS (MAOIS)			
Phenelzine (Nardil)	60–90	■ Hyperadrenergic crisis precipitated by ingestion of pressor amines in foods or sympathomimetic drugs ■ Orthostatic hypotension ■ Sexual dysfunction Insomnia	■ Atypical depression ■ Panic disorder ■ Eating disorders ■ Pain disorders ■ Social phobia (phenelzine)
Tranyl-cypromine (Parnate)	20–60		
OTHER ANTIDEPRESSANTS			
Amoxapine (Asendin)	200–400	■ Antidopaminergic effects such as ■ Parkinsonian symptoms, galactorrhea, and sexual dysfunction ■ Most dangerous in overdose	■ Depression with psychotic features

TABLE 19-6 Antidepressant Agents (Continued)

AGENT (CURRENT OR FORMER BRAND NAME)	ORAL DOSE (MG/DAY)	EFFECTS	CLINICAL USES IN ADDITION TO DEPRESSION
Bupropion (Wellbutrin, Wellbutrin SR [sustained-release form], Wellbutrin XL [extended-release form], Zyban)	200–450 (Wellbutrin) 200–400 (Wellbutrin SR) 150–300 (Wellbutrin XL and Zyban)	■ Norepinephrine and dopamine reuptake inhibition ■ No effect on serotonin ■ Insomnia ■ Seizures ■ Sweating ■ Decreased appetite ■ Fewer adverse sexual effects	■ Refractory depression (inadequate clinical response to other agents) ■ Smoking cessation (Zyban) ■ Seasonal affective disorder ■ Adult ADHD ■ SSRI-induced sexual dysfunction
Mirtazapine (Remeron)	15–45	■ Stimulates release of serotonin and norepinephrine ■ Targets specific serotonin receptors ■ Fewer adverse sexual effects ■ More sedation ■ May increase appetite	■ Refractory depression ■ Insomnia
Nefazodone (Serzone) Discontinued 6/04	300–600	■ Related to trazodone but with less sedation and priapism (persistent erection) ■ Dizziness ■ Fewer sexual side effects	■ Refractory depression ■ Depression with anxiety ■ Insomnia ■ SSRI-induced sexual dysfunction
Trazodone (Desyrel)	200–600	■ Sedation ■ Rarely, causes priapism ■ Hypotension	■ Insomnia

ADHD, attention deficit/ hyperactivity disorder; GAD, generalized anxiety disorder; OCD, obsessive-compulsive disorder; PTSD, post-traumatic stress disorder.

dextroamphetamine sulfate (Dexedrine) may also be used as antidepressants in specific patient populations (see later text). Antidepressants that target other neurotransmitter systems (e.g., antagonists of CRF-1 receptors) are in development.

HCAs

Heterocyclic antidepressants (HCAs), including secondary tricyclic, tertiary tricyclic, and tetracyclic agents, work primarily by blocking the reuptake of norepinephrine and serotonin in the synapse. Secondary tricyclics such as desipramine (Pamelor) are more potent blockers of norepinephrine reuptake, and tertiary agents such as amitriptyline (Elavil) are more potent blockers of serotonin reuptake. Because HCAs also block muscarinic acetylcholine and histamine receptors, they (particularly tertiary agents) cause anticholinergic and antihistaminergic side effects. Coincidental blockade of α-adrenergic receptors by HCAs leads to cardiovascular effects such as orthostatic hypotension and prolonged Q.T interval. HCAs also cause neurologic effects such as tremor, and they have negative effects on sexual function.

MAO inhibitors

There are two subtypes of the enzyme monoamine oxidase: MAO_A and MAO_B. MAO_A is the subtype most closely linked to the breakdown of the neurotransmitters involved in depression. **MAOIs** inhibit the breakdown of norepinephrine and serotonin by MAO_A in the brain in an irreversible reaction, thereby increasing the availability of these neurotransmitters and improving the patient's symptoms. Because MAO also metabolizes tyramine, a precursor of norepinephrine which in turn is a pressor, MAOIs can also cause a potentially fatal reaction when taken in conjunction with tyramine-rich foods (e.g., aged cheese, beer, wine, broad beans, beef or chicken liver, and smoked or pickled meats or fish) or sympathomimetic drugs (e.g., ephedrine, methylphenidate [Ritalin], phenylephrine [Neo-Synephrine], and pseudoephedrine [Sudafed]). This reaction, including elevated blood pressure, sweating, headache, and vomiting (i.e., **a hypertensive crisis**), can lead to stroke and death. Dietary restrictions when taking MAOIs are therefore necessary, although eating in an unfamiliar place such as at a restaurant or a party can lead to unwitting ingestion of these forbidden foods and precipitate such a crisis. A subtype of the MAOIs, **reversible inhibitors of MAOI-A (RIMAs),** permits the ultimate metabolism of norepinephrine and thus does not require dietary restrictions. RIMAs have not yet received FDA approval for treating depression.

MAOIs and SSRIs used together can cause a potentially life-threatening interaction, **the serotonin syndrome,** marked by autonomic instability, hyperthermia, convulsions, coma, and sometimes death. Other adverse effects of MAOIs are similar to those of the heterocyclics, including danger in overdose. MAOIs may be particularly useful in patients with atypical depression (see Chapter 12) or with treatment resistance to other agents.

SSRIs and SSNRIs

Selective serotonin reuptake inhibitors (SSRIs) selectively block the reuptake of serotonin but have little effect on dopamine, norepinephrine, acetylcholine, or histamine systems. They are less cardiotoxic and safer in overdose than heterocyclics or MAOIs. Because of this selectivity for the serotonin receptor, SSRIs cause fewer side effects than other antidepressant agents. The **selective serotonin and norepinephrine reuptake inhibitors (SSNRIs)** block the reuptake of both serotonin and norepinephrine but have little effect on other neurotransmitter systems. In some patients, SSNRIs may work more quickly, have more efficacy, and cause fewer sexual side effects than SSRIs.

Stimulants

In addition to treating attention-deficit hyperactivity disorder (ADHD) (see Chapter 2) and narcolepsy (see Chapter 7), **psychoactive stimulants** such as methylphenidate (Ritalin), pemoline (Cylert), dextroamphetamine sulfate (Dexedrine), and amphetamine/dextroamphetamine combinations (Adderall) are used in the treatment of depression, particularly in patients refractory to other treatments (Table 19-7). These agents work more rapidly than antidepressants and thus may be particularly useful in depressed elderly patients or in depressed patients with life-limiting illnesses. They are also useful in patients at risk for adverse effects of antidepressants. The major disadvantage of the stimulants is their potential for causing tolerance and dependence (see Chapter 23). **Modafinil** (Provigil), a highly selective noradrenergic receptor blocker with stimulant properties, is used in combination with antidepressants for patients with treatment-resistant depression and for narcolepsy and it apparently does not have abuse potential. Atomoxetine (Strattera) is a non-stimulant norepinephrine reuptake inhibitor used to treat ADHD, particularly in adults.

■ MOOD-STABILIZING AGENTS

Mood stabilizers are used to prevent both the manic and depressive phases of bipolar disorder. They include lithium carbonate or citrate and anticonvulsant agents, such as carbamazepine and valproic acid. The atypical antipsychotic olanzapine is also used as a mood stabilizer, particularly in patients with bipolar disorder with psychotic features (Table 19-8).

Lithium

Lithium is used to treat bipolar disorder and to increase the effectiveness of antidepressant agents in depressive illness. It is also used to help con-

TABLE 19-7 Stimulants

AGENT (BRAND NAME)	ORAL DOSE (MG/DAY)	CLINICAL USES	ADVERSE EFFECTS
Amphetamine/ dextroamphetamine (Adderall, Adderall XR [extended release])[a]	5–40	■ Attention-deficit/ hyperactivity disorder ■ Narcolepsy ■ Depression in the elderly and terminally ill ■ Treatment-resistant depression ■ Treatment-resistant obesity	■ Anorexia ■ Insomnia ■ Irritability ■ Aggravation of psychotic symptoms
Dextroamphetamine sulfate (Dexedrine)[a]	10–40		
Methylphenidate (Ritalin, Concerta [extended release])[b]	20–60 (Ritalin) 18–54 (Concerta)		
Pemoline (Cylert)[b]	50–75	discontinued 3/05	

[a]For adults and children over age 3 years.
[b] For adults and children over age 6 years.

trol aggressive behavior. Lithium is administered in oral form and is eliminated by the kidneys. Its mode of action is largely unknown, but certain mechanisms have been suggested (see Table 19-1). Negative and even life-threatening effects of lithium include renal dysfunction, cardiac conduction problems, gastric distress, mild cognitive impairment, tremor, and hypothyroidism. Thus, before prescribing lithium, the physician must perform a thorough physical examination and obtain baseline laboratory values. Because of these side effects, caution must be used in prescribing lithium for elderly or debilitated patients; for patients with chronic diarrhea or organic brain syndromes; or for patients with prior kidney, cardiovascular, or thyroid disease. Because it can cause birth defects, particularly of the cardiovascular system, lithium is usually contraindicated in early pregnancy.

Because of potential toxicity, blood concentrations of lithium must be maintained within a narrow range in all patients. To do this and to monitor other laboratory values, blood tests and urinanalysis should be done initially and in the ongoing care of a patient on lithium therapy (Table 19-9).

TABLE 19-8 Mood Stabilizers

AGENT (BRAND NAME)	ORAL DOSE (MG/DAY)	ADVERSE EFFECTS	CLINICAL USES IN ADDITION TO MOOD STABILIZATION
Lithium (Eskalith)	900–1800 (titrated to a blood level of 0.8–1.2 mEq/L)	■ First trimester congenital abnormalities (especially of the cardiovascular system, e.g., Ebstein's anomaly of the tricuspid valve) ■ Renal dysfunction ■ Cardiac conduction problems ■ Hypothyroidism ■ Tremor ■ Gastric distress ■ Mild cognitive impairment	■ Prophylaxis for both manic and depressive episodes ■ Control of aggressive behavior ■ Enhancement of the activity of tricyclic antidepressants (at blood levels of 0.6–0.8 mEq/L) ■ Premenstrual dysphoric disorder ■ Borderline personality disorder ■ Bulimia nervosa ■ Cluster headaches
Carbamazepine (Tegretol)	400–1000 (titrated to blood level of 4–12 μg/mL)	■ Aplastic anemia ■ Agranulocytosis ■ Sedation ■ Dizziness ■ Ataxia	■ Anticonvulsant ■ Trigeminal neuralgia ■ Mixed episode and rapid cycling bipolar disorder ■ Impulse control disorders ■ Alcohol and benzodiazepine withdrawal
Oxcarbamazepine (Trileptal)	300–1200 (titrated to blood level of 4–12 μg/mL)	■ No blood dyscrasias ■ No autoinduction ■ Dizziness ■ Ataxia ■ Visual disturbances	■ Anticonvulsant ■ Trigeminal neuralgia ■ Mixed episode and rapid cycling bipolar disorder
Valproic acid (Depakene, Depakote [more slowly absorbed])	500–1500 (titrated to blood level of 50–100 μg/mL)	■ Gastrointestinal symptoms ■ Liver problems ■ Congenital neural tube defects ■ Weight gain ■ Alopecia	■ Anticonvulsant ■ Migraine headache ■ Bipolar symptoms resulting from cognitive disorders ■ Mixed episode and rapid cycling bipolar disorder ■ Impulse control disorders ■ Alcohol and benzodiazepine withdrawal

TABLE 19-8 **Mood Stabilizers (Continued)**

AGENT (BRAND NAME)	ORAL DOSE (MG/DAY)	ADVERSE EFFECTS	CLINICAL USES IN ADDITION TO MOOD STABILIZATION
Olanzapine (Zyprexa)	10–20	■ Sedation ■ Weight gain ■ Diabetes	■ Bipolar disorder with psychotic features ■ Adjunct to SSRIs for obsessive-compulsive disorder ■ Refractory depression

SSRIs, selective serotonin reuptake inhibitors.

Anticonvulsants

Anticonvulsant agents such as carbamazepine (Tegretol), oxycarba-mazepine (Trileptal), an isomer of carbamazepine, and valproic acid (De-pakene, Depakote) are used to treat bipolar disorder. The mechanism of action of these agents is unknown but may be related to modulation of the gamma-amino-butyric acid (GABA) system, which leads to reduced neuronal excitability. Anticonvulsants are particularly useful for the **rapid-cycling** (i.e., more than four episodes annually) (see Chapter 15) and

---

CASE 19-1

THE PATIENT A 40-year-old woman is brought to the emergency department by the police after someone reported that she was walking down the street naked. The woman, who is speaking very quickly, tells the doctor that God spoke to her and told her to give her clothing to a homeless woman. She reports that a few weeks ago her family doctor gave her pills because she was "very down." The patient is a supermarket clerk who is married and has two school-aged children. Her history reveals that over the past 5 years, she has had two episodes of major depression for which she did not seek treatment.

COMMENT This patient's past depression, age, and good employment and relationship history suggest that her current psychotic symptoms are an acute manifestation of a manic episode rather than schizophrenia or other psychotic illness. Because antidepressants can precipitate a manic episode in potentially bipolar patients, this episode may have been triggered by the medication (probably an antidepressant) prescribed by her family physician.

TREATMENT The most effective immediate treatment for this patient is hospitalization and administration of an antipsychotic, such as haloperidol or risperidone, to control her hallucinations and delusions. After the patient undergoes laboratory tests of thyroid and renal function, lithium or another mood stabilizer will be used in the long-term treatment of this bipolar patient.

TABLE 19-9	Suggested Laboratory Tests For Patients Taking Lithium

FREQUENCY OF TESTING DURING THE FIRST YEAR OF TREATMENT	MEASURE
At least every week (initially) and then at least every month	■ Concentration of lithium in blood
Every 3 months	■ Serum blood urea nitrogen and creatinine level in blood
Every 3–6 months	■ White blood cell count ■ Triiodothyronine (T_3), thyroxine (T_4), and thyroid stimulating hormone levels in blood ■ Creatinine clearance including urine volume (24-hour urine output)

mixed episode (mania and depression occurring at the same time) types of bipolar disorder. Anticonvulsants are also useful for patients who have not responded to or who have had unacceptable side effects of lithium treatment. Other anticonvulsant agents that appear to have mood-stabilizing effects include **lamotrigine (Lamictal), gabapentin (Neurontin), topiramate (Topamax),** and **tiagabine (Gabitril).** With the exception of lamotrigine, which is useful in both mania and depression, these agents seem to be more effective against the manic than the depressive symptoms of bipolar disorder. They are also used in combination with lithium for treatment-resistant and psychotic bipolar patients.

Valproic acid may be especially useful for treating bipolar disorder with psychotic features, bipolar symptoms resulting from cognitive disorders (see Chapter 14), and substance abuse with a coexisting personality disorder. It is also useful for prophylaxis of migraine headaches. Valproic acid is also effective when used in conjunction with atypical antipsychotics (such as clozapine and risperidone) to treat patients with refractory schizophrenia or bipolar disorder. Adverse effects of valproic acid include gastrointestinal and liver problems, congenital neural tube defects, and alopecia (hair loss).

Carbamazepine, although effective for mood stabilization, is associated with severe adverse hematologic effects, such as aplastic anemia and agranulocytosis, as well as the less severe and reversible leukopenia. It is also associated in some patients with peripheral anticholinergic effects as well as dizziness, sedation, and ataxia.

■ ANTIANXIETY AGENTS

The **antianxiety agents** are also known as anxiolytics or minor tranquilizers. They include benzodiazepines, buspirone, and carbamates. Some of these agents also have antiseizure and muscle-relaxant activity. The more sedating agents, **hypnotics,** are used particularly to treat insomnia (Table 19-10).

TABLE 19-10	Antianxiety Agents (in Order of Duration of Action by Category)			
AGENT (CURRENT OR FORMER BRAND NAME)	ORAL DOSE (MG/DAY)	ONSET OF ACTION	DURATION OF ACTION	CLINICAL USES IN ADDITION TO ANXIETY
BENZODIAZEPINES				
Chlorazepate (Tranxene)	15–60	Short	Short	▪ Adjunctive use in the management of partial seizures
Oxazepam (Serax)	30–120	Inter-mediate	Short	▪ Alcohol withdrawal
Triazolam (Halcion)	0.125–0.25	Inter-mediate	Short	▪ Insomnia
Alprazolam (Xanax)	0.5–6	Short	Short	▪ Depression (adjunct to antidepressants) ▪ Panic disorder ▪ Social phobia ▪ High abuse potential
Lorazepam (Ativan)	2–6	Inter-mediate	Inter-mediate	▪ Psychotic agitation ▪ Acute seizure control ▪ Alcohol withdrawal
Temazepam (Restoril)	15–30	Inter-mediate	Inter-mediate	▪ Insomnia
Chlordiazepoxide (Librium)	15–100	Short	Long	▪ Alcohol withdrawal
Clonazepam (Klonopin)	0.5–4	Short	Long	▪ Seizures ▪ Mania ▪ Social phobia ▪ Panic disorder ▪ Obsessive-compulsive disorder
Diazepam (Valium)	2–60	Short	Long	▪ Muscle relaxation ▪ Analgesia ▪ Seizures of alcohol withdrawal
Flurazepam (Dalmane)	15–30	Short	Long	▪ Insomnia

AGENT (CURRENT OR FORMER BRAND NAME)	ORAL DOSE (MG/DAY)	ONSET OF ACTION	DURATION OF ACTION	CLINICAL USES IN ADDITION TO ANXIETY
NONBENZODIAZEPINES				
Zolpidem (Ambien)	5–10	Short	Short	■ Indicated only for insomnia
Zaleplon (Sonata)	10–20	Short	Short	■ Indicated only for insomnia
Buspirone (BuSpar)	15–60	Very long	Very long	■ Anxiety in the elderly ■ Generalized anxiety disorder ■ Adjunct to antidepressants for major depressive disorder and OCD ■ No abuse potential, sedation or withdrawal symptoms

Benzodiazepines

Benzodiazepines activate binding sites on the $GABA_A$ receptor, thereby decreasing neuron and muscle-cell firing. These agents have a short, intermediate, or long onset and duration of action, and they can be used to treat disorders other than anxiety disorders (Table 19-10). Benzodiazepines commonly cause sedation but have few other adverse effects. Their characteristics of action are related to their clinical indications and to their potential for causing tolerance and dependence with chronic use (see Chapter 23). For example, shorter-acting agents such as triazolam (Halcion) are good hypnotics but have a higher potential for abuse than longer-acting agents.

Flumazenil (Mazicon, Romazicon) is a benzodiazepine receptor antagonist that can reverse the effects of benzodiazepines in cases of overdose or when benzodiazepines (e.g., midazolam [Versed]) have been used to provide sedation for a surgical procedure.

Nonbenzodiazepines

Buspirone (BuSpar), an azaspirodecanedione, is a serotonin $5\text{-}HT_{1A}$ receptor agonist that also is active at $5\text{-}HT_2$ and D_2 receptors. Buspirone is not related to the benzodiazepines and, in contrast to them, is not associated with sedation, dependence, abuse, or withdrawal problems. It is used primarily to treat conditions causing chronic anxiety such as generalized anxiety disorder, in which benzodiazepine dependence can become a problem. However, because buspirone takes up to 2 weeks to work, it may not be acceptable for anxious patients who are accustomed to the fast relief of symptoms provided by benzodiazepines. At high doses, buspirone has antidepressant activity, and it may be used in combination with antidepressants to treat depression.

Zolpidem tartrate (Ambien) and zaleplon (Sonata) are unrelated to benzodiazepines and are used primarily to treat insomnia. Although these agents have less abuse potential than benzodiazepines, they also cause dependence and should therefore not be used for more than a few weeks. Carbamates such as meprobamate are now used rarely because they have a greater potential for abuse and a lower therapeutic index than other antianxiety agents.

■ OTHER PSYCHOACTIVE AGENTS

Naturally occurring substances such as endocrine hormones, as well as antihypertensive agents and enzyme inhibitors, can alter the activity of neurotransmitters and have psychoactive effects.

Endocrine hormones

Thyroid hormones and **sex hormones** have been used in the treatment of mood disorders. Levothyroxine (Synthroid, Levothroid), a synthetic form of thyroxine (T_4), has mood-stabilizing effects in patients with bipolar disorder. Liothyronine (Cytomel), a synthetic form of T_4's metabolically active form triiodothyronine (T_3), can augment the effects of antidepressant medication (Joffe et al., 1996). It is not yet known whether thyroid hormones improve mood by correcting subclinical thyroid abnormalities (Joffe & Marriot, 2000) or by a more general effect on brain function.

Estrogens may improve mood directly and may augment the effects of antidepressants in postmenopausal women. These effects may be mediated by the ability of estrogen to increase monoamine availability by lowering monoamine oxidase concentrations or enhancing the availability of tryptophan, a serotonin precursor (Halbreich & Chakravorty, 1997; Stahl, 1998). By a generally stimulating effect, testosterone and other **androgens** may improve mood and energy level in hypogonadal men and increase libido in both hypogonadal men and postmenopausal women.

Because elevated glucocorticoids may play a role in depression (see Chapter 6), the abortion agent **mifepristone (Mifeprex or RU486),** a glucocorticoid receptor antagonist, is currently being evaluated for antidepressant activity (Belanoff et al., 2002).

Acetylcholinesterase inhibitors

Acetylcholinesterase inhibitors (AChIs) block the enzyme that breaks down acetylcholine (Table 19-11). This improvement in cholinergic transmission decelerates the progression of memory loss and may even result in transient improvement in memory and other cognitive function in about 25% of patients with Alzheimer's disease. AChIs can also be useful in patients with other dementias like Lewy-body dementia (see Chapter 18). The first AChI, tacrine (Cognex), caused gastrointestinal disturbances and had significant hepatic toxicity, which limited its usefulness for many patients. The newer agents donepezil (Aricept), rivastigmine (Exelon), and galantamine (Reminyl) cause fewer adverse side effects than tacrine.

Antihypertensives

Antihypertensive agents, including the **β-antagonists** (β-blockers) such as propranolol (Inderal) and **α_2-adrenergic receptor antagonists** such as clonidine (Catapres) decrease the autonomic hyperarousal associated with some psychiatric conditions. These agents are particularly useful for treating symptoms associated with mild anxiety states and withdrawal from opioids and sedatives.

■ ELECTROCONVULSIVE THERAPY AND RELATED THERAPY

In the film "One Flew Over the Cuckoo's Nest," the main character played by Jack Nicholson is given electroconvulsive therapy (ECT) as punish-

TABLE 19-11	Acetylcholinesterase Inhibitors			
AGENT (BRAND NAME)	ORAL DOSE (MG/DAY)	LENGTH OF ACTION	DOSES PER DAY	ADVERSE EFFECTS
Tacrine (Cognex)	40–160	Short	Four	■ Nausea, vomiting, and diarrhea ■ Hepatic toxicity
Donepezil (Aricept)	5–10	Long	One	■ Nausea, vomiting, and diarrhea ■ Muscle cramps
Rivastigmine (Exelon)	6–12	Intermediate	Two	■ Nausea, vomiting, and diarrhea ■ Anorexia
Galantamine (Reminyl)	16–32	Intermediate	Two	■ Nausea, vomiting, and diarrhea ■ Anorexia

ment whenever he fails to conform to the rules of a psychiatric hospital. This and other unfavorable representations of ECT in the media perpetuate negative stereotypes about what is in fact a safe and effective treatment for some serious psychiatric disturbances.

Uses of electroconvulsive therapy

The primary indication for ECT is depression in major depressive or bipolar disorder. Although it is most commonly used to treat patients who are refractory to or intolerant of antidepressants, ECT may also be indicated for depressive symptoms from any cause, particularly when rapid symptom resolution is imperative because of suicide risk (see Chapter 14). Thus, ECT is a first-line treatment for suicidal, malnourished, catatonic, or psychotic agitated patients. In fact, ECT is more effective for psychotic depression than antidepressants or antipsychotics administered alone or combined.

In some patients (e.g., the elderly and pregnant women), ECT may be safer than long-term use of antidepressant agents. ECT is also useful for patients with mania, mixed manic-depressive states, schizophrenia with prominent affective symptoms, or schizoaffective disorder.

The precise action of ECT on the brain is not known; however, it appears to alter neurotransmitter function in a manner similar to that of antidepressants, namely by increasing the availability of biogenic amines and GABA.

Administration

In ECT, a generalized seizure lasting 25 to 60 seconds is induced by passing an electric current through the brain. Prior to the procedure, an intravenous line is established and the patient is premedicated with a drug such as atropine to prevent bradyarrhythmias and to dry secretions. Next, the patient is given a short-acting general anesthetic such as methohexital (Brevital) and a muscle relaxant such as succinylcholine (Anectine) to prevent injury during the seizure. A bite block protects the teeth and tongue during the seizure. Because succinylcholine also paralyzes breathing muscles, 100% oxygen is administered until spontaneous respiration resumes.

Electroconvulsive therapy can be administered in at least three ways: **bitemporal ECT** (one electrode placed on each temple), **right unilateral ECT** (two electrodes placed on the nondominant hemisphere), and **bifrontal ECT** (one electrode placed above the end of each eyebrow) (Fig. 19-1). In general, unilateral and bifrontal ECT have fewer side effects but are less effective at relieving symptoms than bilateral ECT.

Typically, ECT is given 2 to 3 times per week for 2 to 3 weeks. Improvement in mood begins after a few ECT treatments, with maximum response occurring after 5 to 10 treatments. However, if no other treatment is given, most patients relapse within 6 months of discontinuation of ETC. Biweekly or monthly maintenance ECT or ongoing antidepressant treatment can reduce the relapse rate (Sackeim et al., 2001).

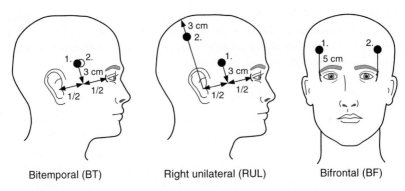

Bitemporal (BT)   Right unilateral (RUL)   Bifrontal (BF)

FIGURE 19-1. Electrode placement for patients receiving electroconvulsive therapy (ECT).

(From Lawson, J.S., Inglis, J., Delva, N.J. et al. (1990). Electrode placement in ECT: Cognitive effects. Psychol Med 20(2):335–334.

Problems associated with ECT

The major adverse effects of ECT are memory disturbances. These occur in three basic types: an acute confusional state, retrograde amnesia, and anterograde amnesia. An **acute confusional state** typically lasts for about 30 minutes after the seizure and then remits. **Anterograde amnesia,** which also occurs after the seizure, is characterized by the inability to put down new memories and invariably resolves within 1 to 2 weeks. In the most problematic type, **retrograde amnesia,** the patient forgets events occurring during the ECT course and about 1 to 2 months prior to it, and these memories rarely return. Other side effects include headache, nausea, and muscle aches caused by the seizure. Despite these adverse effects, ECT is safe; its mortality rate is comparable to that associated with the induction of general anesthesia. ECT is contraindicated in patients with increased intracranial pressure from any cause (e.g., a space-occupying lesion) or recent (within 2 weeks) myocardial infarction (Kellner & Beale, 1994), and should be avoided in patients taking lithium.

Rapid transcranial magnetic stimulation

In **rapid transcranial magnetic stimulation (rTMS),** an electric current is applied to the scalp to generate a magnetic field about 2 cm deep that stimulates cortical interneurons lying parallel to the surface of the brain. Although rTMS currently has no approved psychiatric indication, research suggests that it improves symptoms in some patients with refractory major depressive disorder, psychotic depression, obsessive-compulsive disorder, and post-traumatic stress disorder.

* Disulfiram for alcohol abuse
* Acamprosate; prevents relapse

REVIEW QUESTIONS

1. A 30-year-old woman comes to the emergency department with elevated blood pressure, sweating, headache, and vomiting. Her companion tells you that the patient became ill at a Mexican restaurant where she ate cheese enchiladas and drank sangria. Of the following agents, the one that this patient is most likely to be taking is
   (A) fluoxetine
   (B) clozapine
   (C) nortriptyline
   (D) phenelzine
   (E) haloperidol

2. Which of the following psychoactive agents should the physician avoid in the treatment of a 40-year-old woman with a history of substance abuse?
   (A) Diazepam (Valium)
   (B) Haloperidol (Haldol)
   (C) Fluoxetine (Prozac)
   (D) Buspirone (BuSpar)
   (E) Lithium

3. A 30-year-old male schizophrenic patient is taking an antipsychotic agent that is helping him to be more outgoing and sociable. However, the patient is experiencing seizures, and a blood test reveals agranulocytosis. The antipsychotic agent that this patient is most likely to be taking is
   (A) fluphenazine
   (B) clozapine
   (C) trifluoperazine
   (D) perphenazine
   (E) haloperidol

4. A 42-year-old woman with chronic paranoid schizophrenia who is taking haloperidol has begun to show involuntary chewing and lip-smacking movements. These symptoms are best treated initially
   (A) by changing to an atypical antipsychotic agent
   (B) with an antianxiety agent
   (C) with an antidepressant agent
   (D) with an anticonvulsant
   (E) by stopping the antipsychotic agent

5. A 76-year-old woman is brought to the emergency room by her sister with whom she lives. The woman, who has a history of depression and suicidal behavior, refuses to eat and states that life is not worth living anymore. Consultations with her primary care physician and a consulting psychiatrist reveal that the patient has not responded to at least three different antidepressant medications that she has taken in adequate doses and for adequate time periods in the past 2 years. The most appropriate next step in the treatment of this patient is to recommend

(A) diazepam

(B) electroconvulsive therapy (ECT)

(C) buspirone (BuSpar)

(D) intensive psychotherapy

(E) lithium

ANSWERS AND EXPLANATIONS

1-D. This patient is most likely to be taking phenelzine, a monoamine oxidase inhibitor (MAOI). These agents can cause a hypertensive crisis if certain foods (e.g., aged cheese, smoked meats, beer, and red wine) are ingested. A patient such as this woman, who eats in an unfamiliar place or a restaurant may unwittingly ingest forbidden foods. This patient ate cheese, which may have been aged, and drank sangria, which probably contained red wine. This resulted in a life-threatening hypertensive crisis, including elevated blood pressure, sweating, headache, and vomiting. Fluoxetine, clozapine, nortriptyline, and haloperidol do not interact negatively with food.

2-A. Benzodiazepines such as diazepam are likely to be abused and should be avoided in patients with histories of substance abuse. Antipsychotics such as haloperidol, antidepressants such as fluoxetine, antimanics such as lithium, and nonbenzodiazepines such as buspirone have little or no abuse potential.

3-B. The antipsychotic agent that this patient is most likely to be taking is clozapine. Clozapine, an atypical agent, is more effective against negative symptoms of schizophrenia (e.g., social withdrawal), but it is also more likely to cause seizures and agranulocytosis than traditional agents such as haloperidol, fluphenazine, trifluoperazine, and perphenazine.

4-A. Involuntary chewing and lip-smacking movements indicate that this patient has developed tardive dyskinesia, a serious side effect of treatment with high-potency antipsychotic agents such as haloperidol. Other side effects of high-potency antipsychotic agents include neuroleptic malignant syndrome (high fever, sweating, increased pulse and blood pressure, and muscular rigidity); pseudoparkinsonism (muscle rigidity, shuffling gait, resting tremor, and mask-like facial expression); akathisia (a subjective feeling of motor restlessness); and dystonia (prolonged muscular spasms). Tardive dyskinesia usually occurs after at least 6 months of starting a high-potency antipsychotic and is best treated by changing to an atypical or low-potency agent. Because tardive dyskinesia results from hypersensitivity of dopamine receptors, stopping the antipsychotic medication will exacerbate this patient's symptoms.

5-B. Because this severely depressed elderly patient has not responded to antidepressant medication, the most appropriate next step in treatment is to recommend a course of electroconvulsive therapy (ECT). ECT is a safe, fast, effective treatment for major depression. Diazepam, lithium, buspirone, and psychotherapy are less likely to be effective for this patient.

REFERENCES

Belanoff, J. K., Rothschild, A. J., Cassidy, F., DeBattista, C., Baulieu, E-. E., Schold, C., & Schatzberg, A. F. (2002). An open label trial of C-1073 (mifepristone) for psychotic major depression. *Bio Psychiatry, 52,* 386–392.

Czernansky, J. G., Mahmoud, R., Brenner, R., for the Risperidone-USA-79 Study Group A. (2002). Comparison of risperidone and haloperidol for the prevention of relapse in patients with schizophrenia. *N Engl J Med, 346,* 16–22.

DeBattista, C., & Schatzberg, A. F. (2000). Other biological and pharmacological therapies. In *Comprehensive textbook of psychiatry* (7th ed., Vol. II). Philadelphia: Lippincott, Williams & Wilkins.

Gianfrancesco, F. D., Grogg, A. L., Mahmoud, R. A., Wang, R, & Nasrallah, H. A. (2002). Differential effects of risperidone, olanzapine, clozapine, and conventional antipsychotics on type 2 diabetes: Findings from a large health plan database. *J Clin Psychiatry, 63,* 920–930.

Goode, E. (2002, June 30). Antidepressants lift clouds, but lose "miracle drug" label. *The New York Times.*

Halbreich U, Chakravorty SG. 1997. The influence of estrogen on monoamine oxidase activity. *Psychopharmacol Bull,* 33, 229–233.

Joffe, R. T., & Marriott, M. (2000). Thyroid hormone levels and recurrence of major depression *Am J Psychiatry, 157,* 1689–1691.

Joffe, R. T., Singer, W., Levitt, A. J., & MacDonald, C. (1996). Triiodothyronine augmentation in the treatment of refractory depression. A meta-analysis. *Arch Gen Psychiatry 1996, 53,* 842–848.

Kane, J. M., Carson, W. H., & Anutosh, R. S. (2002). Efficacy and safety of aripiprazole and haloperidol versus placebo in patients with schizophrenia and schizoaffective disorder. *J Clin Psychiatry, 63,* 763–771.

Kellner, C. H., & Beale, M. D. (1994). Cardiovascular complications of ECT. *Am J Psychiatry, 151,* 789–790.

Kellner, C. H, Pritchett, J. T., Beale, M. D., & Coffey, C. E. (1997). Handbook of ETC. Washington, DC: American Psychiatric Press.

Lawson, J.S., Inglis, J., Delva, N.J. et al. (1990). Electrode placement in ECT: Cognitive effects. Psychol Med 20(2):335–334.

McEvoy, J. P., Scheifler, P. L., & Frances, A. (1999). Treatment of schizophrenia 1999. *J Clin Psychiatry, 60,* (Suppl. 11), 1–80.

Meltzer, H. Y., Alphs, L., Green, A. I., Altamura, A. C., Anand, R., Bertoldi, A., et al., for the InterSePT Study Group. (2003). Clozapine treatment for suicidality in schizophrenia: International Suicide Prevention Trial (InterSePT). *Arch Gen Psychiatry, 60,* 82–91.

Pascual-Leone, A., Rubio, B., Pellardae, F., & Fatalaa, M. I. J. (1996). Rapid-rate transcranial magnetic stimulation of left dorsolateral prefrontal cortex in drug-resistant depression. *Lancet, 348,* 233.

Sackeim, S. A., Haskett, R. F., Mulsant, B. H., Thase, M. E., Mann, J. J., Pettinati, H. M., et al. (2001). Continuation pharmacotherapy in the prevention of relapse following electroconvulsive therapy: a randomized controlled trial. *JAMA, 285,* 1299–1307.

Stahl, S. M. (1998). Basic psychopharmacology of antidepressants, part 2: Estrogen as an adjunct to antidepressant treatment. *J Clin Psychiatry, 59,* (Suppl 4), 15–24.

Stahl, S. M. (1999). *Essential psychopharmacology.* New York: Cambridge University Press.

Stahl, S. M. (2001). 670 "hit-and-run" actions at dopamine receptors, part 1: Mechanism of action of atypical antipsychotics. *J Clin Psychiatry, 62,* 923

Culture and Illness **20**

A Chinese-American patient who has chronic heart disease is more likely to die on the fourth than on any other day of the month. This puzzling observation, called "The Hound of the Baskervilles Effect" because of a similar occurrence in the classic Sir Arthur Conan Doyle novel, is attributed to the stress provoked by the similarity in the Chinese language between the words for "four" and "death" (Phillips et al., 2001).

Culture and ethnicity can influence a patient's health also by less dramatic means. Attitudes toward health care providers, compliance with treatment, beliefs about the causes and treatment of illness, and use of specific health practices are significantly affected by culture. While seeming at first to make little sense and even to hamper the delivery of care, cultural beliefs, which are often based on empiric observations over time, can improve health care. For example, curcumin, a component of turmeric, a spice historically used in India to treat burns (see Table 20-4), appears to confer protection from burns caused by radiation therapy (Okunieff et al., 2002). In contrast, when cultural health beliefs are suspected or rejected, the outcome can be tragic. In a true case documented in "The Spirit Catches You and You Fall Down" (Fadiman, 1997), an epileptic child in a Hmong (Laotian) family died because the family's beliefs about her illness and its treatment were not understood or accepted by her American doctors.

Physicians who understand the health beliefs, customs, and characteristics of specific groups of people have acquired "cultural competency," a skill that will help them communicate with, encourage trust in, and ultimately provide the most effective clinical care to their patients.

■ ETHNOCULTURAL ISSUES IN HEALTH CARE

Graduation ceremonies at large American universities and medical schools reveal our great cultural diversity. This country of approximately 285 million people is made up primarily of immigrants and descendants of immigrants from countries outside of the United States.

Although composed of many subcultures, the American culture seems to have certain characteristics of its own. For example, financial and personal independence are valued at all ages, especially in the elderly. Youthfulness and continued sexual interest into old age are also valued. Store shelves crowded with soaps and deodorants for every part of the body demonstrate the almost obsessional American emphasis on personal hygiene and cleanliness.

Culture and illness

The United States has a large, white, middle class that is the major cultural influence, and subcultures including African American, Latino, Asian American, Native American, and Middle Eastern American. Because cultural groups vary in their health beliefs and practices, this diversity poses important challenges for physicians. For example, schizophrenia is seen to about the same extent in all cultures (see Chapter 12), but the presentation of its symptoms (e.g., delusions of persecution) typically differ by culture. For example, although a white patient may fear that the FBI is after her, an Asian American patient may believe that the ghost of a dead relative is torturing her, and an African American patient may believe that someone has put a curse on her (Westermeyer, 1988).

Physician's attitudes

Most folk beliefs and remedies are benign and can be included in the patient's medical treatment plan. For example, a patient who believes that his illness can be cured by eating a certain food should be helped to get the food. Similarly, if the patient believes that an outside influence like a hex or a curse imposed by the anger of another person caused her illness, the doctor should ask the patient who can help to remove the curse and then involve that individual in the patient's treatment. When a folk remedy is potentially harmful or medically contraindicated, the doctor can explain the danger and substitute a similar but safe remedy that harmonizes with the patient's belief system. Whatever the plan, patients tend to be more satisfied with their care and to comply with treatment recommendations when their physicians acknowledge and have a nonjudgmental attitude toward their cultural and religious beliefs and practices.

Speaking with patients

Adult patients are addressed using their correct titles, such as Mr., Ms., or Dr., and family names. Using first or given names to address patients is not appropriate. However, the correct title and family name may not be obvious. For example, in people from certain parts of India, what appears to be the last or family name is actually the given name. Among the Chinese, the family name commonly comes first and is followed by the given name. For example, for someone named Yang Lin Lin, Yang is the family name. Sikh patients are likely to have three names, the first, the religious (typically Singh for men and Kaur for women), and the family name. If it is not clear, the doctor should ask the patient what the family name is and how the patient would like to be addressed.

No matter what the ethnicity or culture, it is essential that the physician speak directly to the patient. For non-English-speaking patients, a professional interpreter should be used to facilitate communication. Using a child or adult child for this role is not appropriate (Salas-Lopez et al., 2002; Case 20-1).

Culture shock

Culture shock is a strong emotional response related to geographic relocation and the need to adapt to unfamiliar social and cultural surroundings. It is reduced when immigrants of a particular culture gather in the same geographic area. Young immigrant men appear to be at higher risk for culture shock, including psychiatric symptoms, such as paranoia and depression, than other sex and age groups. This increased risk has been

---

CASE 20-1

THE PATIENT A 75-year-old Vietnamese man is brought to the emergency room by his daughter with whom he lives, because he has been having difficulty breathing. The patient, who is diagnosed with congestive heart failure, is alert and oriented. He speaks little English, and the doctor communicates the diagnosis and treatment plan to him through his daughter. As she translates for the patient, the daughter uses only a few words to translate the doctor's lengthy explanations of the illness and treatment to the patient.

COMMENT Family members can be important allies for doctors. However, in this instance, the daughter appears to be editing the doctor's statements, perhaps to protect her elderly father from the negative medical diagnosis. Protecting elderly relatives from stressful medical information is seen in several cultural groups, including Asians, Latinos, and Middle Easterners. Because the doctor needs to communicate with his patient directly, it is not appropriate for the doctor to use a relative as an interpreter. His best course is to use a professional interpreter rather than a relative in order to interact directly with his patient (the elderly man in this case).

TREATMENT The continuing treatment regimen for this patient involves several different medications and is quite complex. During hospitalization and after the patient is released from the hospital, the doctor can keep in regular direct contact with him via the interpreter.

attributed to at least two factors. First, young men lose the most status on leaving their culture of origin. Also, unlike others in the cultural group who can stay at home among familiar people, young men often must venture out into the new culture, learn the new language, and earn a living.

Ethnic disparities in health care

Certain racial and ethnic minorities in the United States face significant obstacles to obtaining quality health care. These difficulties lead to higher mortality rates in these groups from some common disorders. For example, African Americans and Latinos have less access to physical and mental health care services than other Americans and, when they do receive care, it is often of poorer quality. These disparities are not caused solely by economic factors or lack of physical access to care. They exist even when incomes and health care insurance are equal. Communication difficulties, overt bias (Flores, 2000), and physician-held negative racial stereotypes about African Americans and Latinos (Smedley et al., 2002) contribute to the poorer health care for these groups. Other elements contributing to ethnic disparities in health care include the typically shorter-term relationships between minority patients and primary care physicians, and the relative scarcity of minority physicians.

■ AMERICAN SUBCULTURES

Illness and hospitalization interrupt an individual's dietary, grooming, and health care routines. Knowledge of that individual's preferences and requirements can help reduce the stress caused by such interruptions. Table 20-1 lists questions the physician can use to identify a patient's specific religious and cultural preferences and requirements.

Although people in ethnic, religious, and cultural groups share some characteristics, there is more variability than sameness among the individuals in the group. Thus, although it is important to understand normative cultural beliefs and behaviors, clinicians must avoid stereotyping their patients by these parameters. With this caveat, examples of dietary, dress, and health practices of specific ethnic and religious groups are given in Tables 20-2, 20-3, and 20-4, respectively. (Also see Figures 20-1 to 20-4.)

African Americans

There are approximately 36 million African Americans, 12.7% of the total U.S. population. The average income of African American families is only about half that of white families. Coupled with other health care disparities (see previous text), financial factors result in decreased access to health care services and increased health risks. When compared with white Americans, African Americans have a shorter life expectancy (see Table 4-1) and higher rates of infant mortality, hypertension, heart disease, stroke, obesity, asthma, tuberculosis, diabetes, prostate cancer, and AIDS.

TABLE 20-1 Questioning Patients about Ethnocultural Issues

SUBJECT	SPECIFIC QUESTIONS FOR THE PATIENT	COMMENT
Items of clothing or ornamentation	■ "Do you wear or prefer to wear any special garments, decorations, or jewelry?" ■ "Are you wearing anything special now?" ■ "Are there any special times when you need to wear these things?" ■ "What would you like me to do with the item after you remove it?"	■ Item may be worn for ceremonial or religious purposes. ■ Item may be worn for protection against evil and ill health. ■ Avoid removal of item unless medically necessary. ■ If required, discuss need for removal with patient or relatives.
Diet	■ "Is there anything special that you like or need to eat or drink to keep healthy or to get better?" ■ "Are there any special times when you need to eat or drink these things?" ■ "What is the best way to obtain these foods or drinks for you?" ■ "Are there any days or times that you cannot or do not want to eat or drink?"	■ Dietary needs and preferences should be followed as closely as medically and practically possible. ■ Many groups fast at times. If possible, use alternative to oral medications at such times. ■ Certain groups like children, expectant and nursing mothers, elderly, and the ill are usually exempt from fasting or other severe food restriction.
Health practices	■ "When you or a family member are ill, do you consult anyone in the community or family who is not a doctor?" ■ "When you or a family member are ill, do you use any treatment or medications not prescribed by a doctor?" ■ Are you currently consulting a folk healer or using a folk remedy?	■ Use of folk healers and folk remedies. ■ Loss of blood (even for a blood test) may have significant meaning. ■ Patients often wish to be visited by their clergyman when they are ill or dying.

TABLE 20-2 Ethnocultural Dietary Practices

RELIGIOUS GROUP (IN ALPHABETICAL ORDER)	DIETARY PRACTICES
Buddhist and Hindu	■ Most are vegetarian
Jewish	■ Meat animals (only animals with cloven hooves which chew their cud) slaughtered according to Jewish law (e.g., Kosher meat) ■ No pork, or pork products ■ Avoid medication, (e.g., insulin) derived from pigs ■ No shellfish (only fish with fins and scales) ■ Milk products and meat products are not served in the same meal ■ Fast on the day of Yom Kippur ■ No bread or other leavened products during the 10 days of Passover
Mormon	■ No tea and coffee ■ No alcohol or tobacco
Muslim	■ Meat animals slaughtered according to Islamic law (e.g., Halal meat) ■ No pork, or pork products ■ Avoid medication derived from pigs ■ No alcohol ■ Fast during the month of Ramadan from sunrise to sunset and other special days during the year; break the fast with fruit (e.g., dates) and water
Roman Catholic	■ Dietary restrictions during Lent (40 days before Easter Sunday) ■ Avoid meat on Fridays ■ Fast or avoid meat on Ash Wednesday and Good Friday
Seventh-Day Adventist	■ Are vegetarian ■ No caffeinated beverages ■ No alcohol ■ No spices (e.g., black pepper)
Sikh	■ Most are vegetarian, but may eat meat other than beef

In fact, African-American men and women are 15 times and five times more likely to have AIDS than white men and women, respectively. African Americans also have higher death rates from heart disease and from all forms of cancer. Although the higher cancer mortality rates among African Americans compared with white Americans had been attributed

TABLE 20-3	Ethnocultural Dress and Adornment
ETHNIC/ RELIGIOUS GROUP	**DRESS AND ADORNMENT**
Asian Indian	■ For weddings, paint designs in henna (orange-red dye) on hands, arms, feet, and legs of bride, attendants, and female guests in the Mehndi (i.e., henna) ceremony (Fig. 20-3).
Chinese	■ Wear jade to prevent evil and illness
Hindu	■ Boys wear sacred thread over the right shoulder and around the body; avoid cutting or removal; if it must be removed, preserve for the patient ■ Married women wear bindi (vermillion forehead ornament) to ensure the longevity of their husbands ■ Married women wear bangle bracelets until widowhood ■ Married women wear mangalsutra (black beads around the neck)
Jewish	■ Orthodox males wear sacred undergarments and Orthodox married women may wear wigs
Latino	■ Wear "mano negro" (black hand), "mano milagroso" (miraculous hand), or "eye beads" (see Fig. 20-4) on one's person (on wrists or ankles of infants) to avoid "mal de ojo," a curse or "evil eye"
Mormon	■ Wear sacred undergarment
Muslim	■ Women covered from head to toe with over garments and head scarves ■ Help in undressing given only by those of the same sex ■ Wear or carry bits of copies of the Koran as protection
Roman Catholic	■ Wear crucifix (cross) or scapular (fabric medallion) or image of a saint on a medal on a chain around the neck
Sikh	■ Men wear the "5 Ks"; kesh (uncut hair) covered by a turban, kangha (comb in hair), kara (steel bangle or ring), kirpan (dagger), kaccha (white shorts as undergarment)

SUBJECT	ETHNIC/ RELIGIOUS GROUP	HEALTH BELIEF

TABLE 20-4　Ethnocultural Health Beliefs and Practices

SUBJECT	ETHNIC/ RELIGIOUS GROUP	HEALTH BELIEF
Blood	African American	■ Patient says she has "high blood" (usually refers to having high blood pressure) or "low blood" (usually refers to having malaise or being tired) ■ Patient says that he has a "touch of sugar" (usually refers to diabetes)
	Chinese Haitian Latino	■ Loss of any blood (even for a blood test) can be life-threatening ■ Drawing blood can cause ill health or bad luck (patient may be suspicious of blood thinners, such as coumadin)
	Jehovah's witness	■ Will not accept blood transfusions or blood products (however, parents cannot refuse needed blood for children [see Chapter 25]) ■ May accept clotting factor, immunoglobulins or plasma expanders
Death and Dying	Roman Catholic	■ Clergyman gives Holy Communion (thin bread wafer) and last rites (a blessing) to the dying; includes prayer and anointing of the forehead with holy oil ■ Baptism (blessing with holy water) for very ill newborns
	Jewish	■ No embalming ■ Autopsies usually not allowed ■ Preference for burial within 24 hours of death
	Muslim	■ Lie with the face toward Mecca when dying or dead ■ Family members prepare the body for burial ■ Non-Muslims cannot touch a dead body unless they wear gloves ■ Family members stay with the body from death until burial ■ Autopsies and organ donation are usually not permitted ■ Preference for burial within 24 hours of death
	Sikh	■ Family member or practicing Sikh recites hymns from the Sikh Holy Book (Guru Granth Sahab) ■ Hair and beard should not be cut after death

TABLE 20-4   Ethnocultural Health Beliefs and Practices (Continued)

SUBJECT	ETHNIC/ RELIGIOUS GROUP	HEALTH BELIEF
Folk Medicine Beliefs and Practices	African American	■ Belief that a person has put a curse or hex on someone using herbs (i.e., "somebody is working roots") causing illness in a patient ■ Afro-Carribean may use magic ("voodoo") to remove illness
	Asian Indian	■ Orange discoloration around wounds and burns from the practice of treating with powdered turmeric (Haldi) spice
	Southeast Asian	■ In "coining," a coin is rubbed on the affected area or down the back of the neck; the resulting bruises are believed to aid the patient ■ In "cupping" or "moxibusion," a vacuum created by heating a glass jar is used to raise a welt on the skin to improve symptoms (Figs. 20-1, 20-2)
	Latino	■ Folk healers, botanical remedies ■ "Empacho": Syndrome of digestive problems caused by dietary errors, which is treated with massage and dietary changes (see Case 20-2) ■ "Mal de ojo": Illness in someone (usually a child) due to a curse from a jealous person

mainly to biological differences between the races, recent studies suggest that this difference is more likely to result from economic factors and co-existing medical conditions affecting African Americans than from genetic factors (Bach et al., 2002). As evidence for this, African-American women under age 50 years have lower breast cancer survival rates than do white women of the same age. However, African-American women and white women aged 65 years and older (who all have Medicare benefits) have equivalent survival rates (see Chapter 27) (Chu, 2003).

America's long and destructive history of racism, fueled by tragic events like the **Tuskegee Institute Study,** in which some African-American men with syphilis were given a placebo instead of an effective medication, has resulted in a general distrust among some African Americans of the white-dominated health care system. This has resulted in low participation in organ donation programs and clinical trials, as well as reluctance to seek routine preventive care for diseases like HIV (Thomas & Quinn, 1991).

Religion plays a major role in social and personal support among many African-Americans. Pastors (leaders of the church) and ministers, either lay or formally trained, are often consulted before physicians, especially for mental health problems. Strong extended family networks also play an important role in social support, and elderly family members are respected and consulted for their health care advice.

The strong church and family support systems may in part explain why the overall suicide rate is lower among African Americans than among white Americans. Unfortunately, suicide in African American teenagers, once relatively uncommon, has more than doubled in the last 20 years. Now, as in white teens, it is the third leading cause of death. The leading cause of death in African American teens is homicide, and accidents are second. In white teenagers, the order of these two is reversed.

Hispanic/Latino Americans

The Federal government uses the term **"Hispanic"** to describe Americans of Spanish-speaking background. Arguably, the term **"Latino"** more correctly describes this group, because it is composed mainly of people from the Spanish-speaking regions of Latin America (e.g., Mexico, the Caribbean, and Central and South America).

With approximately 37 million people, Latinos recently became the largest minority group in the United States, making up 13% of the population and surpassing African Americans in number (Clemetson, 2003). About two thirds of Latinos are of **Mexican** origin and live in the Southern and Western states. The second largest group of Latinos (about 3 million people) are **Puerto Rican Americans,** living mainly in the Northeastern states. **Cuban Americans** number over 1 million and live primarily in the Southeast, especially in Florida.

As a group, Latinos tend to have larger families than non-Latinos. Twelve percent of non-Latino families and 31% of Latino families (those with a Latino head of household) consist of five or more people. Respect for the extended family (**"familismo"**), especially the elderly, is important in this group. Younger people are expected to care for elderly family members, to protect elderly relatives from negative medical diagnoses, and, often, to make medical decisions concerning the care of elderly relatives.

Latino patients may have certain expectations of the doctor-patient relationship. For example, they expect physicians to show **"simpatia"** or kindness, and to be polite and positive when under stress. They also expect physicians to show **"personalismo,"** or friendliness in the form of physical contact, such as handshaking, and **"respeto,"** or respectfulness (Flores, 2000). Physicians also need to be aware that Latino patients can be quite emotional when ill, because many believe that voicing emotion and pain improves the symptoms of the illness.

Latinos may seek health care from folk healers such as **chamanes, curanderos, santeros, and espiritistas.** Treatment provided by these healers, often sought in conjunction with traditional medical care, includes herbal or botanical medicines, magical remedies, and specific changes in diet (Case 20-1). For example, one dietary treatment aims to balance hot and cold influences. A cold food—the designation, not the actual temperature

THE PATIENT   A 35-year-old woman of Puerto Rican background brings her 8-year-old child to the emergency room. The child, who has been complaining of stomach pain and nausea for the past 2 weeks, seems hyperactive and frightened of "monsters" that are trying to hurt him. The patient and child speak English well. The mother tells the doctor that when the child became ill she took him to a santera who diagnosed the child with "empacho" and recommended treatment with wormwood tea. Physical examination of the child reveals tenderness in the lower right quadrant and fever of 100.2°. Blood tests reveal elevated white blood cell count and lead levels in the toxic range (>130 mg/mL).

COMMENT   Most folk remedies are harmless. However, in this case, the mother's choice of a folk healer has both delayed potentially lifesaving traditional treatment for this child. The folk treatment itself also is causing problems. Psychotic symptoms, like this child's delusion that monsters are trying to harm him, can be manifestations of lead toxicity that can occur with the ingestion of wormwood tea.

TREATMENT   Treatment of lead toxicity should be started immediately using intravenous administration of calcium disodium edetate (calcium disodium versenate) daily for 5 days. Coupled with surgery for appendicitis, the child's physical and mental symptoms should resolve. These parents should be encouraged in the future to contact the physician first when the child first becomes ill. The parents also should be cautioned against the possible toxicity of herbal remedies and encouraged to clear such remedies with the physician prior to use.

of the food—such as corn is used to treat a hot illness, e.g., rheumatic fever. The idea that opposing influences can cause and treat illness is seen also in other cultural groups (e.g., yin versus yang in Asian culture). Although the reasons are not clear, Latino women are less likely to get mammograms and are more likely to have cervical cancer than white or African-American women. Obesity is also a problem in Latinos, particularly among Mexican-American adolescents (Ogden et al., 2002) (see Chapter 17).

Asian Americans

Census 2000 figures indicate that with a total of more than 10 million members, the largest groups of Asian Americans are the Chinese (2.4 million), Filipino (1.8 million), and Asian Indian (1.7 million). Other Asian American groups include Vietnamese (1.1 million), Korean (1 million), and Japanese (800,000) Americans. Although many groups are assimilated into the U.S. culture, ethnic differences may still result in different responses to illness among Asian-American groups.

Folk medicine practices such as **coining and cupping,** used by some Asian Americans, can cause injuries that, when seen in children, may be mistaken for abuse (Dinulos & Graham, 1999). The injuries from coining, in which a coin is used to rub oil or ointment into the skin, include linear petechiae and ecchymosis on the neck, back, and chest (Fig. 20-1). Cupping, in which a heated glass cup is applied to the skin, can cause raised, round lesions (Fig. 20-2). Although these acts are aimed at providing relief from symptoms when they cause harm to a child they must be reported to the appropriate state child protective agency.

There are other things to consider when treating Asian American patients. First, as in Latino cultures, adult Asian American children show strong respect for and are expected to care for their elderly parents, protect elderly relatives from negative medical diagnoses, and make medical decisions about elderly relatives' care (Case 20-1). Also, these patients commonly express emotional pain as physical pain. Thus, a patient may report pain in the stomach or head when she is in fact depressed. Finally, in some Asian American groups, particularly the Japanese, the thoracic area rather than the brain is thought to be the spiritual core of the person. Thus, the concept of brain death and organ transplant after brain death (see Chapter 26) are generally not well-accepted.

Native Americans

People of Native-American descent, including American Indians and Eskimos, number about 2.7 million and have their own program of medical care under the direction of the Indian Health Service of the federal government. Native Americans have higher rates of suicide and alcoholism

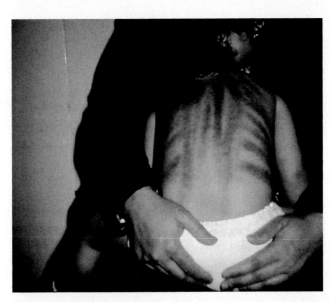

FIGURE 20-1. Coining. The lesions on this child's back were caused by rubbing oil into the skin by abrading it with a coin or other instrument.

(Reprinted with permission from www.ethnomed.org, Harborview Medical Center, Seattle, Washington.)

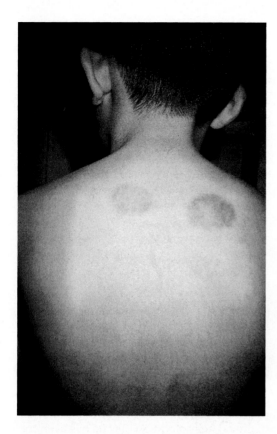

FIGURE 20-2. Cupping. These circular lesions were caused by application of the rim of a cup or other device that had been heated using a flame and then quickly applied to the skin.

(Reprinted with permission from www.ethnomed.org, Harborview Medical Center, Seattle, Washington.)

than white Americans. At least 20% of Native American teenage boys have problems with alcohol by the end of high school. Also, the suicide rate is four times higher and the overall death rate is twice as high in Native American than in other American teens (Duclos and Manson, 1993).

In this group, the distinction between mental and physical illness may be blurred. Health is believed to result from being in harmony with nature, and illness to result from engaging in forbidden behavior and witchcraft.

Americans of European descent

European country of descent can influence a patient's response to illness. **Anglo Americans** (those originating in English-speaking European countries, like Ireland, Scotland, England, and Wales) tend to be less emotional, more stoic, and less vocal about pain and illness than members of groups of **Mediterranean** origin (e.g., Jewish, Greek, and Italian people). The medical implication of this stoicism is that Anglo Americans may delay seeking treatment and thus be very ill when they are finally seen by a physician. Conversely, patients of Mediterranean origin may be labeled complainers by medical personnel and not be taken seriously when they are in fact ill.

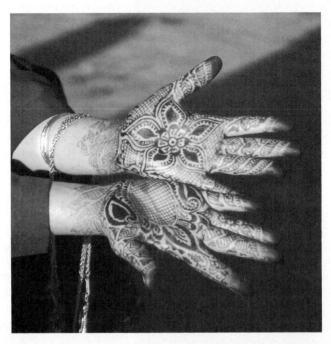

FIGURE 20-3. Design painted on the palms in henna, an orange-red dye. This dye is used in weddings in the Mehndi (i.e., henna) ceremony for the bride and her attendants. As it wears off, the orange coloration may be mistaken for a skin rash.

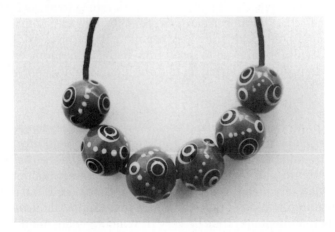

FIGURE 20-4. Eye beads that are strung together and worn to ward off "mal de ojo," the evil eye (bad luck and ill health).

Americans of Middle Eastern descent

People of **Middle Eastern** or North African origin who speak dialects of the Arabic language (e.g., those from Egypt, Saudi Arabia, Kuwait, Bahrain, Iraq, Oman, Qatar, Syria, Jordan, Palestine, and Lebanon) are often referred to as Arabs. Other Middle Eastern peoples include those from Iran (formerly Persia), Afghanistan, and Pakistan.

In the Middle Eastern family, the elders are respected and often are consulted before doctors for advice about health issues. Nevertheless, Middle Eastern families tend to value and have confidence in Western medicine, highly respect physicians, and closely follow medical advice. As in Latino and Asian families, the adult children in Middle Eastern families may try to spare the elderly relative the need to make medical decisions or to hear negative diagnoses.

Although some Middle Eastern people are Christian or Jewish, most are Muslim and follow the dietary, dress, and health practices of this religious group (see Tables 20-2, 20-3, and 20-4). Among Muslim patients, female purity and modesty are valued, and separation of the sexes is maintained if possible. Female patients expect to remain as covered as possible in the examining room and may ask to keep their heads and faces covered by a scarf. In the hospital and for obstetrical and gynecological outpatient care, female patients are often more comfortable with female doctors. If a female patient must be examined or treated by a male physician, the husband may wish to be present.

REVIEW QUESTIONS

1. A 40-year-old Latino woman who has been diagnosed with iron-deficiency anemia tells the physician that an espiritista in her community told her to treat her illness by drinking a quart of goat's milk a day. Goat's milk poses no danger to this patient. She explains that the healer told her that anemia is a "cold" illness and goat milk is a "hot" food. What is the doctor's most appropriate next statement to the patient?

    (A) "There is no medical evidence that goat's milk is beneficial in the treatment of anemia."

    (B) "Folk healers are not trained in modern medicine."

    (C) "Try the goat's milk for a month and if you do not feel better, I will give you medication."

    (D) "There are medical treatments for your condition that can be used along with the espiritista's recommendation."

    (E) "I cannot treat your condition until you stop going to the espiritista."

2. A physician has two 55-year-old male patients, one Jewish and one Muslim. Of the following, both patients are **least likely** to

(A) prepare meat according to religious law

(B) eat pork

(C) fast at certain times

(D) avoid medication derived from pigs

3. Which of the following is most likely to be true about the number of African Americans and Latinos in the United States?

(A) There are twice as many African Americans as Latinos

(B) There are three times as many African Americans as Latinos

(C) There are twice as many Latinos as African Americans

(D) There are three times as many Latinos as African Americans

(E) The numbers of Latinos and African Americans is approximately equal

4. A physician has two 56-year-old male patients. One of them is African American and one is white. When compared with the white patient, the African American patient has a lower likelihood of

(A) stroke

(B) asthma

(C) hypertension

(D) suicide

(E) prostate cancer

5. A 40-year-old woman who recently had back surgery does not complain of pain, although magnetic resonance imagery (MRI) reveals reherniation of the disc with significant nerve involvement. Of the following, this woman is most likely to be of

(A) Welsh descent

(B) Puerto Rican descent

(C) Greek descent

(D) Italian descent

(E) Mexican descent

ANSWERS AND EXPLANATIONS

1-D. People from many cultures use folk healers and folk remedies. As long as the treatment will not harm the patient, the physician should try to work alongside such healers, not separate patients from their cultural beliefs. Because in this case the folk treatment is innocuous, the patient can continue using it along with traditional medicine.

2-B. Jewish and Muslim patients are likely to avoid eating pork or using medication derived from pigs. Both groups prepare meat according to religious law and fast at certain times.

3-E. The percentage of Americans who are African American and Latino is approximately equal.

4-D. Statistically, a middle-aged African-American patient has a lower likelihood of suicide than a white patient of the same age. However, when compared with white patients, African American patients have a higher likelihood of stroke, asthma, hypertension, and prostate cancer.

5-A. Of the listed ethnic groups, this woman is most likely to be of Welsh descent. Anglo Americans tend to be more stoic and less vocal about pain than do Americans of Mediterranean or Latino descent.

REFERENCES

Bach, P. B., Schrag, D., Brawley, O. W., Galaznik, A., Yakren, S., & Begg, C. B. (2002). Survival of blacks and whites after a cancer diagnosis. *JAMA, 287,* 2106–2113.

Brawley, O. W. (2002). Disaggregating the effects of race and poverty on breast cancer outcomes. *J Natl Cancer Inst, 94,* 471–475.

Chu, K. C., Lamar, C. A., & Freeman, H. P. (2003). Racial disparities in breast cancer survival rates: Separating factors that affect diagnosis from factors that affect treatment. *Cancer, 97,* 2853–2860.

Clemetson, L. (2003, January 22). Hispanics now largest minority, census shows. *The New York Times.*

Dinulos, J. G., & Graham, E. A. (1999). *Self teaching module for the influence of culture and pigment on skin conditions in children.* University of Washington: Harborview Medical Center.

Duclos, C. W., & Manson, S. M. (Eds.) (1993). *Calling from the rim: Suicidal behavior among American Indian and Alaska Native Adolescents.* Denver, Colorado: The National Center for American Indian and Alaska Native Mental Health Research.

Fadiman, A. (1997). *The spirit catches you and you fall down.* New York: Farrar, Straus and Giroux.

Flores, G. (2000). Culture and the patient-physician relationship: Achieving cultural competency in health care. *J Pediatrics, 136,* 14–23.

Kirmayer, L. J. (2001). Cultural variations in the clinical presentation of depression and anxiety: Implications for diagnosis and treatment. *J Clin Psychiatr, 62,* 22.

Laffrey, S. C., Meleis, A. I., Lipson, J. G., Solomon, M., & Omidian, P. A. (1989). Arab-American Health Care Needs. *Social Sci Med, 29,* 877–883.

Leary, W. E. (1999, January 21). Study urged on cancer and races: Health panel cites higher rates in poor. *The New York Times,* p. A11.

Ogden, C. L., Flegal, K. M., Carroll, M. D., & Johnson, L. (2002). Prevalence and trends in overweight among US children and adolescents, 1999–2000. *JAMA, 28,* 1728–1732.

Okunieff, P., Xu, J., Hu, D., Liu, W., & Ding, I. (2002). Protective effect of curcumin on radiation induced skin damage involves down-regulation of chemokine gene expression. *Int'l J Radiation Oncology Biology Physics, 54, 2:79.*

Phillips, D. P., Liu, G. C., Kwok, K., Jarvinen, J. R., Zhang, W., & Abramson, I. S. (2001). Hound of the Baskervilles effect: Natural experiment on the influence of psychological stress on timing of death. *Br Med J, 323,* 1443–1446.

Salas-Lopez, D., Cominolli, R., & Soto-Greene, M. (2002). *Bridging language and culture in healthcare communication.* State of New Jersey, Department of Health and Senior Services, Office of Minority and Multicultural Health.

Satcher, D. (2001). *Mental health: Culture, race, and ethnicity.* A supplement to the Surgeon General's Report on Mental Health. Report presented at the annual conference of the American Psychological Association, San Fransisco, CA.

Shaffer, D., Gould, M., & Hicks, R. C. (1994). Worsening suicide rate in black teenagers. *Am J Psychiatry, 151,* (Suppl. 12), 1810–1812.

Smedley, B. D., Stith, A. Y., & Nelson, A. R. (Eds.). (2002). *Unequal treatment: Confronting racial and ethnic disparities in health care.* Washington, DC: National Academy Press.

Soto-Greene, M., & Cominolli, R. (2001). *History and physical exam skills.* 2002 course syllabus, UMDNJ-New Jersey Medical School.

Thomas, B. & Quinn, S. C. (1991). The Tuskegee syphilis study, 1932–1972: Implications for HIV education and AIDS risk programs in the Black community. *Am J Pub Health, 81,* 1503.

Westermeyer, J. J. (1988). Cross-cultural psychiatric assessment. In A. Kleinman (Ed.), *Rethinking psychiatry.* New York: Free Press.

Human Sexuality 21

S exual and relationship problems can hamper recovery from illness and impair quality of life. Although people who have sexual concerns are commonly counseled to consult their family doctors, many physicians are not particularly knowledgeable or at ease addressing these issues. In order to develop competence in dealing with the sexual issues of patients, doctors need to understand not only how sexuality is affected by illness, but the many forms of expression it can take. Perhaps even more importantly, physicians must confront their own feelings about sexuality in order to be effective resources for their patients' sexual concerns.

■ SEXUAL DEVELOPMENT

Physical development

Like all other mammals, the default pattern for sexual development in humans is female. Under the influence of the **testis determining factor (TDF) gene** in fetuses with Y chromosomes, the indifferent gonads assume the characteristic structure of testes. Once formed, sometime around gestational week six to seven, the testes begin to secrete androgenic hormones and Müllerian-inhibiting substance (MIS).

Both male and female embryos possess **Wolffian and Müllerian duct systems,** which have the potential to form the male and female genitalia, respectively. In males, androgens secreted by the developing testes support the development of the Wolffian duct system, which becomes the male internal genitalia (seminal vesicles, vas deferens, and epididymis) and external genitalia (penis and scrotum); MIS suppresses the development of the Müllerian duct system. This combination of hormonal influences results in a normal male genital phenotype. In females, development of the Wolffian duct system is not stimulated, and development of the Müllerian duct system is not inhibited. Therefore, the fallopian tubes, uterus, and top third of the vagina develop in the fetus.

Brain development

Increasing evidence demonstrates that the brain is sexually differentiated by gonadal hormones during prenatal life. In animals, experimental manipulations that alter gonadal hormone levels in developing fetuses affect the display of species-typical sexual and related behaviors in adulthood. When examined as adults, males deprived of androgens as fetuses are neurologically and behaviorally demasculinized, and females exposed to androgens as fetuses are neurologically and behaviorally masculinized (Goy & McEwen, 1980; Berenbaum, 1998).

Brain differentiation occurs later in gestation than does genital differentiation. In humans, it is believed to occur during the second trimester, and it results in gender differences in the hypothalamus, anterior commissure, corpus callosum, and thalamus (see Fig. 5-2) (Halpern, 2000). The significance of these sex differences in the brain is not clear, but they may be related to the expression of **gender identity, gender role,** and **sexual orientation** (Institute of Medicine, 2001) (Table 21-1).

Physical and psychological disorders of sexual development

Experimental hormonal manipulations such as those done in animals obviously cannot be carried out in humans. However, clinical disorders of sexual development can give clues to the effects of gonadal hormones on sexual differentiation of the human brain.

At birth, most infants can be clearly identified as male or female. However, in some rare conditions, phenotypic sex does not accurately reflect genetic sex. One such condition is **androgen insensitivity syndrome (AIS),** formerly known as **testicular feminization.** In AIS, despite an XY genotype and testes that secrete androgen, a genetic defect results in failure of the fetal cells to respond to this androgen. As in normal females, the absence of androgenic stimulation results in a female phenotype. Because individuals with AIS have female external genitalia and a blind vaginal

TABLE 21-1	Gender Identity, Gender Role, and Sexual Orientation	
TERM	**DEFINITION**	**PRESUMED ETIOLOGY**
Gender identity	Sense of self as being male or female	Differential exposure to prenatal sex hormones and genetic influences
Gender role	Expression of one's gender identity in society (e.g., choice of gender-specific clothing)	Societal expectations to conform to sexual norms
Sexual orientation	Persistent and unchanging preference for people of the same sex (homosexual) or the opposite sex (heterosexual) for love and sexual expression	Differential exposure to prenatal sex hormones and genetic influences

pouch, the disorder may not be identified during childhood. At puberty, normal breast development occurs (due in part to conversion of testosterone to estradiol); however, menstruation fails to occur and, in some individuals, the descending testes appear in the inguinal region or labia as masses. Like the body, the behavior of individuals with AIS is feminine; most have a female gender identity and gender role. Most are also heterosexual with respect to their female phenotype (Case 21-1).

In **congenital virilizing adrenal hyperplasia (CAH),** formerly called **adrenogenital syndrome,** the presence of excessive adrenal androgen secretions (resulting from 21-hydroxylase [21-OH] deficiency in more than 90% of cases) in a genetically normal (XX) female results in masculinization of the female genitalia prenatally. At birth, infants with this disorder may have enlarged phalluses and fused labia and are sometimes identified initially as males. As adults, individuals with CAH generally have a female gender identity and adopt a female gender role. The fact that about one third of these individuals have a lesbian sexual orientation suggests that early exposure to androgens may affect sexual orientation (Berenbaum, 1998; Berenbaum, 1999).

Traditionally, parents of children with ambiguous genitalia caused by these or other conditions were advised to have their child sexually reassigned early in infancy. Most such children were assigned to be female because it is easier to surgically form female than male genitalia. However, increasing evidence from these individuals as adults suggests that their gender identity does not necessarily fit with their reassigned sex. This implies that early exposure of the brain to gonadal hormones is a significant factor in gender identity. In addition, this indicates that the nature of hormonal exposure of the brain should be considered before surgically reassigning the gender of an infant.

THE PATIENT An 18-year-old woman comes to the doctor because she has discovered "large swellings" in her labia. Aside from the fact that she has never menstruated, her medical history is unremarkable. Her social history reveals that she has a boyfriend with whom she has a sexual relationship and hopes to marry. Physical observation reveals a tall, slender female with normal breast development and normal female hair distribution. Pelvic examination reveals that the vagina ends in a closed pouch. There are no Barr bodies in the buccal smear.

COMMENT This patient has androgen insensitivity syndrome (AIS). In this condition, the body cells of a fetus with an XY chromosome complement do not respond to the androgen that is produced by the testes. The fetus is not masculinized, and the resulting phenotype is female. While the body cells do not respond to androgen, they do respond to the estrogen produced by the testes and the adrenal glands at puberty, hence breast development and female hair distribution. The "swellings" that the patient has discovered are testes that have descended into the labia. There are no Barr bodies in the buccal smear because there is only one X chromosome. The patient's heterosexual orientation with respect to phenotype is typical of individuals with AIS.

TREATMENT The testes are commonly surgically removed to prevent the development of malignancy; however, there is no specific medical treatment for individuals with AIS. Psychologically, the patient should be reassured that her gender is made up of many factors other than her chromosomes. With a female gender identity and gender role, she is essentially a female and will remain that way. One difficult task facing the physician in this case is to explain to the patient that she is infertile.

Gender identity disorder

In contrast to individuals with AIS or CAH, people with **gender identity disorder (GID)**, commonly called **transgender** or **transsexual** individuals, are physically normal with respect to their biological sex. However, these people have a pervasive and persistent feeling of having been born into the body of the wrong sex. This feeling causes so much discomfort that, in adulthood, people with GID may take sex hormones and seek sex-change surgery. Although the etiology of this disorder is not known, it has been hypothesized that GID is associated with decreased availability of androgens in males and increased availability of androgens in females during the prenatal period of brain sexual differentiation. Recently it has been shown that men with GID are more likely to have older brothers (but not older sisters) than heterosexual men (Green, 2000). The mechanism of this birth order phenomenon, reported also in homosexual men (see later text), is not known. However, it may be related to a progressive maternal immune reaction to fetal testosterone or to a fetal male-specific antigen (e.g., the H-Y antigen), which leads to changes in sexual differentiation of the brain of subsequent fetuses (Blanchard, 1997; Blanchard et al., 2002).

HOMOSEXUALITY

A significant proportion of the population prefers partners of the same sex for sexual and romantic relationships. Estimates of the number of individuals with a gay or lesbian sexual orientation range widely. (There is no overarching agreement on terminology; these individuals are collectively referred to here as homosexual [American Psychological Association, 1991]). Problems with estimation occur because it can be difficult to define who fits into this category. In addition, homosexual individuals may be hesitant to identify themselves because of realistic fears of job and social discrimination. Nevertheless, most estimates are that 5 to 10% of the population (more men than women) have an exclusively homosexual sexual orientation. Many more people have a history of at least one sexual encounter leading to sexual arousal with a person of the same sex. True bisexuality—the absence of a preference for romantic and sexual relationships with people of one sex or another—is uncommon. Most people have a sexual preference.

The etiology of homosexuality

There are no ethnic differences in the occurrence of homosexuality, and social factors are not believed to play a significant role in its etiology. Some psychoanalytically oriented theories speculate that homosexuality is related to social and family factors during development; however, they currently have little clinical or research support. The most pervasive current belief is that homosexual individuals are born and not made.

Although sex hormone levels in adulthood are generally no different between homosexual and heterosexual people, early chemical influences may play a role in the etiology of homosexuality. Anatomic changes in hypothalamic nuclei resulting from alterations in levels of prenatal sex hormones in both male and female homosexuals (LeVay, 1993), and a preponderance of older brothers (see previous text) in male homosexuals has been reported. Finally, genetic factors may be involved; both markers on the X chromosome and higher concordance rates for homosexuality in monozygotic than in dizygotic twins have been demonstrated (Whitam et al., 1993).

Social considerations

In the 1970s, homosexuality was removed from the American Psychiatric Association's Diagnostic and Statistical Manual of Mental Disorders. Today, homosexuality is considered by most clinicians to be a normal variant of sexual expression. This view is supported by several factors, including absence of evidence that the homosexual population has more emotional problems or psychiatric abnormalities than the heterosexual population.

Many homosexual individuals have been married in the past and have had children. Their sexual orientation can become a legal issue in custody decisions. In particular, homosexuals have been denied custody or even access to their own children in states with laws that consider some of their sexual practices (e.g., anal sex) forms of criminal behavior (Carter &

McGoldrick, 1999). In a landmark decision in 2003, the United States Supreme court struck down all such criminal "sodomy" laws.

■ THE BIOLOGY OF SEXUALITY IN ADULTS

Men and women go through significant physical and psychological changes when they think about sex or engage in sexual activity. In the late 1960s, in groundbreaking laboratory studies, William Masters and Virginia Johnson scientifically documented the physiological changes that take place in the human male and female during sexual stimulation. The information gained from these studies has helped physicians to understand the biological events associated with sexual response, giving them tools they can use to help patients deal with sexual difficulties.

The sexual response cycle

Masters and Johnson proposed a four-stage model for sexual response in both men and women. The proposed stages of the sexual response cycle included excitement, plateau, orgasm, and resolution. The more recent Diagnostic and Statistical Manual of Mental Disorders, 4th Edition-Text Revision (DSM-IV-TR) categorizations of sexual response show similarities and differences when compared with Masters and Johnson's stages (Table 21-2). In the DSM scheme, "desire," including interest and sexual fantasies, is the first stage. The second stage, "excitement," has characteristics of the Masters and Johnson excitement and plateau stages combined. In both schemes, orgasm and resolution are the final stages. Because most sexual dysfunctions can be linked to difficulty with aspects of this cycle, understanding the physiological events of each stage can help establish a clinical perspective for these dysfunctions.

Hormonal influences on sexuality in adults

Medical conditions or medical treatments that alter circulating levels of the major gonadal hormones can have significant effects on sexual behavior in both women and men. However, the hormones that might be expected to affect sexuality are not always the ones that do. For example, in women, estrogen is only minimally involved in sexual interest. As evidence for this, menopause, which involves cessation of ovarian estrogen production, is usually not associated with a reduced sex drive if a woman's general health is good. Estrogen is, however, involved in maintaining the physiological condition of the vagina and external genitalia. Thus, menopause can result in vaginal thinning and dryness, making sexual activity uncomfortable or even painful. This can lead to avoidance of sexual activity. Although estrogen or estrogen-progesterone replacement therapy (ERT) can reverse these vaginal problems and reduce the incidence of hot flashes, it apparently provides little or no overall benefit to health-related quality of life (Hays et al., 2003). Furthermore, association

TABLE 21-2 Stages of the Sexual Response Cycle

DESIRE (DSM-IV-TR MODEL)

- Interest in sexual activities
- Presence of sexual fantasies
- Problems in this stage are associated with hypoactive sexual desire disorder and sexual aversion disorder

EXCITEMENT

- Penile and clitoral erection
- Labial swelling
- Vaginal lubrication (watery exudate caused by vasocongestion)
- Tenting effect (rising of the uterus in the pelvic cavity)
- Nipple erection (both sexes)
- Increased pulse, blood pressure, and respiration (both sexes)
- Problems in this stage are associated with female sexual arousal disorder and male erectile disorder

PLATEAU (MASTERS AND JOHNSON MODEL)

- Increased size and upward movement of the testes
- Secretion of a few drops of sperm-containing fluid
- Flushing of the chest and face (both sexes)
- Contraction of the outer third of the vagina, forming the orgasmic platform (enlargement of the upper third of the vagina)
- Further increase in pulse, blood pressure, and respiration (both sexes)
- Problems in this stage are associated with premature ejaculation

ORGASM

- Forcible expulsion of seminal fluid
- Contractions of the uterus and vagina
- Contractions of the anal sphincter (both sexes)
- Further increase in pulse, blood pressure, and respiration (both sexes)
- Problems in this stage are associated with male and female orgasmic disorder

RESOLUTION

- Muscle relaxation
- In men, a refractory, or resting, period (length varies by age and physical condition) when restimulation is not possible; little or no refractory period in women
- Return of the sexual, muscular, and cardiovascular systems to the prestimulated state over 10–15 minutes

DSM-IV-TR, Diagnostic and Statistical Manual of Mental Disorders, 4th Edition-Text Revision.

of ERT with increased risk of breast cancer (when combined with progesterone) (Chlebowski et al., 2003; and see Chapter 3) and a slightly increased risk of dementia (Rapp et al., 2003) limits the use of hormone replacement therapy for symptoms of menopause for most women. At least one of the antidepressants, paroxetine (Paxil), may be effective in reducing postmenopausal symptoms such as hot flashes (Stearns et el., 2003).

Testosterone, secreted by the adrenal glands (as well as the ovaries and testes) throughout adult life, appears to play a major role in sexual interest and drive in women as well as in men. Addition of testosterone to ERT or use of testosterone alone may improve sexual functioning in some postmenopausal women (Vastag, 2003).

In men, testosterone levels generally are higher than necessary to maintain normal sexual functioning. Psychological and physical stress, however, can decrease these levels. Availability of testosterone can also be reduced via hypothalamic feedback mechanisms by medical treatment with hormones (e.g., estrogens, progesterone, or antiandrogens) that are used in the treatment of prostate and other androgen-dependent cancers.

Circulating gonadal hormones can also have significant effects on emotion in women and in men. For example, some women experience depression, anxiety, irritability, lethargy, and food cravings during the premenstrual phase but not at other times during the menstrual cycle. This symptom picture, called **premenstrual dysphoric disorder** (PMDD) in the appendix of the DSM-IV-TR, is commonly known as **premenstrual syndrome** or **PMS.** Postulated hormonal causes of PMS include alterations in the estrogen/progesterone ratio and hormonal effects on neurotransmitters such as serotonin. At least two selective serotonin reuptake inhibitors (SSRIs), fluoxetine (Sarafem) and sertraline (Zoloft), have been approved for the treatment of PMS (see Chapter 19), but they may have negative effects on sexual function (see later text). In men, normal temporal fluctuations in testosterone levels are associated with changes in emotions. In addition, people who take androgenic steroids to increase muscle mass can show not only increased irritability and aggressiveness, but also confusion and even psychosis. Withdrawal from these agents can result in severe depression.

■ SEXUAL DYSFUNCTION

Biological, psychological, and interpersonal factors or a combination of these elements can lead to sexual problems. Biological factors include unidentified general medical conditions such as diabetes, or post-surgical complications such as pelvic adhesions. Psychological causes of sexual dysfunctions include relationship problems, stress related to employment, or underlying mood or anxiety disorders. In some cases, sexual dysfunction results from a traumatic sexual experience, such as rape or sexual abuse in childhood. Rarely, sexual dysfunctions are primary; that is, they are pervasive and have always been present. Most commonly, they are secondary and occur after an interval when sexual functioning has been relatively normal.

Taking a sexual history

The greatest impediment to helping patients with their sexual problems is that the doctor may never find out about the problems. It is not surprising that practicing physicians who are uncomfortable about sexual issues have very few patients reporting sexual problems. Patients are often ill at ease about bringing up sexual issues; they may instead visit the doctor to report vague physical symptoms, such as fatigue or headache. Whenever a patient's complaint could be associated in some way with sexuality, it is the charge of the doctor to initiate a discussion with the patient.

Because talking about sexuality is difficult for most people, the physician should establish a comfortable relationship with the patient before asking specific questions about sexuality. It is also important, if possible, to allow such questions to arise in the course of the clinical interview. In asking patients about current and past relationships, questions about sexuality naturally follow. It is usually better to start with general questions and then proceed to specific ones. For example, the doctor might reflect on something the patient has just said: "You say that you have been married for 20 years. Tell me about how these years have been for you and your spouse overall." Later on the doctor can move to questions such as, "How has your sexual relationship been over these years?"

No matter what their own sexual beliefs, physicians must avoid being judgmental. Patients quickly notice this negative attitude and then fail to reveal important information. In addition, physicians should not assume anything about a patient's sexuality. The middle-aged woman being questioned about her preferred contraceptive method may in fact have never had sexual intercourse.

Homosexual patients will be a part of every doctor's medical practice and are as likely as heterosexual patients to have relationship problems. Questions about sexual orientation pose a particular challenge for many doctors. Generally, until you know someone's sexual orientation, it is best to use neutral terms such as "partner" or "relationship" to describe a person's significant other. When asking specific questions about sexual orientation, it is usually best to ask patients to describe their close relationships and then ask if they have been sexually active with men, women, or both.

Homosexuality itself is not a dysfunction and there is no "treatment." Most individuals are comfortable with their sexual orientation, but some are not. In the DSM-IV-TR, sexual disorder not otherwise specified (NOS) includes persistent and marked distress about sexual orientation. Although some psychiatrists believe that sexual orientation can be changed with intensive therapy, most agree that, like gender identity, sexual orientation is pervasive and unchangeable. Therefore, the most effective psychological intervention for individuals unhappy with their homosexuality is aimed at helping them become more comfortable with and accepting of their sexual orientation.

Classification of sexual dysfunctions

DSM-IV-TR classifications of sexual dysfunctions include disorders of desire, arousal, and orgasm. They are used only when the individual has no identifiable physiological or relationship problem that could explain the symptoms. The sexual desire disorders are **hypoactive sexual desire** and **sexual aversion;** the sexual arousal disorders are **female sexual arousal disorder** and **male erectile disorder;** the orgasmic disorders are **male and female orgasmic disorders** and **premature ejaculation.** Sexual dysfunctions also include the sexual pain disorders **dyspareunia** and **vaginismus** (Table 21-3).

Drugs and sexuality

Substances, both legal and illicit, cause changes in sexual function via their action on neurotransmitter systems. For example, because dopamine has stimulatory effects on sexuality, agents that decrease its availability, such as dopamine 2 (D_2) receptor antagonists (antipsychotics), have negative effects on sexual functioning. In addition, because dopamine normally inhibits prolactin release, treatment with antipsychotics results in increased prolactin, which in turn has negative effects on sexuality, such as suppression of libido and erectile difficulties. Stimulants such as amphetamines and cocaine increase sexual interest and performance primarily by stimulating dopaminergic systems.

Serotonin tends to have negative effects on sexuality. Antidepressants (particularly the SSRIs) that increase serotonin availability decrease sexual interest and have the specific and often uncomfortable effect of delaying orgasm in both men and women. On a positive note, this side effect makes the SSRIs useful in the treatment of premature ejaculation.

Norepinephrine also affects sexual functioning. Antihypertensives that act by either increasing central norepinephrine α (α-adrenergic agonists) or decreasing norepinephrine β (β-adrenergic blockers) reduce libido and cause erectile dysfunction. When compared with these antihypertensive agents, the angiotensin-converting enzyme inhibitors (e.g., captopril [Capoten]) are less likely to cause sexual problems. Alterations in libido, erection, orgasm, ejaculation, and other sexual functions by prescription drugs that affect neurotransmitter systems are described in Table 21-4.

In the short term, drugs of abuse such as alcohol and marijuana can decrease psychological inhibitions and enhance sexual interest and performance. However, with long-term use, most drugs of abuse ultimately decrease sexual functioning. For example, because the liver degrades circulating estrogens, liver damage caused by long-term alcohol use ultimately results in increased estrogen availability and concomitant sexual dysfunction in men. Chronic use of marijuana may reduce testosterone

TABLE 21-3 Characteristics of the DSM-IV-TR Sexual Dysfunctions

DISORDER	CHARACTERISTICS
Hypoactive sexual desire	■ Decreased interest in sexual activity ■ May be normal individual variation in desire
Sexual aversion disorder	■ Aversion to and avoidance of sexual activity
Female sexual arousal disorder	■ Inability to maintain vaginal lubrication until the sex act is completed despite adequate physical stimulation ■ Reported in as many as 20% of women
Male erectile disorder (commonly called "impotence")	■ Lifelong or primary (rare): Has never had an erection sufficient for penetration ■ Acquired or secondary (the most common of all male sexual disorders): Current inability to maintain erections despite normal erections in the past ■ Situational (common): Difficulty maintaining erections in some situations, but not others ■ In men with erectile disorder, the presence of morning erections, erections during masturbation, or erections during rapid eye movement sleep suggests a psychological rather than a physical cause
Orgasmic disorder (male and female)	■ Lifelong: no previous orgasm ■ Acquired: Current inability to achieve orgasm despite adequate genital stimulation (normal orgasms in the past) ■ Reported in more women than men
Premature ejaculation	■ Ejaculation before the man would like it to occur ■ Short or absent plateau phase of the sexual response cycle ■ Usually accompanied by anxiety ■ Second most common of all male sexual disorders
Vaginismus	■ Painful spasm of the outer third of the vagina ■ Makes intercourse or pelvic examination difficult
Dyspareunia	■ Persistent pain associated with sexual intercourse ■ Much more common in women; can occur in men

DSM-IV-TR, Diagnostic and Statistical Manual of Mental Disorders, 4th Edition-Text Revision.
Adapted from Fadem, B. (2000). *Behavioral science* (3rd ed.) (p. 179). Philadelphia: Lippincott, Williams & Wilkins.

TABLE 21-4	Effects of Some Prescription Drugs on Neurotransmitter Activity and Sexuality	
EFFECT	DRUG TYPE (REPRESENTATIVE AGENT)	ASSOCIATED NEUROTRANSMITTER (↑ INCREASED OR ↓ DECREASED AVAILABILITY)
Reduced libido	Antidepressant (fluoxetine) Antihypertensive (propranolol) Antihypertensive (methyldopa)	↑ Serotonin ↓ Norepinephrine β ↑ Central norepinephrine α
Increased libido	Antiparkinsonian (l-dopa)	↑ Dopamine
Erectile dysfunction	Antihypertensive (propranolol) Antihypertensive (methyldopa) Antidepressant (fluoxetine) Antipsychotic (thioridazine)	↓ Norepinephrine β ↑ Central norepinephrine α ↑ Serotonin ↓ Dopamine
Vaginal dryness	Antihistamine (diphenhydramine) Anticholinergic (atropine)	↓ Histamine ↓ Acetylcholine
Inhibited orgasm (in men and women)	Antidepressant (fluoxetine)	↑ Serotonin
Priapism	Antidepressant (trazodone)	↑ Serotonin
Inhibited ejaculation	Antidepressant (fluoxetine) Antipsychotic (thioridazine)	↑ Serotonin ↓ Dopamine

Adapted from Fadem, B. (2000). *Behavioral science* (3rd ed.) (p. 183). Philadelphia: Lippincott Williams & Wilkins.

levels in men and pituitary gonadotropin levels in women. Opiates such as heroin and, to a lesser extent, methadone are associated with suppressed libido, retarded ejaculation, and failure to ejaculate.

▪ TREATMENT OF SEXUAL DYSFUNCTION

In the past, patients with sexual problems were commonly referred to sex therapists for treatment. In recent years, a growing trend is for physicians to treat the sexual problems of their patients rather than to refer them. Treatments available to physicians include behavioral, medical, and surgical techniques.

Behavioral techniques

Behavioral techniques used to treat sexual dysfunctions are aimed primarily at decreasing the performance anxiety often associated with sexual activity. For example, in one type of behavioral technique, **sensate-focus exercises,** patients are instructed to concentrate on and to learn nongenital means of sexual arousal. To do this, stimulation of the sensations of touch, sight, smell, and sound rather than of genital sensations are employed during sexual activity. At the same time, psychological pressure to achieve an erection or orgasm is decreased (Case 21-2). Relaxation techniques, hypnosis, and systematic desensitization (see Chapter 9) are also used to reduce anxiety associated with sexual performance. Masturbation is another treatment technique that may be recommended to help the patient learn what stimuli and techniques are most effective in achieving sexual arousal and orgasm. The patient can then instruct his or her partner in these techniques.

In a behavioral method used to treat premature ejaculation (the **squeeze technique**), a man is taught to concentrate on and identify the sensations that just precede orgasm. Once he can identify these sensations, the man asks his partner to exert pressure on the coronal ridge of the glans on both sides of the penis. This pressure results in reduction in the erection by about one-third, and the man gains more time until orgasm.

Medical and surgical treatment

Medical and surgical treatment techniques are effective in treating sexual problems. For example, as noted, SSRIs are useful to treat premature ejaculation because they delay orgasm. Systemic administration of opioid antagonists (e.g., naltrexone) and vasodilators (e.g., yohimbine) have been used to treat erectile dysfunction.

Sildenafil citrate (Viagra), a pharmacologic agent that has revolutionized the treatment of erectile dysfunction, is now being used to treat at least 11 million American men. The drug works by blocking phosphodiester (PDE) 5, an enzyme that destroys cyclic guanosine monophosphate (cGMP), a vasodilator secreted in the penis with sexual stimulation. Thus, the degradation of cGMP is slowed and the erection persists. Sildenafil has not shown efficacy in treating female sexual arousal disorder. Although sildenafil has a good safety profile, it is contraindicated in men who take nitrates because of synergistic hypotensive effects. Newer PDE-5 inhibitors with greater potency and selectivity than sildenafil, such as **vardenafil (Levitra, Nuviva)** and **tadalafil (Cialis)** have recently been developed. Another new agent, apomorphine hydrochloride (**Uprima**), works to increase sexual interest and performance by increasing the availability of dopamine in the brain.

Techniques such as intracorporeal injection of vasodilators (e.g., papaverine, phentolamine) and prostaglandin E_1 have also been used to treat erectile dysfunction. Erectile dysfunction in men who do not respond to these interventions can be treated using surgical implantation of prosthetic

THE PATIENT   A man in his mid-50s tells his physician that, for the first time in his life, he is having trouble maintaining an erection during sexual intercourse with his wife of 20 years. Physical examination and laboratory values are all within the normal range. In discussing the history of the problem, the man reveals that the problem began 6 weeks previously after an office party at which he had "too much to drink." Since then he has had erectile difficulty even when he has not had a drink.

COMMENT   This patient has secondary or acquired erectile disorder. Although drinking alcohol caused his initial problem, he now has problems with erection even when he is not drinking. By classical conditioning (see Chapter 9), this man has associated sexual activity with erectile dysfunction. The resulting anxiety due to this negative association now leads to difficulty maintaining an erection.

TREATMENT   The doctor should help the patient reduce the performance anxiety he has developed with respect to sexual intercourse. One way to do this is to instruct the patient to forego actual intercourse and concentrate on nongenital, pleasurable physical sensations in romantic situations with his wife (e.g., sensate focus exercises). Sildenafil (Viagra) may also be used to demonstrate to the patient that he is able to maintain an erection.

devices, e.g., penile implants. However, in diabetic men, who form a large percentage of patients with erectile dysfunction, surgical treatment is complicated by greater difficulties in wound-healing and greater susceptibility to infection.

■ SEXUALITY IN PHYSICAL ILLNESS AND AGING

Physical illness and sexual function

Common medical illnesses, such as heart disease and diabetes, more common in middle aged and elderly people, often have effects on sexuality.

Men who have a history of myocardial infarction (MI) are likely to experience erectile dysfunction, and both men and women who have a history of MI commonly show decreased sexual interest. Although this decreased interest can be a side effect of cardiac medication, it also results from the realistic fear that sexual activity will provoke another heart attack. Generally, post-MI patients are counseled that if exercise that raises the heart rate to 110 to 130 beats per minute (i.e., exertion equal to climbing two flights of stairs) can be tolerated without severe shortness of breath or chest pain, sexual activity can be resumed after a heart attack. Sexual positions that produce the least exertion in the patient (e.g., the partner in the superior position) are the safest after MI.

Diabetic patients also are likely to have sexual problems. Up to one half of diabetic men (more commonly older patients) have erectile dysfunction. Orgasm and ejaculation are less likely to be affected than erection in these patients. Sexual problems generally occur several years after diabetes is diagnosed, but they may be the first symptoms of the disease. The major causes of erectile dysfunction in men with diabetes are vascular changes and diabetic neuropathy caused by damage to blood vessels and nerve tissue resulting from hyperglycemia. Poor metabolic control of diabetes is related to an increased incidence of sexual problems; patients who carefully control their blood sugar levels have fewer sexual problems. Psychological discomfort associated with repeated "failure" to gain an erection may exacerbate the erectile problems associated with diabetes.

Spinal cord injuries in men commonly cause erectile and orgasmic dysfunction, retrograde ejaculation (into the bladder), reduced testosterone levels, and decreased fertility. As with other physical functions, sexual function is associated with the level of spinal cord injury. Injuries higher up on the cord cause more dysfunction than lower-level injuries. Although women are much less likely then men to sustain spinal cord injuries, such injuries can cause decreased vaginal lubrication and pelvic vasocongestion, and decreased likelihood of orgasm. In addition, when compared to men, spinal cord injuries in women are less likely to adversely affect fertility.

Aging and sexuality

Although there is a belief in our youth-oriented culture that elderly people are asexual, this is far from true. Despite negative physical changes, societal attitudes, and loss of sexual partners due to illness or death, sexual interest does not invariably decrease with age. Rather, many older people are interested in sexuality and, when partners are available, engage in romantic, social, and physical relationships.

As in younger people, continuing social and sexual relationships are associated with good mental and physical health in old age. However, the physical changes of aging alter sexual functioning. In men, these alterations include slower erection, diminished intensity of ejaculation, and longer refractory period. The aging man may also need more direct genital stimulation to achieve erection and orgasm than he did in the past. In aging women, the vaginal dryness and discomfort associated with the absence of estrogen can be relieved with local application of moisturizing agents.

HIV and sexuality

More than 33 million people in the world are infected with HIV, a number that continues to increase. About 95% of HIV-infected people live in Africa, Asia, and Eastern Europe; less than 1 million infected people live in North America. Fewer than 2 million infected people live in Latin America and the Caribbean, and approximately 0.5 million live in Western Europe.

An important source of HIV infection is sexual activity. Of different sexual practices, anal intercourse is riskiest for transmitting HIV (Table

21-5) because of the increased likelihood of tissue tearing leading to contact with the blood supply, Patients who are HIV positive must protect their sexual partners from infection. If they fail to do so (e.g., do not use condoms) and refuse to inform their partners of the risk, the physician can inform threatened partners (see also Chapter 26).

Progression of HIV-associated illness is different between men and women. If all other conditions are equal, a woman with the same HIV viral load as a man is likely to develop the symptoms of AIDS sooner than the man (Sterling et al., 2001).

■ PARAPHILIAS

Paraphilias involve the preferential use of unusual objects of sexual desire or engagement in unusual sexual activity (Table 21-6). To fit DSM-IV-TR criteria, the behavior must continue over a period of at least 6 months and cause impairment in occupational or social functioning.

A person has a paraphilia when he has acted on his desires, is preoccupied about them, or has problems forming close relationships with others because of them. Fantasies are not paraphilias; rather, they often are normal components of human sexuality.

TABLE 21-5	Route of Contact and Chance of Contracting HIV
INFECTION ROUTE	**APPROXIMATE CHANCE OF CONTRACTING HIV**
Sexual activity with an HIV-infected Person	
Anal intercourse	1 in 10 to 1,600
Vaginal intercourse with an infected man	1 in 200 to 2,000
Vaginal intercourse with an infected woman	1 in 700 to 3,000
Direct contact with blood of an HIV-infected person	
Transfusion	1 in 1.05 (95 in 100)
Needle sharing	1 in 150
Needle stick	1 in 200
HIV-positive mother to fetus	
Mother to fetus (mother not taking AZT)	1 in 4
Mother to fetus (mother taking AZT)	<1 in 10

AZT, zidovudine.
Adapted with permission from Royce, R.A., Seña, R. A., Cates, W., & Cohen, M. S. (1997). Sexual transmission of HIV. *N Engl J Med, 336,* 1072–1078.

TABLE 21-6 DSM-IV-TR Paraphilias

PARAPHILIA	SEXUAL GRATIFICATION OBTAINED BY
Exhibitionism	■ Revealing one's genitals to unsuspecting women ■ Shocking unsuspecting women
Fetishism	■ Contact with certain inanimate objects, such as shoes or rubber sheets. ■ In transvestic fetishism (exclusive to heterosexual men), wearing women's clothing, particularly underclothing
Frotteurism	■ Rubbing the penis against a woman ■ The woman is not consenting and not aware
Pedophilia	■ Engaging in fantasies or actual behaviors with children under age 14 years, of the opposite or same sex ■ The pedophile must be at least 16 years of age and 4 or 5 years older than the victim ■ Most common paraphilia
Sexual masochism	■ Receiving physical pain ■ Being humiliated
Sexual sadism	■ Giving physical pain or humiliation
Voyeurism	■ Secretly watching other people (often with binoculars) undressing or engaging in sexual activity
Paraphilias not otherwise specified	■ Coprophilia: Engaging in sexual activity involving feces ■ Klismaphilia: Engaging in sexual activity involving enemas ■ Necrophilia: Having sexual activity with dead bodies ■ Partialism: Engaging in sexual activity involving only parts of the body ■ Telephone scatologia: Making phone calls to unsuspecting women in order to involve them in conversations of a sexual nature ■ Urophilia: Engaging in sexual activity involving urine ■ Zoophilia: Engaging in sexual activity with animals

DSM-IV-TR, Diagnostic and Statistical Manual of Mental Disorders, 4th Edition-Text Revision.

The etiology of the paraphilias includes developmental psychological disturbances and possibly genetic and hormonal influences. Paraphilias are seen almost exclusively in men.

Pharmacologic treatment includes antiandrogens and female sex hormones for paraphilias characterized by excessive sexual interest and activity.

REVIEW QUESTIONS

1. A 40-year-old woman has been taking a selective serotonin reuptake inhibitor (SSRI) for treatment of depression for the past 4 months. Her mood is now normal but she reports that she is having sexual problems. Which of the following sexual dysfunctions is this woman most likely to report?

   (A) Desire disorder

   (B) Sexual aversion

   (C) Vaginismus

   (D) Dyspareunia

   (E) Orgasmic disorder

2. A 20-year-old male college student says that he has always felt as if he was "really a woman inside." He relates that he played with girls' toys and games as a child and always played the bride in "marriage games." The student states that he is sexually attracted to heterosexual men but is definitely not gay. He states that he wants to have his penis and testicles removed as soon as possible and have surgery to create a vagina and breasts. Physical examination and laboratory tests reveal no abnormalities. The final diagnosis for this patient is most likely to be

   (A) adrenogenital syndrome

   (B) androgen insensitivity syndrome

   (C) gender identity disorder

   (D) transvestic fetishism

   (E) homosexuality

3. A 72-year-old married patient reports erectile dysfunction. The man, who is in the early stages of Alzheimer's disease, has mild hypertension that does not require pharmacological treatment. He also has Parkinson's disease that is well controlled with L-dopa. The patient also relates that he drinks two martinis each evening and smokes two packs of cigarettes a day. His sexual dysfunction is most likely to be associated with his

   (A) Alzheimer's disease

   (B) hypertension

   (C) L-dopa

   (D) alcohol drinking

   (E) cigarette smoking

4. Contractions of the anal sphincter are most likely to occur in which stage of the sexual response cycle and in men, women, or both men and women?

   (A) Excitement phase: men only

(B) Plateau phase: men only

(C) Orgasm phase: men only

(D) Excitement phase: men and women

(E) Plateau phase: men and women

(F) Orgasm phase: men and women

(G) Excitement phase: women only

(H) Plateau phase: women only

(I) Orgasm phase: women only

5. A 45-year-old man states that he recently developed a penile discharge and has begun to experience discomfort with urination. He states that he is concerned that he acquired an infection from a recent sexual encounter. To identify this patient's sexual orientation, which of the following is the best question?

   (A) "Are you heterosexual or homosexual?"

   (B) "Are you mainly gay or mainly straight?"

   (C) "Are you exclusively gay or exclusively straight?"

   (D) "Do you have sex with men, women, or both men and women?"

   (E) "Would you describe yourself as homosexual?"

ANSWERS AND EXPLANATIONS

1-E. Although they may be associated with loss of libido, selective serotonin reuptake inhibitors (SSRIs) are most commonly linked to delayed or absent orgasm (orgasmic disorder). The sexual pain disorders dyspareunia and vaginismus are not specifically associated with SSRI treatment.

2-C. The final diagnosis for this patient who has always felt as if he was really a woman in a normal male body is most likely to be gender identity disorder. Adrenogenital syndrome is caused by excessive exposure to adrenal androgens developmentally; transvestic fetishists are heterosexual men who wear women's underclothing for sexual pleasure. People with androgen insensitivity syndrome are genetic males with female bodies (with which they are content) and sexual interest in men. Homosexual men have sexual interest in men but have a male gender identity and no desire to change their physical sex.

3-D. This patient's sexual dysfunction is most likely to be associated with his alcohol drinking. Cigarette smoking is less likely than alcohol to affect sexual function. The medications used to treat hypertension, rarely the condition itself, cause erectile problems. This patient is not taking antihypertensive medication. Alzheimer's disease has little effect on sexuality in the early stages; patients often retain their sexual ability long into the illness. L-dopa tends to increase rather than decrease sexual interest and performance by elevating dopamine availability.

4-F. Anal sphincter contractions occur during the orgasm phase of the sexual response cycle in both men and women.

5-D. The most correct way to determine the sexual orientation of this patient is to ask him, "Do you have sex with men, women, or both?"

REFERENCES

American Psychiatric Association. (2001). *Diagnostic and statistical manual of mental disorders* (4th ed., text revision) (pp. 535–582). Washington, DC: American Psychiatric Association.

American Psychological Association. Committee on Lesbian and Gay Concerns. (1991). Avoiding heterosexual bias in language. *Am Psychol, 46,* 973–974.

Berenbaum, S. A. (1998). How hormones affect behavioral and neural development: Introduction to the special issue on "gonadal hormones and sex differences in behavior." *Dev Neuropsychol, 14,* 175–196.

Berenbaum, S. A. (1999). Effects of early androgen on sex-typed activities and interests in adolescents with congenital adrenal hyperplasia. *Horm Behav, 35,* 102–110.

Blanchard, R. (1997). Birth order and sibling sex ratio in homosexual versus heterosexual males and females. *Annu Rev Sex Res, 8,* 27–67.

Blanchard, R., Zucker, K. J., Cavacas, A., Allen, S., Bradley, S. J., & Schachter, D. C. (2002). Fraternal birth order and birth weight in probably prehomosexual feminine boys. *Horm Behav, 41,* 321–327.

Carter, E. A., & McGoldrick, M. (1999). *The expanded family life cycle: Individual, family, and social perspectives* (3rd ed.) (p. 541). Boston: Allyn and Bacon.

Chlebowski, R. T., Hendrix, S. L., Langer, R. D., Stefanick, M. L., Gass, M., Lane, D., et al., for the WHI Investigators. (2003). Influence of estrogen plus progestin on breast cancer and mammography in healthy postmenopausal women. The Women's Health Initiative Randomized Trial. *JAMA,* 289:3243–3253.

Goy, R. W., & McEwen, B. S. (1980). *Sexual differentiation of the brain.* London: Oxford University Press.

Green, R. (2000). Birth order and ratio of brothers to sisters in transsexuals. *Psychol Med, 30,* 789–795.

Halpern, D. F. (2000). *Sex differences in cognitive abilities* (3rd ed.). Mahwah, NJ: Lawrence Ehrlbaum Associates.

Hays, J. H., Ockene, J. K., Brunner, R. L., Kotchen, J. M., Manson, J. E, Patterson, R. E., et al., for the Women's Health Initiative Investigators. (2003). Effects of estrogen plus progestin on health-related quality of life. *N Engl J Med, 348,* 1839–1854.

Institute of Medicine. (2001). Exploring the biological contributions to human health: Does sex matter? Washington, DC: National Academy Press.

LeVay, S. (1993). *The sexual brain.* Cambridge, Massachusetts: MIT Press.

Leiblum, S. R., & Rosen, R. C. (2000). *Principles and practices of sex therapy* (3rd ed.). New York: Guilford Press.

Masters, W., & Johnson, V. (1966). *Human sexual response.* Boston: Little, Brown.

Rapp, S. R., Espeland, M. A, Shumaker, S. A., Henderson, V. W., Brunner, R. L., Manson, J. E., et al., for the WHIMS Investigators. (2003). Effect of estrogen plus progestin on global cognitive function in postmenopausal women: the Women's Health Initiative Memory Study: A randomized controlled trial. *JAMA, 289,* 2663–2672.

Rotheram-Borus, M. J. (1999). HIV risk among homosexual, bisexual and heterosexual male and female youths. *Arch Sex Behav, 28,* 159–177.

Rowland, D., Greenleaf, W., Dorfman, L., & Davidson, J. (1993). Aging and sexual function in men. *Arch Sex Behav, 22,* 545–557.

Seña, R. A., Cates, W., & Cohen, M. S. (1997). Sexual transmission of HIV. *N Engl J Med, 336,* 102–107.

Stearns, V., Beebe, K. L., Iyengar, M., & Dube, E. (2003). Paroxetine controlled release in the treatment of menopausal hot flashes: A randomized controlled trial. *JAMA, 289,* 2827–2834

Sterling T. R., Vlahov, D., Astemborski, J., Hoover, D. R., Margolick, J. B., & Quinn, T. C. (2001). Initial plasma HIV-1 RNA levels and progression to AIDS in women and men. *N Engl J Med, 344,* 720–725.

Vastag, B. (2003). Many questions, few answers for testosterone replacement therapy. *JAMA, 289,* 971–972.

Whitam, F. L., Diamond, M., Martin, J. (1993). Homosexual orientation in twins: A report on 61 pairs and 3 triplet sets. *Arch Sex Behav, 22,* 187–206.

Violence, Impulse Control Disorders, and Abuse

22

T he catastrophic events of September 11, 2001 have led to increased public understanding that all citizens are potential victims of violence. This awareness has resulted in heightened interest in identifying the variables that influence and strategies that can reduce the likelihood of not only terrorism, but also of more common examples of violent behavior such as fighting and abuse.

There are significant distinctions between types of violent behavior. **Fighting** is physical or psychological aggression that occurs between people presumed to be equally matched. In contrast, **abuse** is physical or psychological aggression (or neglect) carried out by people with physical, social, or financial power over weaker or more vulnerable individuals, such as children or the elderly. Whatever the type of violence, physicians and other health professionals play a central role in dealing with its physical and emotional consequences.

DETERMINANTS OF VIOLENCE

Developing methods to predict which individuals will ultimately show violent behavior is of significant public interest. One way to do this is to identify the social and biological factors associated with the display of aggression.

Social determinants of violence

Certain social factors in childhood can predict violence in adulthood. Children at risk for showing aggressive behavior in the future are likely to have had repeated household moves and school changes. Their parents are also likely to have shown criminal behavior, to have abused drugs and alcohol, and to have physically or sexually abused these children. These children also typically have a history of harming animals, have low intelligence, and have trouble delaying gratification.

For many years, it has been noted that children exposed to violence on television are more likely to be violent toward others in adulthood. It was recently demonstrated that the childhood television–future violence association exists even when environmental characteristics such as neglectful parenting (associated with both aggressive behavior and excessive television viewing) are controlled (Johnson et al., 2002).

A significant predictor of future violence is the previous display of violence. Individuals who have assaulted others or who have been arrested for violent behavior are therefore at higher risk. Poverty is also associated with violent behavior. Homicide occurs more often in low socioeconomic populations (see Chapter 20) and, in the 15- to 24-year-old age group, it is the leading and second-leading cause of death in African-American and white males, respectively. Availability of firearms is also a risk factor for violence. At least half of all homicides result from guns.

Biological determinants of violence

In most animal species, males are more aggressive than females. This sex difference is associated with higher levels of androgenic steroids in males (Briganti et al., 2003; Goy & McEwen, 1980). The effects of androgens on aggression in humans are not as clear. However, men, particularly those in their teens or early twenties, are more likely to be violent than women. Most perpetrators and victims of homicide are men. Women are responsible for fewer than 7% of homicides that occur during the commission of a crime (felony murder) and for about 36% of homicides involving an intimate partner (Table 22-1).

Irregularities in the brain have been associated with aggressive behavior. Violent people commonly have a history of head injury or show abnormal electroencephalogram (EEG) readings. Lesions of the temporal lobes, frontal

TABLE 22-1 Gender and Homicide

| | VICTIMS | | OFFENDERS | |
	MALE	FEMALE	MALE	FEMALE
All Homicides	76.4%	23.6%	87.9%	12.1%
Victim/offender relationship				
Intimate	37.9%	62.1%	63.7%	36.3%
Family	52.5%	47.5%	70.2%	29.8%
Infanticide	54.5%	45.5%	61.2%	38.8%
Eldercide	58.3%	41.7%	85.4%	14.6%
Circumstances				
Felony murder	77.9%	22.1%	93.4%	6.6%
Sex related	19.1%	80.9%	93.4%	6.6%
Drug related	90.1%	9.9%	95.8%	4.2%
Gang related	94.4%	5.6%	98.4%	1.6%
Argument	78.3%	21.7%	85.2%	14.8%
Workplace	78.3%	21.7%	92.3%	7.7%
Weapon				
Gun homicide	82.4%	17.6%	90.4%	9.6%
Arson	56.5%	43.5%	79.6%	20.4%
Poison	54.5%	45.5%	63.0%	37.0%
Multiple victims or offenders				
Multiple victims	62.5%	37.5%	93.7%	6.3%
Multiple offenders	85.4%	14.6%	91.7%	8.3%

Reprinted with permission from U.S. Department of Justice. (2002). *Uniform crime reports. Crime in the United States, 1976–2000. Homicide trends.* Washington, DC: Bureau of Justice Statistics.

lobes, and hypothalamus, as well as abnormal activity in the prepiriform area and amygdala, are associated with increased aggression. As further evidence of a role for the amygdala, damage to this structure results in the Klüver-Bucy syndrome, which includes decreased display of aggression (see Table 5–2).

Among the neurotransmitters, dopamine is associated with increased aggression. Patients with mental illnesses associated with elevated availability of dopamine may show increased aggressive behavior. For example, psychotic schizophrenic patients may become violent when they are experiencing "command" hallucinations or paranoid delusions (see Chapter 12), and bipolar patients typically show irritability and rage during manic episodes (see Chapter 13). Gamma-aminobutyric acid (GABA) and serotonin are associated with decreased aggression. Low levels of the serotonin metabolite 5-hydroxyindoleacetic acid (5-HIAA) are seen in the body fluids of impulsively violent people (see Chapter 4).

The effects of substances of abuse on the likelihood of violent behavior may be explained in part by these neurotransmitter effects (see also Chapter 23). For example, stimulants such as cocaine, which increase dopamine availability, can precipitate combative, violent behavior. In contrast, sedatives such as benzodiazepines and barbiturates, which increase levels of GABA, tend to inhibit aggression. The relaxation and absence of violence associated with the use of d-lysergic acid diethylamide (LSD) may be due in part to the drug's ability to increase serotonin availability.

Other drugs of abuse may affect aggressive behavior through their effects on peptide neurotransmitters. Specifically, opiates tend to reduce aggressiveness; heroin users are unlikely to be violent when intoxicated. In contrast, phencyclidine (PCP) use is associated with increased aggression, an effect that may be attributable to increased activity of the excitatory neurotransmitter glutamate.

■ IMPULSE CONTROL DISORDERS

The impulse control disorders include intermittent explosive disorder, pyromania, kleptomania, pathological gambling, and trichotillomania. They are characterized by irresistible urges to commit harmful or illogical acts. Most impulse control disorders are chronic and lifelong, and some lead to serious financial and legal problems.

Not all impulse control disorders involve violent behavior. The group is discussed here because, like many people who show violent behavior, patients with impulse control disorders cannot resist engaging in negative behavior. These patients are also likely to have experienced family dysfunction in childhood and life stress in adulthood. In these disorders, increased tension usually exists before the behavior occurs, followed by relief or pleasure after the behavior is completed.

Intermittent explosive disorder

Intermittent explosive disorder (IED) is characterized by episodes in which an individual loses self-control and attacks another person without adequate cause. This disorder, formerly called "episodic dyscontrol syndrome," is more common in men, and it usually begins in the late teens or early twenties.

The differential diagnosis of IED includes alcohol or drug intoxication, psychosis, and dementia. In contrast to patients who are violent because of substance abuse, patients with IED often show **soft neurological signs** (minor neurological findings such as poor balance or mild incoordination) and other nonspecific evidence of cerebral dysfunction. Unlike the psychotic or demented patient, in IED, there is no loss of touch with reality.

Other differential diagnoses of IED include conduct disorder/antisocial personality disorder (see Chapter 25) or dissociative disorder (see Chapter 18). A single episode of explosive behavior occurring in conjunction with dissociative symptoms characterizes a syndrome that has been described in several cultural groups. This syndrome has been referred to as **amok** in persons native to some Southeast Asian countries, **cathard** in Polynesia, **mal de pelea** in Puerto Rico, and **iich'aa** in the Navajo (DSM-IV-TR, 1999).

Pyromania

Pyromania is characterized by repetitive fire setting and an overwhelming interest in and attraction to fires. The disorder must be distinguished from setting fires for insurance or other gain, as well as normal curiosity about fire. It must also be distinguished from impaired judgment caused by another mental condition, such as mental retardation. Pyromania is more common in males and in children with conduct disorder (see Chapter 6). Frequently, individuals with pyromania seek situations where they can be involved with fires (e.g., they become volunteer firefighters).

Kleptomania

Kleptomania is the impulse to take things without paying for them despite the fact that they are affordable. For the person with kleptomania, taking rather than having the object is the intent. The differential diagnosis of kleptomania includes stealing for actual gain and then faking the disorder to avoid prosecution for stealing (malingering). Kleptomania must also be differentiated from a general failure to follow rules during a manic episode and from antisocial personality disorder and its disregard for rules. In contrast to patients with kleptomania, patients with these disorders have many other behavioral problems. The presence of kleptomania in approximately 25% of patients with bulimia nervosa (see Chapter 17) suggests that patients with both disorders have difficulty with impulse control.

Pathological gambling

Pathological gamblers have an overwhelming need to gamble despite the behavior negatively affecting family and work relationships. It is seen in 1 to 3% of adults of both sexes but has a later age of onset in women than in men. **Pathological gambling** must be distinguished from a manic episode; in the latter, obvious mood elevation is seen. Gamblers Anonymous, a 12-step program modeled after Alcoholics Anonymous, may be effective for treating compulsive gambling.

Trichotillomania

Trichotillomania is a condition in which there is a strong need to pull out one's own hair. This behavior, which often starts in childhood, is more common in women and can lead to obvious hair loss. Some patients with this disorder also engage in **trichophagia** (hair eating) that can result in **trichobezoars** (hairballs) which can cause intestinal obstruction and malnutrition. The differential diagnosis of trichotillomania includes alopecia caused by a medical condition and a compulsion of obsessive-compulsive disorder (OCD). However, unlike trichotillomania, OCD commonly includes other compulsions.

Biological treatment of impulsive and aggressive behavior

Both impulsive and aggressive behavior are associated with decreased serotonergic function (see Chapter 5). It is not surprising, therefore, that antidepressants that increase serotonergic function, such as the selective serotonin reuptake inhibitors (SSRIs), are useful in treating impulse control disorders (Chong and Low, 1996). Other agents used to treat impulsive and aggressive behavior include benzodiazepines, antipsychotics (particularly atypical agents such as clozapine and olanzapine), and mood stabilizers, such as lithium and anticonvulsants (see Chapter 19).

■ ABUSE AND NEGLECT OF CHILDREN AND THE ELDERLY

Because they must depend on others for care, children and the impaired elderly are particularly vulnerable to abuse. Unfortunately, the supposed loved one or caretaker is often the abuser (Quayhagen et al., 1997).

CASE 22-1

THE PATIENT   A 29-year-old man is arrested for leaving his car and physically attacking another motorist while waiting for a red light. When the man is brought to the emergency room with injuries he sustained in the fight, he reports that the motorist cut in front of him at the previous light. The attacker has had two previous arrests for fighting; the first occurred when someone pushed him on the checkout line in the supermarket. On the other occasion, a waiter accidentally spilled a glass of water on him in a restaurant. In neither case did he know the person he assaulted. The patient reports that he has held a full-time job as a construction supervisor for more than 6 years, is happily married, and has two young children. The patient is remorseful over the incident and says that he sometimes "loses it" for little reason. Physical and psychiatric examination of the patient show no evidence of another mental disorder, substance abuse, or medical illness.

COMMENT   This case illustrates several aspects of intermittent explosive disorder. First, the patient has shown repeated, discrete episodes of explosive temper with minimal provocation. Between episodes, he shows essentially normal behavior, can hold a job, and has a good relationship with his wife. His behavior cannot be accounted for by substance abuse or another psychiatric condition, such as personality disorder, psychotic disorder, or bipolar disorder.

TREATMENT   Treatment that includes both psychotherapy and pharmacotherapy is most likely to be effective for this patient. Lithium and anticonvulsants such as carbamazepine (Tegretol), and phenytoin (Dilantin), as well as fluoxetine (Prozac) and other SSRIs are useful in controlling the outbursts of violent behavior in some patients with IED.

Types of abuse

Types of child and elder abuse include **physical abuse** (e.g., the "battered child syndrome"), **emotional or physical neglect,** and **sexual abuse.** The elderly also may be exploited for monetary gain. Characteristics of the abused and abuser in child and elder abuse are listed in Table 22-2.

Injuries of abuse

Injuries resulting from abuse (Table 22-3) must often be differentiated from injuries obtained during normal activity. For example, abuse-related injuries in children include damage to areas not commonly injured during play, such as the buttocks or back (Fig. 22-1) as well as brain and eye injuries caused by shaking an infant to stop it from crying ("the shaken baby syndrome") (Fig. 22-2) (Peinkofer, 2002). Injuries in children that do not suggest abuse include bruises and scrapes on bony prominences, such as the chin, forehead, knees, and elbows. In the elderly, excessive skin bruising caused by abuse are seen on the inner surfaces of the limbs (Fig. 22-3), whereas bruising caused by accidents or normal aging are more likely to be seen on extensor surfaces. Also, to avoid detection, abusers tend to avoid injuring areas not normally hidden by clothing. Signs that indicate child and elder neglect and abuse are listed in Table 22-3.

TABLE 22-2	Characteristics of the Abused and Abuser in Child and Elder Abuse	
	CHARACTERISTICS OF THE ABUSED	**CHARACTERISTICS OF THE ABUSER**
Child abuse	■ Prematurity or low birth weight ■ Hyperactivity or mild physical disability ■ Perceived as slow or different ■ Colicky or "fussy" infant ■ Most are younger than 5 years of age (one-third of cases); one-fourth of the cases are 5–9 years of age	■ Substance abuse ■ Poverty and social isolation ■ The closest family member (e.g., the mother) is most likely to abuse ■ Personal history of victimization by caretaker or spouse
Elder abuse	■ Some degree of dementia ■ Physical dependence on others ■ Does not report the abuse, but instead says that he fell and injured himself ■ Is incontinent	■ Substance abuse ■ Poverty and social isolation ■ The closest family member (e.g., spouse, daughter, son, or other relative with whom the person lives and often supports financially) is most likely to abuse

TABLE 22-3	Signs of Child and Elder Physical Abuse	
CATEGORY	CHILD ABUSE	ELDER ABUSE
Neglect	■ Lack of needed nutrition ■ Poor personal care (e.g., diaper rash, dirty hair)	■ Lack of needed nutrition ■ Poor personal care (e.g., urine odor in incontinent person), lack of medication, or health aids (e.g., eyeglasses, dentures)
Bruises	■ Bruising in areas not likely to be injured during normal play, such as buttocks or lower back ■ Bruising of soft tissue which is not over bony prominences ■ Bruising of an infant (who is not yet mobile) ■ Belt or belt buckle shaped bruises	■ Often bilateral and on the inner surface of the arms from being grabbed ■ Bruising of soft tissue which is not over bony prominences
Burns	■ Cigarette burns ■ Burns on the hands, feet, or buttocks caused by immersion in hot water	■ Cigarette and other burns
Fractures	■ Fractures (e.g., skull, rib, spinal, clavicular) at different stages of healing ■ Spiral fractures caused by twisting the limbs ■ "Bucket-handle" fractures (on the edge of bone between the metaphysis and epiphysis)	■ Fractures at different stages of healing ■ Spiral fractures caused by twisting the limbs
Other signs	■ Internal abdominal injuries (e.g., ruptured spleen) ■ Wrist rope burns caused by tying to a bed or chair ■ Injuries of the mouth caused by forced feeding ■ Petechiae (pinpoint hemorrhages on skin) caused by excess pressure ■ "Shaken baby" syndrome, e.g., retinal (in 50–100% of cases) and brain injuries caused by shaking the infant to stop it from crying	■ Internal abdominal injuries (e.g., ruptured spleen) ■ Wrist rope burns caused by tying to a bed or chair ■ Injuries of the mouth caused by forced feeding ■ Evidence of depleted personal finances (their money was spent by the abuser and other family members)

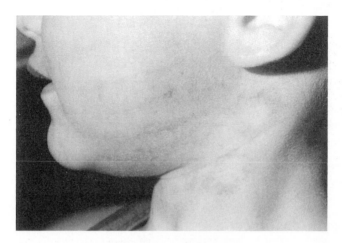

FIGURE 22-1. A young child with a hand print on the face and neck showing the outline of the fingers of the abuser.

(Reprinted with permission from Reece R. M., & Ludwig, S. (Eds.) (2001). Child abuse: Medical diagnosis and management (2nd ed., p. 28). Baltimore: Lippincott Williams & Wilkins.)

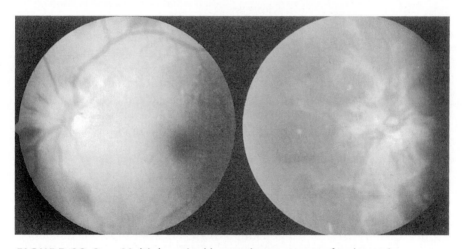

FIGURE 22-2. Multiple retinal hemorrhages seen on funduscopic examination of the eyes of an infant with the shaken baby syndrome. The eye on the right shows a more severe hemorrhage that almost certainly indicates a shaking injury.

(Reprinted with permission from Reece, R. M., & Ludwig, S. (Eds.) (2001). Child abuse: Medical diagnosis and management (2nd ed., p. 98). Baltimore: Lippincott, Williams & Wilkins.)

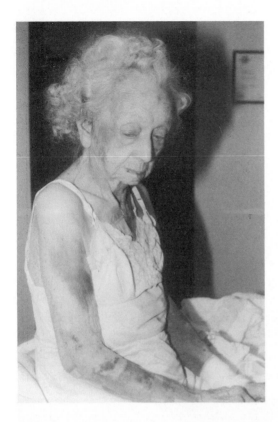

FIGURE 22-3. Bruises that suggest abuse on the arms and face of an elderly woman.

(Photo provided courtesy of National Center on Elder Abuse Library/National Association of State Units on Aging, Washington, DC.)

Identification of abuse

Abused children and elderly persons are often not identified by health care professionals for several reasons. First, because of their young age or the infirmities of old age, the abused may not be able to speak or otherwise communicate effectively. Second, the abused child or elderly person may be afraid to verbalize the abuse because of misplaced loyalty or a realistic fear of retribution.

Sexual abuse of children

An estimated 500,000 American children are sexually abused per year. Approximately 20% of women and 5 to 10% of men report sexual abuse at some time during their childhood and adolescence (Finkelhor & Wells, 2003). Most sexually abused children are 8 to 13 years of age; however, approximately 25% are younger than age 8 years.

Despite extensive media coverage of abduction, sexual abuse, and murder of children by strangers, 70 to 90% of incidents of sexual abuse are committed by someone known to the child. About 90% of these individuals are men (Finkelhor & Wells, 2003). About half of all such incidents are committed by relatives (e.g., uncle, father, or mother's boyfriend) and

THE PATIENT   The grandparents of a 4-month-old male infant bring the child to the emergency room after visiting his home and finding him in an unresponsive state in his crib. The parents, who come in 30 minutes later, demand that they be allowed to take the child home. The child has no obvious external injuries, but physical examination reveals a subdural hematoma and multiple retinal hemorrhages.

COMMENT   Subdural hematoma and retinal hemorrhage are signs of the "shaken baby syndrome," a form of child abuse in which an adult shakes a child to stop its crying. The rapid acceleration and deceleration of the head during shaking causes the brain to move within and strike the inside of the skull, resulting in shearing of intracranial veins leading to subdural, epidural, interhemispheric, and subarachnoid hemorrhage and cerebral edema. Eye injuries caused by shaking include retinal detachment as well as hemorrhage, macular scarring, optic nerve atrophy, optic-nerve sheath and vitreous hemorrhage, and amblyopia. It is not uncommon for the shaken child to have no obvious external injuries.

TREATMENT   The first goal of the physician in cases of child abuse is to protect the child. After hospitalizing and medically stabilizing the child, the physician must report her suspicion of abuse to the appropriate child protective agency. She does not have to inform the parents that she suspects abuse. The doctor also does not have to get the parents' permission to treat or to hospitalize the child (Peinkofer, 2002).

---

about half are committed by family acquaintances, such as teachers or neighbors. Sexually abused children may not reveal the abuse by someone they know because of fear of withdrawal of affection or retribution from the abuser or because of shame and inappropriate guilt.

Although sexual abusers occasionally are true pedophiles who prefer children to appropriate sexual partners (see Chapter 21), most are people with marital problems and no appropriate alternate sexual partners. Alcohol and drugs are commonly used by sexual abusers.

Evidence of sexual abuse

Any sexually transmitted diseases (STD) in a child indicates sexual abuse. Children do not contract these diseases through casual contact with an infected person or via bedclothes, towels, or toilet seats. Genital or anal trauma and recurrent urinary tract infections are also signs of sexual abuse. Because young children have only vague knowledge about sexual activities, specific knowledge about sexual acts, such as fellatio, can indicate that the child has been sexually abused. Also, although children normally play games such as "doctor," which involves sexual exploration (see Chapter 1), excessive initiation of these games or of similar activities are other indications that the child may have been sexually abused.

Psychological sequelae of child abuse

Adults who were abused as children are at high risk for psychological disorders, such as dissociative disorders (e.g., dissociative identity disorder; see Chapter 18), borderline personality disorder (see Chapter 24), posttraumatic stress disorder and other anxiety disorders (see Chapter 15), depression (see Chapter 13), and substance abuse disorders (see Chapter 23). Girls who were sexually abused in childhood are more likely to show sexual disorders in adulthood, such as dyspareunia and vaginismus (see Chapter 21).

Those abused in childhood are also at substantially greater risk for exhibiting violent behavior in adulthood, particularly for abusing their own children. The risk for future violent behavior may be influenced by an interaction between psychological and genetic factors. Abused children (particularly boys) who have inherited a version of the gene for monoamine oxidase A, which results in lower brain concentrations of neurotransmitters such as serotonin, are more likely than children without this gene to show violent behavior as young adults (Caspi et al., 2002). Treatment of abused children involves decreasing the risk of future abuse, developing trust in the child, decreasing feelings of responsibility and guilt for the abuse, and reducing behavioral problems associated with the abuse (Faller, 1993). Group, individual, and family therapy (if appropriate) can all be useful in the treatment of abused children (see Chapter 11).

■ ABUSE OF DOMESTIC PARTNERS

Nearly 25% of women who visit hospital emergency rooms do so because they were purposely injured by their male domestic partners. Like other forms of abuse, physical evidence of **domestic abuse** includes bruises and broken bones. A depressed or sad affect in the victim, an irrational explanation of how the injury occurred, and delay in seeking treatment also indicate that these injuries are caused by domestic abuse. Furthermore, injured women who are accompanied by a partner who is overly assertive or hostile toward the doctor or who interferes in the doctor's care of the patient are also likely to have been abused by that partner.

Not every episode of domestic violence involves men injuring (i.e., **battering**) women. However, in the absence of a weapon, the injuries that women inflict tend to be medically insignificant compared with those inflicted by men. The incidence of domestic violence among gay and lesbian couples is believed to be similar to that of heterosexual couples. It may be even more difficult for doctors to identify these victims of abuse because they may be even more reluctant than heterosexual patients to disclose the abuse. This is true in part because of societal beliefs that such behavior constitutes fighting between "equals" rather than abuse and as such does not require intervention by others (Lundy, 1994).

Typically, domestic abuse occurs in a cycle, starting with a build-up of tension in the abuser over a period of days or weeks. The battering then takes place. This abuse is followed by apologetic and loving behavior by the abuser toward the victim. Typically, there is more than one type of abuse in a family (e.g., a spouse abuser is likely to also be a child abuser).

Many in the lay public do not understand why abused partners do not report the abuse to the police or leave the abuser. This failure to act occurs for several reasons. First, the abused person typically wants to believe that the partner's apology is sincere and that he will never do it again. Also, the abused person commonly has nowhere to go; she is likely to have poor self-esteem after years of battering, and little social, economic, or legal support. Finally, the abuser may have threatened to kill the abused if he is reported or abandoned. The danger to the abused is real; her risk of being killed by the abusive partner is greatly increased if she leaves the relationship.

Pregnant women have a higher risk of being abused by their domestic partners than other women. Often, their injuries are around the breasts and abdomen, the so-called **"baby zone."** Abused pregnant women also commonly have a history of miscarriage and pre-term labor from prior incidents of abuse. Table 22-4 summarizes the characteristics of domestic abusers and their abused partners.

TABLE 22-4	Characteristics of the Abuser and Abused in Physical and Sexual Abuse of Domestic Partners
Characteristics of the abuser	■ Is almost always male ■ Often uses alcohol or drugs ■ Is impulsive and angry ■ Has a low tolerance for frustration ■ Has threatened to kill the abused if she reports or leaves ■ Has a family history of domestic violence ■ Shows apologetic and loving behavior after the abuse
Characteristics of the abused	■ Is financially or emotionally dependent on the abuser ■ Is often pregnant and injuries are to the breasts and abdomen ■ Delays seeking medical care ■ Has an illogical explanation of injuries ■ Shows depression or other mental disorder ■ Has a recent diagnosis of HIV ■ Has a family history of domestic violence ■ Blames herself for the abuse ■ May not report to the police or leave the abuser
Characteristics of both the abused and abuser	■ Low self-esteem

■ ROLE OF THE PHYSICIAN IN SUSPECTED ABUSE

Child and elder abuse

According to laws in every state, physicians must report suspected physical or sexual abuse of a child or elderly person (particularly if the elderly person appears to be physically or mentally impaired) to the appropriate state child- or adult-protective service before, or in conjunction with, treatment of the patient. The physician is not required to tell the suspected abuser of the child or impaired elder that she suspects abuse, nor does she need family consent to hospitalize the abused child or elderly person for protection or treatment.

Domestic partner abuse

Direct reporting by the physician of domestic partner abuse is rarely appropriate because the victim is usually a competent adult. A physician who suspects domestic partner abuse should do the following:

- Document the abuse.
- Ensure the safety of the abused person.
- Develop an emergency escape plan for the abused person.
- Provide emotional support to the abused person.
- Refer the abused person to an appropriate shelter or program.
- Encourage the abused person to report the case to law enforcement officials.

The physician should not insist that the abused person terminate the relationship with the abuser. The abused person must make this decision (Rodriquez, 1999).

In cases of domestic abuse, couples counseling may be considered if both members of the couple want to maintain the relationship and if the abuser accepts responsibility for and seeks to change the abusive behavior.

■ RAPE AND RELATED CRIMES

Legal considerations

Rape is a crime of violence, not of passion. Legally, rape is considered "sexual assault" or "aggravated sexual assault" because it involves sexual contact without consent. While vaginal penetration by a penis, finger, or other object may occur, erection and ejaculation do not have to occur for the crime of rape to have been committed. **Sodomy** is defined as the insertion of the penis into the oral or anal orifice of a male or female victim.

In the past, the presence of semen in the vagina was necessary evidence of rape. Now, because some rapists use condoms to avoid contracting HIV or being identified via DNA, semen may not be present in the vagina of a rape victim. In addition, semen may be absent because some rapists have difficulty with erection or ejaculation.

In past years, conviction of a suspected rapist required that the victim prove that she resisted his advances and that she did not encourage his behavior by wearing seductive clothing or engaging in seductive behavior. This proof is no longer needed. A rapist now can be convicted even if no evidence of a struggle exists, and even if the victim asks him to use a condom. Also, in contrast to past years, certain information about the victim (e.g., previous sexual activity, type of clothing worn at the time of the attack, and so on) now is generally not admissible as evidence in rape trials.

It is illegal to force anyone to engage in sexual activity. In almost every state, husbands can be prosecuted for raping their wives. Also, even if a woman consents to go on a date with a man and agrees to engage in some type of sexual activity, a man can be prosecuted for rape, so-called **"date rape,"** if he forces her to have sexual activity with him. Even consensual sex may be considered rape (**"statutory rape"**) if the victim is younger than 16 or 18 years old (depending on state law) or is physically or mentally disabled. Table 22-5 lists typical characteristics of the rapist and victim.

The psychological and physical sequelae of sexual assault

The length of the emotional recovery period after sexual assault varies. Sexual assault is a psychologically and physically traumatic experience that can cause symptoms of post-traumatic stress disorder for at least 1 year (see Chapter 14). Despite the serious nature of sexual crimes, most rapes and other forms of sexual assault are not reported to the police for several reasons including shame, fear of retaliation, the difficulties involved in substantiating the charges, and the tendency of others to blame the victim.

The role of the physician in sexual assault cases

Immediately after the sexual assault, the physician should take the patient's history in a supportive manner and encourage the patient to notify the police. The doctor is not required to notify the police if the woman is

TABLE 22-5	Characteristics of the Rapist and Victim
Characteristics of the rapist	■ Usually younger than age 25 ■ Usually the same race as the victim ■ Usually known to the victim ■ Alcohol use
Characteristics of the victim	■ Usually between 16 and 24 years of age ■ Usually occurs inside the victim's home ■ Vaginal injuries may be absent, particularly in parous women (those who have had children)

TABLE 22-6	Physician's Role in the Follow-Up of a Rape Victim

IMMEDIATELY AFTER THE INCIDENT

- Take the patient's history (be supportive and nonjudgmental).
- Do not question the patient's veracity or judgment.
- Perform a general physical examination.
- Conduct laboratory tests (e.g., cultures for sexually transmitted diseases from the vagina, anus, and pharynx; pregnancy test; test for presence of semen).
- Prescribe prophylactic antibiotics and postcoital contraceptive measures (e.g., diethylstilbestrol) if appropriate.
- Encourage the patient to notify the police.

1–2 AND 7 DAYS LATER

- Interview the patient and discuss emotional and physical sequelae of the rape (e.g., suicidal thoughts, vaginal bleeding).
- Allow the patient to express her anger.
- Refer the patient for counseling.
- Follow up on legal matters.

6 WEEKS LATER

- Reevaluate the patient's physical status.
- Repeat tests for sexually transmitted diseases.
- Repeat laboratory test for pregnancy.
- Refer the patient for long-term counseling if appropriate (the most effective type of counseling is group therapy with other rape victims).

Adapted from Fadem, B., & Simring, S. (2003). *High-yield psychiatry* (2nd ed.). Baltimore: Lippincott Williams & Wilkins.

a competent adult. Other aspects of the doctor's role and a timeline for caring for victims of sexual assault are presented in Table 22-6.

REVIEW QUESTIONS

1. A 3-year-old girl is brought into the emergency room with a 2-inch-long scalp laceration. Her parents, both attending physicians at the hospital, relate that the child fell down the stairs the previous day. The child is underweight and has bruises on both arms. There are no other physical findings, and laboratory tests are unremarkable. After stabilizing the child, the emergency department physician should

(A) contact the state child-protective service agency

(B) question the parents to determine if they have abused the child

(C) inform the parents that he suspects that they have abused the child

(D) obtain the parents' permission to hospitalize the child

(E) obtain the parents' permission to call a pediatric neurologist

2. A 4-year-old girl tells the physician that "when my daddy was in my room, he wet my bed." Physical examination of the child is unremarkable. The next thing that the physician should do is to

(A) contact the state child-protective service agency

(B) ask the mother's permission to call a child psychiatrist

(C) speak to the father about the child's remark

(D) contact a child psychiatrist to determine if the child is telling the truth

(E) question the child further to determine if she is telling the truth

3. Which of the following injuries in a 3-year-old child is most likely to be the result of abuse?

(A) Cut on the eyebrow

(B) Bruised knees

(C) Scraped forehead

(D) Cut elbow

(E) Damaged liver

4. A 79-year-old, mildly demented woman lives in her own home and has been cared for 6 days a week for the last 5 years by a private-duty nurse. On Sundays, a home health aide cares for the patient. One Sunday morning, the patient sustains an injury to her hand and is brought to the emergency room by the home health aide. During the examination, the emergency room physician notices extensive bruising on the woman's lower back. The woman states that the private-duty nurse hits her and pinches her if she wets or soils the bed. It is most likely that the patient

(A) has imagined that the nurse abused her

(B) has been abused by the home health aide

(C) was injured in the course of ordinary physical care

(D) has been abused by the private-duty nurse

(E) is lying to get the nurse into trouble

5. A 30-year-old well-known singer is caught taking a portable CD player from a store without paying for it. The man has not been in legal trouble for any other reason, but this is the fourth time he has been caught in an offense of this type. The man states that he did not realize that he had the device in his pocket when he walked out of the store. The most likely explanation for this man's behavior is that he

(A) has a dissociative disorder

(B) is faking kleptomania to avoid prosecution for stealing

(C) has the impulse to take things without paying for them

(D) is seeking attention from others

(E) has an antisocial personality disorder

6. In evaluating the risk of leaving abused children with their parents, which of the following is associated with a decreased risk that the child will be abused again?

(A) Young age of the child (e.g., an infant who is unable to walk)

(B) Parents willing to enter marital therapy

(C) Intelligent parents

(D) No history of abuse in the parents' own childhoods

(E) Employment of the parents in law enforcement

7. A 34-year-old woman who is an alcoholic visits a physician. This woman's injuries suggest that she has been abused by her husband. What is the most appropriate question for the physician to ask at this time?

(A) Do you think your drinking has a negative effect on your husband?

(B) Why do you think that your husband abuses you?

(C) Is it safe for you to return home to your husband?

(D) Would you like to talk about your problem with alcohol?

(E) Did your father abuse your mother?

ANSWERS AND EXPLANATIONS

1-A. After stabilizing the child, the emergency department physician should contact the state child-protective service agency to report suspected child abuse. The delay in seeking treatment, signs of neglect (underweight), and bruising indicate that the child has been abused. Parents commonly make up some explanation for the injuries, such as "the child fell." This example illustrates at least two significant facts. First, child abuse happens at all socioeconomic levels. Second, doctors are in a unique position to identify child abuse early and save a child's life. The physician must report any suspicion of abuse to the appropriate authority, but he or she does not have to question the parents or inform them of his suspicions. Similarly, when a physician suspects child physical or sexual abuse, he or she does not need a parent's permission to examine, hospitalize, or treat the child or to consult with a specialist.

2-A. This case demonstrates that a child may show no physical signs of sexual abuse. The doctor's responsibility is to protect the child; she does not need to talk to the child at length, consult a child psychiatrist, or talk to the father to confirm the child's story. The state agency will handle these matters. The physician must assume that patients (even young ones) are telling the truth.

3-E. In a young child such as this one, an internal injury such as a damaged liver is likely to be the result of abuse. Injuries on bony prominences, such as eyebrows, knees, forehead, and elbows, are more likely to have been obtained during normal play.

4-D. Unrelated people such as caretakers are much less likely than close relatives to abuse an elderly person. However, the most likely abuser is the individual who has the most responsibility for a patient's care. In this case, that person is the private-duty nurse.

5-C. This man is showing evidence of kleptomania, the impulse to take things without paying for them. He can easily afford the CD player, so it is unlikely that he is seeking attention or faking kleptomania to avoid prosecution for stealing. The persistent nature of this behavior and absence of other psychiatric symptoms indicate that the singer has kleptomania rather than a dissociative disorder or antisocial personality disorder.

6-D. In evaluating the risk of leaving abused children with their parents, a history of abuse in the parents' own childhoods is associated with an increased risk that the child will be abused again. Intelligence of the parents, employment of the parents in law enforcement, and whether the parents are willing to enter marital therapy are not associated with decreased risk of child abuse. Children who are very young are also more, not less, likely to be abused.

7-C. The most important thing for the physician to do for this woman who has been abused by her husband is to first ensure her safety. Therefore, questioning her about whether it is safe for her to return home is the most important initial intervention. Questions implying that her behavior (e.g., her drinking) or her parents' behavior caused the abuse are not appropriate.

REFERENCES

Albert, D. J., Walsh, M. L., & Jonik, R. H. (1993). Aggression in humans: What is its biological foundation? *Neurosci Biobehav Rev, 17,* 405–425.

Briganti, F., Della Seta, D., Fontani, G., Lodi, L., & Lupo, C. (2003). Behavioral effects of testosterone in relation to social rank in the male rabbit. *Aggress Behav, 29,* 269–278.

Caspi, A., McClay, J., Moffitt, T. E., Mill, J., Martin, J., Craig, I. W., et al. (2002). Role of genotype in the cycle of violence in maltreated children. *Science, 297,* 851–854.

Chong, S. A., & Low, B. L. (1996). Treatment of kleptomania with fluvoxamine. *Acta Psychiatr Scand, 93,* 314.

Faller, K. C. (1993). *Child sexual abuse: Intervention and treatment issues.* U.S. Department of Health and Human Services: National Clearinghouse on Child Abuse and Neglect.

Finkelhor, D., & Wells, M. (2003). Improving national data systems about juvenile victimization. *Child Abuse Neglect, 27(1),* 77–102.

Goy, R. W., & McEwen, B. S. (1980). *Sexual differentiation of the brain.* London: Oxford University Press.

Johnson, J. G., Cohen, P., Smailes, E. M., Kasen, S., & Brook, J. S. (2002). Television viewing and aggressive behavior during adolescence and adulthood. *Science, 295,* 2468–2471.

Lewin, T. (2001, July 17). Child well-being improves, U.S. says. *The New York Times.*

Lion, J. R. (1992). The intermittent explosive disorder. *Psychiatr Ann, 22,* 64.

Lundy, S. (1994). Abuse that dare not speak its name: Assisting victims of lesbian and gay domestic violence in Massachusetts. *N Engl Law Rev, 28,* 273.

Mann, J. J. (1995). Violence and aggression. In F. E. Bloom & D. J. Kupfer (Eds.), *Psychopharmacology: The fourth generation of progress.* New York: Raven Press.

McCauley, J., Kern, D. E, Kolodner, K., Dill, L., Schroeder A. F., DeChant H. K., et al. (1995). The "battering syndrome:" Prevalence and clinical characteristics of domestic violence in primary care internal medicine practices. *Ann Intern Med, 123,* 737.

Peinkofer, J. R. (2002). *Silenced angels: The medical, legal and social aspects of shaken baby syndrome.* Westport, CT: Auburn House.

Quayhagen, M., Quayhagen, M., Patterson, T., Irwin, M., Hauger, R., & Grant, I. (1997). Coping with dementia: Family care giver burnout and abuse. *J Ment Health Aging, 3,* 357–364.

Renzetti, C. M., & Miley, C. H. (Eds.) (1996). *Violence in gay and lesbian domestic partnerships.* New York: Harrington Park Press.

Rodriquez, M., Bauer, H. M, McLoughlin, E., & Grumbach, K. (1999). Screening and intervention for intimate partner abuse: Practices and attitudes of primary care physicians. *JAMA, 282,* 468.

Substance Abuse **23**

S ubstance abuse is an increasing public health concern in the United States. The number of people who self-reported substance dependence or abuse (based on the Diagnostic and Statistical Manual of Mental Disorders, Fourth Edition-Text Revision [DSM-IV-TR] criteria) (Table 23-1) within a year of the 2001 National Household Survey on Drug Abuse were as follows:

■ Alcohol: 13.4 million
■ Marijuana and hashish: 3.5 million
■ Nonmedical use of psychotherapeutic agents (e.g., opioids, sedatives): 1.4 million
■ Cocaine: 1.0 million
■ Heroin: 0.2 million

Because these figures were obtained from self-reports, the actual numbers of abusers are likely to be much higher.

For the individual, the abuse of substances leads to family, health, and legal problems. For society, the cost of substance abuse in the short- and long-term runs into billions of dollars. Illegal substance abuse is more common among young adults aged 18 to 25 years, and it is about twice as common in males.

TABLE 23-1	DSM-IV-TR Definitions
TERM	**DEFINITION**
Substance abuse	A pattern of abnormal substance use that leads to impairment of occupational, physical, or social functioning
Substance dependence	Substance abuse plus withdrawal symptoms, tolerance, or a pattern of repetitive use
Withdrawal	Development of physical or psychological symptoms after the reduction or cessation of intake of a substance
Tolerance	Need for increased amounts of the substance to achieve the same positive physical and psychological effects
Cross-tolerance	Development of tolerance to one substance because of using another substance

It was once believed that substance abuse resulted primarily from a lack of self-control. In the last few decades, however, it has become clear that abuse and addictive illnesses are complex disorders involving social factors as well as genetic, molecular, and cellular modifications in the brain itself. Once effected, these alterations may be difficult or even impossible to reverse; thus substance abuse tends to be chronically relapsing. Such findings about the nature of addiction have led to changes in both the attitudes of health care providers and in the design of treatment interventions. The development of new, often multifocal treatment programs can be expected to improve the historically negative outcomes of treatment for individuals affected by addictive illnesses.

■ OVERVIEW OF SUBSTANCE ABUSE

Biology of abuse

Drugs of abuse have immediate and long-term effects on the brain. The immediate effect of most abused substances is to increase the availability of neurotransmitters that signal the nervous system to feel pleasure. The most important of the "feel good" neurotransmitters is dopamine. Dopamine is produced in the neurons of the mesolimbic dopaminergic tract in the area of the ventral tegmentum of the brain. These neurons project forward through the medial forebrain bundle and, when stimulated, release dopamine toward the nucleus accumbens (NA) and frontal cortex (see Fig. 5-2).

Empirical evidence shows the rewarding nature of dopamine's action on the NA. Laboratory animals will work to receive electrical stimulation of the NA, and the use of opioids, among the most addicting of substances, causes release of dopamine from the NA. Other neurotransmitters, such as serotonin and glutamate, are associated with the positive effects of drugs as well. Glutamate is associated specifically with the maintenance of addictive behavior (Nestler & Aghajanian, 1997). Agents that block its activity, such as acamprosate (Campral), reduce drug cravings. As such, these agents, or agents that prevent glutamate from acting through its major receptor N-methyl-D-aspartate (NMDA receptor blockers), may provide a new avenue for treatment of alcohol, cocaine, and heroin addiction (Wickelgren, 1998).

Although the precise mechanisms are not known, long-term exposure to drugs of abuse most likely induces changes in neurotransmitter receptors. These changes appear to play a major role in the development of physical addiction and psychological dependence. They explain why repeated use of many substances of abuse ultimately leads to both a compulsion to continue using (dependence) and a need for increased doses of the drug to repeat the positive effect (tolerance). DSM-IV-TR definitions of **substance abuse, substance dependence, withdrawal, tolerance,** and **cross-tolerance** are listed in Table 23-1.

Classification of abused substances

Most abused substances can be classified categorically as sedatives, opioids, stimulants, or hallucinogens and related agents. Summaries of the effects of use and withdrawal of these groups can be found in Table 23-2, and a more detailed discussion follows.

Abused drugs can be administered by many routes. Drug abusers tend to use routes that provide fast access to the bloodstream and hence the brain, such as injection (which requires special equipment and expertise), sniffing into the nose (snorting), and inhaling (smoking).

Treatment of substance abuse

Because of the neurologic changes effected by use, once dependency develops, abrupt absence of some abused substances can lead to psychological and physical **withdrawal** symptoms. Psychological withdrawal symptoms can range from mild irritability to severe depression. Physical withdrawal symptoms can range from the uncomfortable but benign headache associated with withdrawal from stimulants to the life-threatening seizures and cardiovascular collapse associated with withdrawal from barbiturates. Treatment of the withdrawal symptoms of substance abuse includes immediate treatment or **detoxification** and extended treatment to prevent relapse or **maintenance** (Table 23-3).

Some substance abusers also have mental disorders. Patients with diagnoses of both mental illness (e.g., major depression) and substance abuse (so-called **dual diagnosis** or **mentally ill–chemically addicted** [**MICA**] patients) require treatment for both substance abuse and the comorbid psychiatric illness. This treatment must often be provided in a special unit in the hospital.

TABLE 23-2	Effects of Use and Withdrawal of Psychoactive Substances	
CATEGORY	EFFECTS OF USE	EFFECTS OF WITHDRAWAL
Sedatives Alcohol Benzodiazepines Barbiturates	■ Mood elevation ■ Decreased anxiety ■ Sedation ■ Behavioral disinhibition ■ Respiratory depression (particularly the barbiturates)	■ Mood depression ■ Increased anxiety ■ Insomnia ■ Delirium (including psychotic symptoms) ■ Seizures ■ Cardiovascular collapse
Opioids Heroin Methadone Opioids used medically	■ Mood elevation ■ Decreased anxiety ■ Sedation ■ Analgesia ■ Respiratory depression ■ Constipation ■ Pupil constriction	■ Mood depression ■ Increased anxiety ■ Autonomic instability ■ "Flu-like" symptoms (e.g. muscle aches) ■ Piloerection ■ Yawning ■ Stomach cramps and diarrhea ■ Pupil dilation
Stimulants Amphetamines Cocaine Caffeine and nicotine (minor stimulants)	■ Mood elevation ■ Insomnia ■ Decreased appetite ■ Increased cardiovascular, neurological, and GI activity ■ Psychotic symptoms ■ Pupil dilation ■ Hallucinations (often tactile)	■ Mood depression ■ Lethargy ■ Increased appetite ■ Decreased cardiovascular, neurological and GI activity ■ Fatigue ■ Headache
Hallucinogens and related agents Marijuana Hashish LSD PCP Psilocybin Mescaline	■ Mood elevation ■ Altered perception (e.g., hallucinations) ■ Cardiovascular symptoms ■ Hyperthermia and sweating ■ Tremor ■ Nystagmus (PCP)	■ Few, if any, withdrawal symptoms

LSD, lysergic acid diethylamide; PCP, phencyclidine.

TABLE 23-3	Treatment (in order of utility, highest to lowest) of Abuse of Sedatives, Opioids, Stimulants and Hallucinogens and Related Agents	
CATEGORY	**IMMEDIATE TREATMENT/ DETOXIFICATION**	**EXTENDED TREATMENT/ MAINTENANCE**
Sedatives Alcohol Benzodiazepines Barbiturates	▪ Hospitalization ▪ Substitution of long-acting barbiturate (e.g., phenobarbital) or benzodiazepine (e.g., chlordiazepoxide [Librium]) in decreasing doses ▪ Intravenous diazepam (Valium), lorazepam (Ativan), or phenobarbital if seizures occur ▪ Specifically for alcohol: thiamine, restoration of nutritional state	▪ Education for initiation and maintenance of abstinence ▪ Specifically for alcohol: Alcoholics Anonymous or other peer support group (12-step program), disulfiram (Antabuse; 125–500 mg/day), psychotherapy, behavior therapy ▪ Acamprosate (compral) ▪ Naltrexone ((ReVia)
Opioids Heroin Methadone Opioids used medically	▪ Hospitalization and naloxone (Narcan) for overdose ▪ Clonidine to stabilize the autonomic nervous system during withdrawal ▪ Substitution of long-acting opioid (e.g., methadone) in decreasing doses to decrease withdrawal symptoms	▪ Methadone and LAMM maintenance program ▪ Naloxone, naltrexone (ReVia), or buprenorphine (Temgesic) used prophylactically to block the effects of abused opioids ▪ Narcotics Anonymous or other peer support program
Stimulants Amphetamines Cocaine	▪ Benzodiazepines to decrease agitation ▪ Antipsychotics to treat psychotic symptoms ▪ Medical and psychological support	▪ Education for initiation and maintenance of abstinence

TABLE 23-3 Treatment (in order of utility, highest to lowest) of Abuse of Sedatives, Opioids, Stimulants and Hallucinogens and Related Agents (Continued)

CATEGORY	IMMEDIATE TREATMENT/ DETOXIFICATION	EXTENDED TREATMENT/ MAINTENANCE
Minor Stimulants Caffeine and nicotine	■ Eliminate or taper from the diet ■ Analgesics to control headache due to withdrawal	■ Substitute decaffeinated beverage ■ Nicotine-containing gum, patch, or nasal spray ■ Antidepressants (particularly bupropion [Zyban]) to prevent smoking ■ Peer support group ■ Support from family members or nonsmoking physician ■ Hypnosis to prevent smoking
Hallucinogens and related agents Marijuana Hashish LSD PCP Psilocybin Mescaline	■ Calming or "talking down" of the patient ■ Benzodiazepines to decrease agitation ■ Antipsychotics to treat psychotic symptoms	■ Education for initiation and maintenance of abstinence

LAMM, l-alpha-acetylmethadol acetate; LSD, lysergic acid diethylamide; PCP, phencyclidine.

■ SEDATIVES

Sedatives are central nervous system depressants and include alcohol, barbiturates, and benzodiazepines. Although dopaminergic systems are also involved, sedative agents work primarily by increasing the activity of the inhibitory neurotransmitter gamma-aminobutyric acid (GABA). The increase in GABA activity results in reduced anxiety and sedation.

Alcohol

Alcohol is the most abused substance in the world. In the United States, there is a 10 to 13% lifetime prevalence of alcohol abuse or dependence. Some ethnic groups (e.g., Native Americans) are more likely to abuse alcohol than others, and men are twice as likely to be abusers as females.

The etiology of **alcoholism** includes genetic and developmental-environmental factors. For example, adopted children tend to show the drinking patterns characteristic of their biological rather than their adoptive parents (see Chapter 5), and behavior problems such as attention-deficit/hyperactivity disorder and conduct disorder correlate with alcoholism in adulthood (see Chapter 2).

Acute use of alcohol is associated with a variety of societal problems, including, but not limited to, suicide (see Chapter 14), traffic accidents, homicide, child physical and sexual abuse, elder abuse, domestic violence, and rape (see Chapter 22). **Fetal alcohol syndrome,** which includes facial abnormalities, reduced height and weight, mental retardation, and other problems, is seen in the offspring of women who drink during pregnancy.

Chronic, heavy use of alcohol results in several serious physical disorders. These include Wernicke and Korsakoff syndromes (see Chapter 14) as well as liver dysfunction and gastrointestinal problems, such as ulcers and pancreatitis.

Although the dangers of heavy drinking are well established, moderate use of alcohol may have positive effects on health (Rimm et al., 1996). In a long-term study of more than 50,000 male health professionals, those who had up to four alcoholic drinks (in any form) at least three days a week had fewer heart attacks than nondrinkers or those who drank only one or two days a week (Mukamal, 2003).

Barbiturates and benzodiazepines

Barbiturates are used medically as sleeping pills, sedatives, antianxiety agents (tranquilizers), anticonvulsants, and anesthetics. Because of their abuse potential and low safety margin, barbiturates are less commonly prescribed than hypnotic benzodiazepines as sleep medications. Frequently used and abused barbiturates include amobarbital, pentobarbital, and secobarbital.

In contrast to barbiturates, **benzodiazepines** have a high safety margin unless taken with another sedative, such as alcohol. The medical uses of benzodiazepines are similar to those of barbiturates.

Withdrawal from alcohol and other sedatives

The withdrawal symptoms associated with long-term heavy use of sedative agents can be severe (see Table 23-2 and see "delirium tremens" in later text). Hospitalization is prudent because seizures and cardiovascular symptoms with life-threatening potential can occur. Treatment of these patients includes preventing seizures by substitution of long-acting barbiturates, such as phenobarbital or benzodiazepines, for the more commonly abused short-acting types (see Table 23-3).

Delirium tremens

Alcohol withdrawal delirium (also called **delirium tremens** or "the DTs") is commonly first observed on about the third day of withdrawal in patients who have been drinking heavily for at least 5 years (Case 23-1). Alcohol withdrawal delirium is a life-threatening condition with a mortality rate of approximately 20%. Emergency treatment of the DTs includes oral and intravenous fluids for dehydration, as well as benzodiazepines such as chlordiazepoxide, diazepam, and lorazepam (see Case 23-1 and Chapter 19) for withdrawal symptoms. Lorazepam is used particularly to detoxify alcoholic patients who have liver failure.

Long-term treatment of alcohol abuse

In some ways, efforts to stop drinking alcohol are more difficult than for other abused substances because alcohol is legal, cheap, and readily available. Although some alcohol abusers may be able to learn to drink in moderation, the goal of treatment for most people is complete abstinence. Methods of maintaining abstinence include peer support programs, such as Alcoholics Anonymous, and pharmacologic treatments, such as disulfiram (see Table 23-2).

Peer support or leaderless therapy groups (see Chapter 11) are gatherings in which people with similar concerns support each other in an effort to eliminate or reduce an addiction or behavioral problem. These pro-

---

CASE 23-1

THE PATIENT   A very thin, 63-year-old woman is brought to the hospital after a fall outside of a neighborhood bar. Radiologic studies indicate that the patient has a fractured hip, and surgery is performed immediately. Two days later, the patient begins to show an intense hand tremor and tachycardia. She tells the doctor that she has been "shaky" ever since her admission and that the shakiness is getting worse. The patient states that although she feels very frightened, she is comforted by the fact that the nurse who is treating her is an old friend (she has never met the nurse before). She also reports that she has started to see ants crawling on the walls and can feel them crawling on her arms. The doctor notes that the patient's speech seems to be drifting from one subject to another.

COMMENT   The most likely cause of the patient's symptoms, which includes tremor, tachycardia, illusions (believing the nurse is an old friend), and tactile hallucinations (e.g., formication, the feeling of insects crawling on the skin), is alcohol withdrawal delirium. This patient is most likely a heavy drinker who is experiencing withdrawal because of hospitalization. Delirium tremens during alcohol withdrawal are more common in physically ill or undernourished patients such as this one.

TREATMENT   Ideally, this patient's heavy prior alcohol use would have been identified on the first day of hospitalization. If at that time she had received a benzodiazepine such as chlordiazepoxide (Librium) every 2 to 4 hours, the severe symptoms of withdrawal may have been attenuated. Because the severe symptoms have already appeared, higher doses of chlordiazepoxide (e.g., 25 to 50 mg every 2 to 4 hours) or lorazepam given intravenously are now needed. Thiamine, supportive treatment for the patient's anxiety, and therapy to restore her fluid and nutritional status are also indicated.

grams are considered by many to be the most, if not the only, effective long-term treatment for alcohol abuse. The first and best known of these groups, **Alcoholics Anonymous (AA),** is so named because participants are identified to each other only by their first names.

Alcoholics Anonymous uses a hierarchy of measures known as the **12 steps to recovery.** The steps range from the first, in which the alcoholic admits that he has been unable to remedy his problem with alcohol on his own, to the twelfth and final step in which he pledges to help other alcoholics (Table 23-4). Because some people find the references to God

TABLE 23-4	The Twelve Steps of Alcoholics Anonymous
STEP	**WE:**
1	Admitted we were powerless over alcohol—that our lives had become unmanageable
2	Came to believe that a Power greater than ourselves could restore us to sanity
3	Made a decision to turn our will and our lives over to the care of God *as we understood Him*
4	Made a searching and fearless moral inventory of ourselves
5	Admitted to God, to ourselves, and to another human being the exact nature of our wrongs
6	Were entirely ready to have God remove all these defects of character
7	Humbly asked Him to remove our shortcoming
8	Made a list of all persons we had harmed, and became willing to make amends to them all
9	Made direct amends to such people wherever possible, except when to do so would injure them or others
10	Continued to take personal inventory and when we were wrong promptly admitted it
11	Sought through prayer and meditation to improve our conscious contact with God, *as we understood Him,* praying only for knowledge of His will for us and the power to carry that out
12	Having had a spiritual awakening as the result of these steps, we tried to carry this message to alcoholics and to practice these principles in all our affairs

or a higher power in the AA 12 steps objectionable, other programs based on the 12-step model avoid such references. Twelve-step programs for other addictions or for behavioral problems patterned on this model include Narcotics Anonymous (NA), Gamblers Anonymous (GA), and Overeaters Anonymous (OA).

Other treatments to prevent alcohol use include daily ingestion of disulfiram (Antabuse), accomprosalic (campral) or naltrexone (ReVia). After taking disulfiram, which blocks the breakdown of alcohol and results in acetaldehyde accumulation, ingestion of alcohol results in intense nausea, headache, and flushing, which act as aversive stimuli (see Chapter 11). After taking naltrexone, the positive effects of alcohol are blunted, an action that seems to be more effective for moderate users than for heavy users (Krystal, 2002). Both of these agents appear to decrease the likelihood of alcohol use in the future.

Psychotherapy alone has had limited success for treating alcoholism, but it may be useful in combination with other treatments. MICA patients in particular need a combined treatment approach, such as psychotherapy plus a 12-step program, to have a successful outcome.

OPIOIDS

Opioids (i.e., narcotics) are drugs derived from opium, a substance obtained from the pods of blossoming poppies. These drugs include agents used medically as analgesics, such as morphine, and drugs of abuse, such as heroin. Although most opium poppies are grown in countries such as Afghanistan, Pakistan, and Myanmar, production in Colombia and Mexico has increased, and these areas now provide the opium for most of the heroin used in the United States. The increased availability of heroin has led to a decrease in price, which has in turn led to increased use. From 1992 to 2002, the number of heroin addicts in the United States increased by at least 40% (Forero & Weiner, 2003).

All opioids have the potential to cause physical and psychological dependence. Some opioids also have the capacity to significantly improve mood (i.e., cause a "high"). When compared with medically used opioids such as morphine, abused opioids such as heroin have more of this euphoric action. Abused opioids also are more potent, cross the blood-brain barrier more quickly, and have a faster onset of action.

Addiction to abused opioids such as heroin (street names include smack and junk) is associated with serious health problems. The intravenous (IV) injection method of drug use employed by heroin addicts often involves sharing contaminated needles, thus contributing to the spread of blood-borne viruses (e.g., HIV and hepatitis B and C) and bacteria (e.g., staphylococcus) that can infect organs such as the heart and lungs. Up to one-third of all patients with HIV are heroin users who contracted the infection by injection with contaminated equipment.

Treatment of opioid abuse

The classic clinical triad of opioid overdose is coma, respiratory depression, and miosis (pinpoint pupils). Patients also show bradycardia, hypotension, and hypothermia. Because respiratory arrest is the most common cause of death from opioid overdose, emergency treatment includes establishing an airway and supplying mechanical ventilation. Opioid receptor antagonists, such as naloxone (Narcan) or its longer-acting form naltrexone (ReVia), rapidly precipitate withdrawal symptoms and are used to reverse the opioid's effects.

Physical withdrawal symptoms of opioids include "flu-like" effects, such as sweating, fever, and rhinorrhea, as well as muscle aches and autonomic instability. However, in contrast to barbiturate withdrawal, which may be fatal, death from withdrawal of opioids is rare unless a serious physical illness is present. The effects of use and withdrawal of some opioids are listed in Table 23-2. Because they share a blood supply with their mothers, newborns of opioid (e.g., heroin or methadone) dependent mothers are born addicted to the drug and must be detoxified after birth.

For detoxification of opioid addicts, a synthetic opioid such as **methadone** (see later text) can be given over a period of weeks in decreasing doses. Some symptoms of abrupt withdrawal, such as autonomic instability, can be mediated by **clonidine** (Catapres). Although the major symptoms of physical withdrawal from heroin are over in approximately 1 week, the recidivism rate in detoxified heroin users is extremely high. An effective way to prevent a return to the physical and legal dangers of heroin use is substitution of methadone or another synthetic opioid (e.g., **l-alpha-acetylmethadol acetate [LAMM]**).

Like heroin, methadone and LAMM cause physical dependence and tolerance. In contrast to heroin, these agents are legal and are dispensed to registered addicts by federal health authorities. Although methadone and LAMM are physically addicting, they have several advantages over heroin. First, they can be taken orally (eliminating the health risks of injection) and have a longer duration of action (24 hours for methadone and 48 to 72 hours for LAMM). They also cause less euphoria and drowsiness, allowing people on maintenance regimens to keep their jobs and avoid the criminal activity that is necessary to maintain a costly heroin habit. Other long-term treatments for opioid abuse include prophylactic use of opioid receptor antagonists such as naloxone to block the euphoric action of heroin, and 12-step programs such as Narcotics Anonymous.

Buprenorphine (Temgesic, Subutex) is an opioid-receptor partial agonist that has actions similar to both methadone and naltrexone in the treatment of opioid addiction. At lower doses, like methadone, it decreases withdrawal symptoms and drug cravings. At the same time, like naloxone, it occupies receptors and thus blocks the euphoric action of opioids. At higher doses, buprenorphine antagonizes its own opioid-like effects and is thus less likely than other opioids to cause respiratory depression.

■ STIMULANTS

Stimulants are agents that activate the central nervous system. These agents include the commonly used minor stimulants, such as caffeine and nicotine, as well as the major stimulants, such as amphetamines and cocaine. In general, stimulants work by increasing the availability of dopamine (DA) in the synapse. This is accomplished either by stimulating the release of DA (e.g., the amphetamines) or by blocking the reuptake of DA (e.g., cocaine). The hyperdopaminergic state induced by these agents can also result in psychotic symptoms, such as hallucinations and delusions, which may have to be distinguished from those seen in psychotic disorders (see Chapter 11) (see Table 23-3).

Caffeine

Caffeine is found in brewed coffee (125 mg/cup), instant coffee (75 mg/cup), tea (65 mg/cup), and cola (45 mg/12 oz), as well as in nonprescription stimulants (150 mg/tablet) and diet agents (150 mg/tablet). The average caffeine intake of Americans is about 200 mg/day, but many people consume more. Ingestion of more than 250 mg a day of caffeine is associated with symptoms of intoxication, including restlessness, agitation, flushing of the face, and tachycardia.

Nicotine and cigarette smoking

Nicotine, a toxic substance found in cigarettes and other tobacco products, has effects and withdrawal symptoms similar to those of caffeine. Although not necessarily associated with nicotine, well-established links exist between long-term cigarette smoking and serious illnesses, such as cancer of the lung, pharynx, and bladder, as well as chronic lung and cardiovascular diseases. Evidence also shows that smokers, especially women, are more likely than nonsmokers to have depressive illnesses. In the United States, cigarette smoking is associated yearly with at least 430,000 deaths and costs to the economy of at least 70 billion dollars. Despite these risks, smoking rates, particularly among the young, have historically been high. Approximately 25% of American adults smokes cigarettes, and, from 1993 to1997, smoking rates in college students rose 28%. Recent studies suggest, however, that government anti-smoking campaigns have been successful. The percentage of high-school seniors who smoke daily decreased from 25% in 1997 to 21% in 2001 (USDHHS, 2001).

Most adult smokers want to stop smoking. Resources that physicians can use to help patients achieve this goal include behavioral treatment techniques, peer support groups, and medications such as bupropion (Zyban) (Table 23-3).

Amphetamines

Like opioids, amphetamines are used both clinically and as drugs of abuse. The most common clinically used amphetamines are **dextroamphetamine** (Dexedrine), **methamphetamine** (Desoxyn), and a related compound, **methylphenidate** (Ritalin). These agents are indicated medically for the treatment of attention-deficit hyperactivity disorder (ADHD) (see Chapter 2) and narcolepsy (see Chapter 7). They are also used to treat depression in patients who do not respond to or are intolerant of standard antidepressants, as well as in some elderly and terminally ill patients (see Chapter 19). Because amphetamines decrease appetite, they are also useful in treating obesity.

Abused amphetamine compounds have street names such as **"speed,"** **"ice,"** **"pink,"** **"blue,"** **"crystal,"** and **"crank."** Amphetamines are used most commonly by people in jobs where staying awake is important or in situations where energy levels must remain high (e.g., performing on stage). **"Ecstasy"** (methylenedioxymethamphetamine [MDMA]) is a combination of amphetamine and hallucinogen. This drug is used primarily by adolescents and young adults at dance parties or **"raves."** Sometimes, users of heroin (or other depressant) counteract its sedating effect by mixing it with a stimulant such as cocaine. This combination is known as a **"speedball"** and the practice is known as "speedballing."

Cocaine

Cocaine can be sniffed into the nostrils (i.e., **"snorted"**) or smoked **"freebase."** **"Crack"** is a smokable form of cocaine that is less pure and thus less expensive than other forms. Cocaine has a rapid mood-elevating effect that dissipates quickly. The "high" is often followed by mood depression, a change that can occur in less than 1 hour. Some people who use cocaine show psychotic symptoms such as a sensation of bugs crawling on the skin (**"cocaine bugs"**), a tactile hallucination. Hyperactivity and growth retardation are seen in newborns of mothers who used cocaine during pregnancy.

Treatment of stimulant abuse

Because dopamine stimulates the cardiovascular and gastrointestinal systems as well as the brain, the use of some stimulants, particularly cocaine, is associated with cardiovascular problems and even sudden death. Therefore, treatment of stimulant abuse includes medication to prevent or to treat possible cardiac symptoms as well as interventions to prevent seizures. Benzodiazepines (e.g., diazepam) are used to treat the agitation, and antipsychotics (e.g., haloperidol) are used to treat the psychotic symptoms that can be associated with stimulant use. Withdrawal from stimulants is associated with depression, headache, hunger, and insomnia, but it is not commonly accompanied by significant physical symptoms (see Table 23-2).

■ HALLUCINOGENS AND RELATED AGENTS

Hallucinogens and related agents include lysergic acid diethylamide (LSD); phencyclidine (PCP, "angel dust"); cannabis (tetrahydrocannabinol, marijuana, hashish); psilocybin (from mushrooms); and mescaline (from cactus) and ketamine (**"Special K"**). Hallucinogens promote altered states of consciousness ("trips") that are usually pleasurable but can also be frightening (**"bad trips"**) (Case 23-2). The effects of use and withdrawal of hallucinogens and related agents are listed in Table 23-2.

No specific treatment exists for abuse of hallucinogens and related agents, although benzodiazepines and psychological support can be helpful when patients who have used these agents become fearful or agitated.

Marijuana

Marijuana is the most commonly used illegal psychoactive substance. Currently, marijuana use is increased in individuals aged 12 to 25 years. Although marijuana use is illegal in the United States, a few states permit limited medical use to treat glaucoma and cancer-related nausea and vomiting.

Tetrahydrocannabinol (THC) is the primary active compound found in marijuana. In low doses, marijuana increases appetite and relaxation

---

CASE   23-2

THE PATIENT   At 9:00 AM on a Sunday morning, a 15-year-old boy is brought to the emergency room by his father. The father states that he found his son on the roof of their house bragging that he could fly. The boy is a good student and has friends, and there is no history of bizarre behavior. When questioned, the patient tells the doctor that he is floating in space and that the lights in the emergency room are huge glaring suns in the sky. He says that his vision and sense of smell are more acute than they have ever been. He reports that he has not used any drugs but that the previous evening he went to a party where he ate a piece of "dream cake" given to him by a friend.

COMMENT   This patient most likely has taken a hallucinogenic agent. Because LSD is active when ingested, it is likely that LSD was in the cake that the patient ate at the party. Although the cake was eaten the previous evening, the effects of LSD can last 12 hours.

TREATMENT   There is no specific treatment for hallucinogen use. However, this patient must be protected from harming himself when having delusional beliefs such as his ability to fly. Reassurance and support in the form of "talking down" the patient and use of benzodiazepines to control his anxiety are useful. With no preexisting psychiatric condition, there should be no long-term sequelae of this experience for the teenager. However, he may experience disturbing "flashbacks" in which he relives this experience when not using LSD, sometimes even months later.

---

and causes conjunctival reddening. Chronic users of marijuana experience lung problems associated with smoking and a decrease in motivation (**"amotivational syndrome"**) characterized by decreased desire to work and increased apathy.

LSD and PCP

The most commonly used hallucinogens and related agents are **LSD** and **PCP.** Although both substances alter perception, there are differences in the methods of use, neurotransmitter systems affected, and behavioral effects. First, while LSD is usually ingested, PCP is smoked in a marijuana or other cigarette. In addition, the effects of LSD are associated with increased availability of serotonin, whereas PCP is known to bind with NMDA receptors of glutamate-gated ion channels. Finally, in contrast to LSD use, PCP use is associated with episodes of violent behavior.

In the emergency room, patients who have used PCP show hyperthermia and nystagmus (vertical or horizontal abnormal eye movements). In addition, PCP is toxic; consumption of more than 20 mg (two to four times the usual dose) can cause convulsions, coma, and death.

■ SUMMARY OF CLINICAL FEATURES OF SUBSTANCE ABUSE

In the emergency room, changes in the pupils of the eyes and presence or absence of psychotic symptoms can quickly narrow the search for the substance responsible for patients' symptoms (Table 23-5). Laboratory findings can then confirm the identity of the abused substance (Table 23-6).

TABLE 23-5	Rapid Emergency Department Identification of Abused Substances	
OBSERVATION	**SEEN WITH USE OF:**	**SEEN WITH WITHDRAWAL FROM:**
Pupil constriction	■ Opioids	■ Stimulants
Pupil dilation	■ Stimulants ■ LSD	■ Opioids ■ Alcohol and other sedatives
Psychotic symptoms (e.g., hallucinations or delusions)	■ Stimulants ■ Alcohol ■ Hallucinogens and related agents	■ Alcohol and other sedatives

LSD, lysergic acid diethylamide.

TABLE 23-6	Laboratory Findings For Selected Drugs of Abuse	
CATEGORY	ELEVATED LEVELS IN BODY FLUIDS	LENGTH OF TIME AFTER USE THAT SUBSTANCE CAN BE DETECTED
Sedatives	■ Alcohol (legal intoxication is 0.08–0.15% BAC, depending on state laws; coma occurs at BAC of 0.40–0.50% in nonalcoholics) Gamma-glutamyltransferase	7–12 hours
	■ Specific barbiturate or benzodiazepine or its metabolite	1–3 days
Opioids	■ Heroin	1–3 days
	■ Methadone	2–3 days
Stimulants	■ Cotinine (nicotine metabolite)	1–2 days
	■ Amphetamine	1–2 days
	■ Benzoylecgonine (cocaine metabolite)	1–3 days in occasional users; 7–12 days in heavy users
Hallucinogens and related agents	■ Cannabinoid metabolites	3–28 days
	■ PCP	7–14 days in heavy users
	■ Serum glutamic-oxaloacetic transaminase level and creatinine phosphokinase (reflecting muscle damage associated with PCP use)	

BAC, blood alcohol concentration; PCP, phencyclidine.

REVIEW QUESTIONS

1. A 19-year-old man is brought to the emergency department by a friend. The patient is speaking rapidly in an excited fashion and says he is "on top of the world" because he is communicating mentally with the President. Physical examination reveals dilated pupils, erythema of the mucous membranes of the nose, and tachycardia. When seen by a physician 1 hour later, the patient seems depressed and

shows little response to her presence. What is the major mechanism of action of the agent this patient has abused on neurotransmitter systems in his brain?

(A) Blocks reuptake of dopamine

(B) Blocks release of dopamine

(C) Blocks reuptake of serotonin

(D) Blocks release of serotonin

(E) Blocks release of norepinephrine

2. A 24-year-old woman complains of intense hunger as well as tiredness and headache. She states that she has been studying for final exams over the last few weeks and took the last exam yesterday. This woman is most likely to be withdrawing from which of the following substances?

(A) Alcohol

(B) Amphetamines

(C) Benzodiazepines

(D) Phencyclidine (PCP)

(E) Heroin

3. Six hours after birth, an infant begins to show excessive salivation and lacrimation. The child is also sweating, has a rapid heart rate, and appears restless and agitated. Of the following, what is the most likely cause of this picture?

(A) Exposure to alcohol

(B) Alcohol withdrawal

(C) Exposure to heroin

(D) Heroin withdrawal

(E) Amphetamine withdrawal

4. A 50-year-old man who has been taking diazepam in moderate doses daily over the past 5 years finds that he has forgotten to take the pills with him when he goes on vacation. Two days later, he calls his physician to report which of the following symptoms?

(A) Somnolence

(B) Lethargy

(C) Respiratory depression

(D) Sedation

(E) Tremor

5. When a 45-year-old smoker fills out a form to obtain a life insurance policy, he checks the box marked "never smoked." He is denied the policy when the insurance company tests his urine sample and finds elevated levels of which of the following?

(A) Benzoylecgonine

(B) Gamma-glutamyltransferase

(C) Serum glutamic-oxaloacetic transaminase

(D) Cotinine

(E) Creatinine phosphokinase

ANSWERS AND EXPLANATIONS

1-A. The fact that this patient has gone from euphoric and psychotic (the hallucination about the President) to depressed and unresponsive in only 1 hour, combined with the findings of dilated pupils and erythema (redness) of the nose (from snorting the drug), indicate that this patient has used cocaine. The major mechanism of action of cocaine is to block reuptake of dopamine, thereby increasing its availability in the synapse. Increased availability of dopamine is involved in the "reward" system of the brain and accounts for some of the euphoric effects of stimulants such as cocaine.

2-B. Tiredness and headache are seen with withdrawal from stimulants. Although increased appetite can be seen in withdrawal from all stimulants, intense hunger is most commonly seen in withdrawal from amphetamines. Withdrawal from sedatives such as alcohol and benzodiazepines or opioids such as heroin do not include these symptoms. There are no significant physical withdrawal symptoms from PCP.

3-D. This constellation of symptoms, including excessive salivation, lacrimation (tearing eyes), sweating, rapid heart rate, restlessness, and agitation, indicate that the child's mother is a heroin addict and that the child is in withdrawal after birth.

4-E. Withdrawal from benzodiazepines is associated with tremor, insomnia, and anxiety. Respiratory depression and sedation are associated with use of, not withdrawal from, sedative agents.

5-D. Elevated levels of cotinine, a metabolite of nicotine, are found in the urine of smokers. Benzoylecgonine is a cocaine metabolite, and elevated gamma-glutamyltransferase is found in the body fluids of heavy alcohol users. Elevated levels of serum glutamic-oxaloacetic transaminase and creatinine phosphokinase, reflecting muscle damage, may be found with use of PCP.

REFERENCES

Alcoholics Anonymous. (1990). *The AA group: The A.A. Grapevine, Inc.* New York: Alcoholics Anonymous World Services, Inc.

American Psychiatric Association. (2001). *Diagnostic and statistical manual of mental disorders* (4th ed., text revision) (pp. 191–295). Washington, DC: American Psychiatric Association.

Brody, J. (2001, December 11). An old enemy, smoking, hangs tough. *The New York Times.*

Forero, J., & Weiner, T. (2003, June 8). Latin American poppy fields undermine U.S. drug battle. *The New York Times.*

Grigson, P. S. (2002). Like drugs for chocolate: Separate rewards modulated by common mechanisms? *Physiol Behav, 76,* 345–346.

Krystal, J. H., Cramer, J. A., Krol, W. F., Kirk, G. F., & Rosenheck, R. A. (2001). Naltrexone in the treatment of alcohol dependence. *N Engl J Med, 345,* 1734–1739.

Leshner, A. I. (1999). Science-based views of drug addiction and its treatment. *JAMA, 282,* 1–3.

McHugh, P. F., Kellogg, S., Bell, K., Schluger, R. P., Leal, S. M., & Kreek, M. J. (2002). Potentially functional polymorphism in the promoter region of prodynorphin gene may be associated with protection against cocaine dependence or abuse. *Am J Med Genet, 114,* 4.

Mukamal, K. J., Conigrave, K. M., Mittleman, M. A., Camargo, C. A., Stampfer, M. J., Willett, W. C., & Rimm, E. B. (2003). Roles of drinking pattern and type of alcohol consumed in coronary heart disease in men. *N Engl J Med, 348,* 109–118.

National Institute on Drug Abuse (NIDA). 2001 National Household Survey on Drug Abuse. *www.samhsa.gov.* Table H.57.

Nestler, E. J., & Aghajanian, G. K. (1997). Molecular and cellular basis of addiction. *Science, 278,* 58–63.

ONDCP: Drug Policy Information Clearinghouse 2003. Street terms: Drugs and the drug trade. *http://www.whitehousedrugpolicy.gov*

Rimm, E. B., Klatsky, A., Grobbee, D., & Stampfer, M. J. (1996). Review of moderate alcohol consumption and reduced risk of coronary heart disease: Is the effect due to beer, wine, or spirits? *Br Med J, 312,* 731–736.

United States Department of Health and Human Services (USDHHS). (2001). 2001 monitoring the future survey released: Smoking among teenagers decreases sharply and increase in ecstasy use slows. HHS News. December 19,2001.

Wickelgren, I. (1998). Teaching the brain to take drugs. *Science, 280,* 2045–2047.

Doctor– **24**
Patient
Communication

P
rofessionals must often establish relationships with and elicit personal information from their clients. This may be problematic for
at least two reasons. First, the professional is essentially a stranger
to the client. Second, in some professions, such as accounting and
law, clients must reveal sensitive information to the professional, which
can be uncomfortable for the client.

Doctors must also establish relationships with and elicit personal information from clients (i.e., patients). Only in medicine, however, must
the practitioner also obtain information about that client's most personal
space—his or her own body. This task is made more difficult by the fact
that medical practitioners often have to obtain this information under
stressful or even life-threatening circumstances.

Establishing effective communication between doctor and patient is
the first step in establishing the essential alliance that will allow the doctor to help the patient. This step is influenced by many factors. For example, a patient's previous experiences with medical care can influence how
he or she responds to the doctor. A doctor's unconscious countertransference reactions based on past relationships can influence how he or she relates to the patient (see Chapter 8). Other factors that influence the doctor–
patient relationship include the patient's physical and mental condition,
personality style and coping mechanisms (see later text), use of defense
mechanisms (see Chapter 8), and cultural belief system (see Chapter 18).

Establishing an effective interaction with a patient can take time, but it is well worth the effort. Patient satisfaction with the physician and compliance with medical advice are closely related to the quality of the doctor–patient relationship.

■ GETTING INFORMATION FROM PATIENTS

The clinical interview is the most important tool a physician has for obtaining information about patients. An effective interview starts with establishing trust in and rapport with the patient. Doing this involves maximizing the physical placement of the doctor and patient to facilitate effective and safe interaction (Fig. 24-1) and then gathering the physical, psychological, and social information needed to identify the patient's problem.

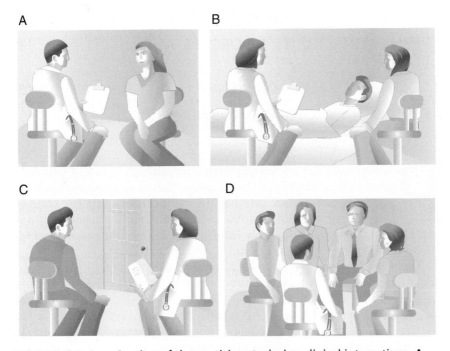

FIGURE 24-1. Seating of the participants during clinical interactions. **A.** Physician and patient interaction in the office. Note that there is no desk or other obstacle between the participants. **B.** Physician, patient, and patient's relative interaction in the patient's hospital room. Note that the three participants sit in a triangular fashion, with the doctor to one side of the patient's bed and the relative to the same side so that the bed is not an obstacle between any two individuals. **C.** Physician and potentially violent patient in the office. Note that there is no obstacle between the physician and patient and that both participants have clear access to the door. **D.** Physician and patient's family in the hospital waiting room. Note that the participants, including the doctor, sit in a circle.

The clinical interview

The **clinical interview** is used to obtain the patient's medical and psychiatric history (see Table 10-3) and to gather other relevant information. The two major categories of questions used in the clinical interview are open-ended and direct. **Open-ended questions** are nonstructured, do not close off potential areas of pertinent information, and allow for a variety of responses. These questions are used in the interview to facilitate conversation and obtain information. **Direct questions** are those that can be answered with "yes," "no," or a few simple words. They are used to clarify the information obtained from open-ended questions. For example, an open-ended question such as "Describe the pain" is used to get an overview of the patient's distress. "Does the pain wake you at night?" is a direct question about a specific area of interest.

Direct questions are also used to elicit information quickly in an emergency or when a patient has a cognitive disorder (see Chapter 18). This type of question may also be preferred when a patient is sexually provocative toward the doctor or overly talkative. Whatever the situation, doctors should avoid using **leading questions** that suggest an answer, such as, "You really feel better, don't you?"

Specific strategies and techniques, such as **support**, **empathy**, **validation**, **facilitation**, **reflection**, **silence**, **confrontation**, and **recapitulation**, that are used in interviewing patients are described in Case 24-1.

Defense mechanisms in illness

People unconsciously use **defense mechanisms** to protect themselves from realities that cause conflict and anxiety (see Chapter 8). The need for such protection is intensified by illness. A patient's use of defense mechanisms can act as a barrier to the physician in obtaining information and in gaining patient compliance.

Two of the most common defense mechanisms used by people when they are ill are denial and regression (see Table 8-2). In **denial,** a patient unconsciously refuses to admit to being ill or to acknowledge the severity of the illness. Use of this defense mechanism can be helpful initially because it can protect the individual from the physical and emotional consequences of intense fear. However, denial can be destructive in the long term if it hinders the patient from seeking treatment. For example, if a patient in the initial stages of a myocardial infarction attributes his severe chest pain to a minor problem like indigestion, his physiological fear responses (e.g., increased heart rate and blood pressure) will be attenuated. However, if he persists in this denial and fails to seek treatment, the patient can die.

In **regression,** the ill patient reverts to a more childlike pattern of behavior that may involve a desire for more attention and time from the physician. This response can make it more difficult for the physician to interact with and treat the patient effectively.

THE PATIENT Ms. Gardner, an 80-year-old nursing home patient, is brought to the hospital after a fall. The emergency room physician introduces himself to the patient by saying, "Ms. Gardner, I am Dr. Smith." He then outlines what he will do: "I am going to ask you a few questions now and then I will examine you." Dr. Smith then pulls a chair up to the bed and sits down. As he begins to talk to her, Dr. Smith notes that Ms. Gardner is oriented and alert, but seems suspicious and agitated. She also appears to be in pain. Dr. Smith asks, "Ms. Gardner, how are you feeling?" The patient says that she is "fine" and then starts crying.

COMMENT Dr. Smith correctly addresses the patient by her family name and sits at eye level with her during the interview. Although the patient says she is "fine," her behavior suggests that she is not. Before confronting this discrepancy, however, the doctor must establish a relationship with this patient. Although this situation is an emergency, the doctor can express interest and concern for the patient using support and empathy and give credence to her feelings using validation. For example, to show **support** and **empathy**, he can say, "That fall must have been a frightening experience for you." He can use **validation** to confirm to the patient that her feelings are normal and to be expected under the circumstances by stating, "Many people would feel scared if they had been injured as you were."
Once a relationship has been established, the doctor can maximize information gathering by encouraging the patient to elaborate on her responses using interview techniques such as facilitation and reflection. An example of **facilitation** would be a simple statement like," Tell me more." **Reflection** entails using what the patient has just said to encourage her to continue talking, such as asking, "You said that your pain increased during the ambulance trip?" Both techniques can increase the flow of information from the patient. Silence is the most powerful interview technique for obtaining information from patients. Therefore, when this patient begins to cry, the physician should remain attentive and concerned but should not speak. This use of **silence** allows the patient to gather her thoughts and composure so that the conversation can continue. Effective use of silence requires practice on the part of the physician. It is a natural human response to try to make a person feel better when he or she shows evidence of sadness. However, statements such as "Everything will be okay" or "Don't worry," which are used in ordinary conversation, are not usually appropriate in a doctor-patient interview because they stop the flow of conversation from the patient. These comments also may not be true and can be interpreted as patronizing.

TREATMENT Prior to treating Ms. Gardner, Dr. Smith must clarify the information he has received from her. Information can be clarified by calling the patient's attention to inconsistencies in her responses or body language using confrontation and by summarizing the information obtained during the interview using recapitulation. However, the doctor should be careful not to judge a patient who is not forthcoming. In **confrontation**, the doctor might say, "Ms. Gardner, you say that you feel fine but you seem to be in pain." A statement such as this allows the patient to confirm or correct the doctor's observation. The final step in an interview is for the doctor to use **recapitulation** to summarize what the patient has said. For example, the doctor can say, "Let's go over what happened this morning. You fell in the shower and hurt your leg. When you realized that you could not move it, the emergency squad was called. The paramedics then brought you to the hospital where I met you. Have I gotten it right?" This gives the patient the opportunity to either confirm the doctor's comprehension or correct his misunderstanding of the story.

Interviewing children

Like adults, children and adolescents respond best during a clinical interview when they feel comfortable with the doctor. In contrast to adults, the type of questions most effective in interviews with adults may not be appropriate for children. For example, young children may have difficulty responding to open-ended questions. A 6-year-old child may not know how to respond to a question such as "Tell me about yourself," but she may be able to answer a specific question such as, "What grade are you in?" Other children may not respond well even to direct questions. Methods of obtaining information from these children (if they are old enough to understand and comply) include asking the child to draw a picture (e.g., "Can you draw a picture of yourself?") and asking questions in the third person (e.g., "Why do you think the little boy in the picture looks sad?") Getting the child to use his imagination can be fun for the child and can provide information for the doctor (e.g., "Let's pretend that you have two wishes. What would they be?") Gaining parental permission to speak to teachers and babysitters can also be helpful in getting information about a child.

Typically, adolescents worry about appearance, hetero- and homosexuality, sexually transmitted diseases, and substance abuse, concerns they may find difficult to discuss with their parents. Often, all that is required of the doctor is that she be nonjudgmental and able to reassure the adolescent that his or her thoughts are normal and common in people in this age group. With the exception of certain breaches of confidentiality (see Chapter 26), it is also appropriate for the doctor to reassure the patient that such information will not be shared with his or her parents. Parents usually understand this need for privacy.

■ GIVING INFORMATION TO PATIENTS

Patients are understandably reticent to ask questions about issues that are potentially embarrassing, such as sexual problems, or potentially fear-provoking, such as laboratory results. A doctor should anticipate such unspoken questions, verbalize them, and then answer them truthfully and completely (Case 24-2).

Giving information to adult patients

In the United States, it is customary for adult patients to be told the complete truth about the diagnosis and prognosis of their illness. For example, if a dying patient asks the doctor how long he has to live, the doctor should answer truthfully. An accurate statement such as, "I do not know for sure, but most people at this stage of the illness usually live from 1 to 3 months," is an appropriate response. A falsely reassuring response to this patient's question (e.g., "Do not worry, we will take good care of you") is not appropriate (see Case 24-1). The doctor should also avoid philo-

THE PATIENT During his regular office visit, a 54-year-old male patient who has been taking propranolol (Inderal) for hypertension for the past 6 months says to the doctor, "Could you please tell me again the side effects of the medication I am taking for my blood pressure?" The patient then stops speaking.

COMMENT Some antihypertensives cause sexual difficulties, such as erectile dysfunction (see Table 21–4). This patient is most likely uncomfortable mentioning his sexual problems. The doctor should raise the issue with a statement such as, " Sexual side effects are common with antihypertensive medication. Please tell me about the effects you have been experiencing." The doctor should not simply repeat the known side effects or tell the patient that the side effects are not medically significant.

TREATMENT If the doctor determines that this patient is experiencing sexual dysfunction because of the antihypertensive medication, she can recommend switching to a medication with fewer sexual side effects. Among the antihypertensives, angiotensin converting enzyme (ACE) inhibitors (e.g., captopril) are less likely than beta blockers, such as propranolol, to cause sexual side effects (see Chapter 21).

sophical or religious statements that could be interpreted as patronizing (e.g., "No matter how long you live, you have had a very productive life"). Table 24-1 provides a six-step strategy for giving bad news to patients (Baile et al., 2000).

In some cultural groups, adult children protect elderly relatives from negative medical diagnoses and make medical decisions about their care (see Chapter 20). In the United States, information about a competent patient's illness should be given directly to the patient and not relayed through relatives. With the patient's permission, the physician can tell relatives this information in conjunction with or after telling the patient, especially because relieving the fears of close relatives can bolster the patient's support system.

Sometimes, a doctor must reconcile the wishes of patients with those of their families. For example, relatives may want an elderly patient to be cared for in a long-term care facility, such as a nursing home, before the patient is ready to do this (see Chapter 27). In such a circumstance, the role of the doctor is to evaluate the need for such placement, encourage communication between the patient and family members, and perhaps provide recommendations for interventions that will allow the patient to live at home safely.

Giving information to ill children

Children should be told about their illness and treatment in an age-appropriate way in terms that they can understand. It is up to the parents to decide if, how, and when this information will be given. In the

TABLE 24-1 SPIKES: A Six-Step Protocol For Giving Patients Bad News

STEP	TECHNIQUES
Setting up the interview	■ Arrange for privacy ■ Involve significant others at the patient's request ■ Sit down and maintain eye contact with the patient ■ Touch the patient's arm or hand (if comfortable for the patient) ■ Silence your pager and do not respond to the phone
Perception of the patient	■ Find out what the patient understands about the medical situation ■ Determine if the patient is using denial or wishful thinking ■ Determine if the patient has unrealistic expectations about the diagnosis
Invitation	■ Find out how the patient would like to receive the diagnosis and related information ■ Find out how much detail the patient wishes to have ■ Offer to answer questions in the future ■ Offer to talk to a relative or friend
Knowledge	■ Prepare the patient for bad news ■ Give the positive news first ■ Present bad news clearly and unambiguously ■ Give information in small doses and check the patient's understanding regularly ■ Use nontechnical words of explanation if possible ■ Avoid conveying hopelessness
Emotions/ Empathy	■ Observe the patient's emotions ■ Ask the patient about his feelings ■ Connect the patient's emotion with the reason for it (e.g., news about the illness) ■ Tolerate the patient's distress ■ Stay near the patient and wait silently for him to speak ■ Ask if anyone should be called
Strategy/ Summary	■ Ask the patient if he is ready to discuss treatment ■ Evaluate the patient's understanding, expectations, and hopes for the future ■ Share decision-making responsibility with the patient ■ Understand the goals of the patient (e.g., pain control) ■ State immediate plans for care ■ Schedule a follow-up visit

Adapted from Baile, W. F., Buckman, R., Lenzi, R., Glober, G., Beale, E. A., & Kudelka, A. P. (2000). SPIKES—A six-step protocol for delivering bad news: Application to the patient with cancer. *Oncologist, 5,* 302–311.

unlikely event that parents do not want their child to know the diagnosis or prognosis, the doctor cannot tell the child. However, if the child asks the doctor about his or her condition, it is appropriate for the doctor to ask the child a question like, "What have your parents told you about your illness?"

If the doctor needs to do a procedure on a child that will cause pain (e.g., an injection), the doctor should describe to the child what to expect in an age-appropriate manner. For example, a 5-year-old child would be told, "This will feel like a bug bite, but it will stop stinging after we count from one to five together."

Making decisions for patients

Under certain circumstances, it is difficult for patients to make health care decisions. At such times, patients may ask their doctors, "What would you do if this happened to you or your family member?" Doctors need to remember that their role is not to decide what patients should do, but rather to provide the information patients need to make their own decisions. For example, the parents of a pregnant teenager who wants to keep her baby may expect the doctor to convince the girl to give her child up for adoption. Although he may agree with the parents, the doctor's role is to furnish the teenager with the information she needs to help her make an informed decision. This includes providing her with details about the responsibilities of raising a child. The doctor's role also involves facilitating discussion between the teenager and her parents so that they all participate in and ultimately agree on the decision.

Abandonment

It is inappropriate to refer patients to other doctors because the patients are annoying, seductive, or angry. Referrals of patients should be reserved for patients with medical and psychiatric problems outside the range of expertise of the treating physician. Referrals are also appropriate for patients who require services that the treating physician does not wish to perform. For example, if a doctor does not perform abortions for personal reasons and her patient wants the procedure, rather than abandon the patient, the doctor should arrange for the abortion to be done by a physician who does the procedure.

■ PERSONALITY TRAITS, DISORDERS, AND COPING STYLES

Personality traits and coping styles are individuals' unique ways of responding to the environment and interpersonal relationships. These characteristics are influenced by genetic make-up (see Chapter 5) and life experiences, and they are important determinants of how people react to illness. Understanding these characteristics can help doctors predict the responses of individual patients and can help them gain patients' compliance with recommended medical treatment.

Everyone has personality traits. However, if these traits lead to personal distress or to problems in social or occupational functioning, the person may have a personality disorder. For example, it is normal for a patient to be skeptical about having a medical test or procedure. However, if a patient is so skeptical of the physician's motives for ordering the test that she refuses it, her paranoid personality trait can have life-limiting consequences.

Personality disorders

Personality disorders (PDs) are chronic and lifelong. The Diagnostic and Statistical Manual of Mental Disorders, Fourth Edition-Text Revision (DSM-IV-TR) classifies PDs on Axis II, separating them from the Axis I psychiatric disorders, and it places each into either **Cluster A** (paranoid, schizoid, schizotypal), **Cluster B** (histrionic, narcissistic, antisocial, borderline), or **Cluster C** (avoidant, obsessive-compulsive, dependent) based on certain shared characteristics and genetic associations. Table 24-2 provides examples of patients, differential diagnoses, and genetic or familial associations of the PDs with other psychiatric disorders. Individuals with atypical personality traits or mixtures of abnormal personality traits are diagnosed with **personality disorder not otherwise specified (NOS).** Passive-aggressive PD is currently NOS and in the appendix of the DSM-IV-TR.

Characteristics of the personality disorders

Histrionic, borderline, dependent, antisocial, and schizotypal PD may be somewhat more common (each occurring in 2 to 3% of the population) than obsessive compulsive, narcissistic, avoidant, and schizoid PD (each occurring in 1% or less of the population). For the DSM-IV-TR diagnosis, a PD must be present by early adulthood. Antisocial PD cannot be diagnosed until 18 years of age; prior to age 18, the diagnosis is conduct disorder (see Chapter 2).

Treatment of the personality disorders

Typically, patients with PD have no insight and lack awareness that they are the cause of their own relationship problems. Thus, they rarely seek psychological help unless compelled by others. Patients with PD do not show frank psychosis and, unless the PD brings the person into conflict with others, they do not show disabling psychiatric symptoms, such as anxiety or depression.

Pharmacologic treatment has no proven usefulness in PDs. Medications can, however, be used when patients with PDs also show depression and anxiety. Individual and group psychotherapy and self-help groups may also benefit patients with PDs.

Personality traits and coping styles

Even if a patient does not have a diagnosable personality disorder, his or her personality characteristics can affect the way he or she copes with

TABLE 24-2 Characteristics and Patient Examples of the DSM-IV-TR Personality Disorders

PERSONALITY DISORDER	CHARACTERISTICS	INTERACTIONS WITH DOCTORS	PATIENT EXAMPLE
CLUSTER A: Hallmarks: Acts peculiar or avoids social relationships but is not psychotic GENETIC OR FAMILIAL ASSOCIATION: Psychotic illnesses DIFFERENTIAL DIAGNOSES: Disorders with frank psychotic symptoms like schizophrenia (Chapter 11), delusional disorder (Chapter 12), mood disorder with psychotic features (Chapter 13), and, particularly for schizoid PD, a pervasive developmental disorder such as Asperger disorder (Chapter 1).			
Paranoid	■ Distrustful ■ Suspicious ■ Litigious ■ Attributes responsibility for own problems to others ■ Interprets motives of others as malevolent	■ Blames the physician for the illness ■ Is overly sensitive to a perceived lack of attention or caring from the physician	A 45-year-old woman who has been a heavy smoker for more than 25 years and has a persistent cough refuses to have a chest radiograph recommended by her doctor. She states that she is sure that the doctor is just trying to make extra money by recommending tests she does not need. She reports that when her previous doctor made a similar recommendation, she filed a complaint against him with the state.
Schizoid	■ Longstanding pattern of voluntary social withdrawal without psychosis ■ Detached ■ Restricted emotions	■ Shows little emotional connection with the doctor ■ Becomes even more withdrawn during illness	The parents of a 26-year-old man tell the doctor that they are concerned about him because he has no friends and spends most of his time hiking in the woods. The interview reveals that the man is content with his solitary life, and there is no evidence of a formal thought disorder.

TABLE 24-2 Characteristics and Patient Examples of the DSM-IV-TR
Personality Disorders (Continued)

PERSONALITY DISORDER	CHARACTERISTICS	INTERACTIONS WITH DOCTORS	PATIENT EXAMPLE
Schizotypal	■ Peculiar appearance ■ Magical thinking ■ Odd thought patterns and behavior without psychosis	■ Behaves strangely and even more inappropriately when ill	An oddly dressed 32-year-old woman tells the doctor that she has 35 cats that can sense her feelings. She says that she never goes out on Thursdays because they are "unlucky days," and she has few friends.

CLUSTER B: Emotional, inconsistent, or dramatic
GENETIC OR FAMILIAL ASSOCIATION: Mood disorders, substance abuse, and somatoform disorders
DIFFERENTIAL DIAGNOSES: Hypomanic episode (Chapter 13) and substance abuse (Chapter 23)

Histrionic	■ Attention-seeking ■ Extroverted ■ Emotional ■ Sexually provocative ("life of the party") ■ Shallow, vain ■ Unable to maintain intimate relationships ■ In men, "Don Juan" dress and behavior	■ Dramatic reporting of symptoms ■ Approaches the physician in an inappropriate sexual fashion during illness	A 28-year-old female patient comes to the physician's office dressed in a low-cut, red satin dress. She reports that she feels so warm that she "must have a fever of at least 106" and then places the doctor's hand on her chest so that he can "feel how hard my heart is beating."
Narcissistic	■ Pompous; has sense of special entitlement and lacks empathy for others ■ Feels superior to others	■ Has a perfect self-image that is threatened by illness ■ Often demanding when ill	A 38-year-old male patient asks the doctor to refer him to a physician who graduated from an Ivy League medical school. He says he knows that the doctor will not be offended because the doctor

PERSONALITY DISORDER	CHARACTERISTICS	INTERACTIONS WITH DOCTORS	PATIENT EXAMPLE
			understands that the patient is "better" than the doctor's other patients .
Antisocial	■ Refuses to conform to social norms ■ Dishonest ■ Associated with conduct disorder in childhood and criminality in adulthood ■ Are known in lay terms as "psychopaths" or "sociopaths"	■ Has no concern for others ■ Fails to learn from experience	A 35-year-old man brags to his physician that he has been sexually assaulting women ever since high school but has never been caught. He has often been unemployed and has been arrested for shoplifting several times. After he leaves, the doctor notices that a prescription pad is missing and that a nurse cannot find the wallet she left in her desk.
Borderline	■ Erratic, unstable behavior and mood ■ Boredom ■ Feelings of aloneness ■ Impulsiveness ■ Suicide attempts ■ Self-injury (e.g., cutting, burning) ■ Often comorbid with mood and eating disorders	■ May show "mini-psychotic" episodes (i.e., brief periods of loss of contact with reality) ■ Overidealizes and then overreacts to perceived rejection by the doctor	A 20-year old female college student tells the physician that, because she was afraid to be alone again, she tried to commit suicide after she asked her former doctor out and he refused. After the interview, she tells the physician that all of the other doctors she has seen were terrible and that he is the only doctor who has ever understood her problems (use of "splitting" as a defense mechanism; see Table 8-1).

TABLE 24-2	Characteristics and Patient Examples of the DSM-IV-TR Personality Disorders (Continued)		
PERSONALITY DISORDER	CHARACTERISTICS	INTERACTIONS WITH DOCTORS	PATIENT EXAMPLE
CLUSTER C: Fearful and anxious **GENETIC OR FAMILIAL ASSOCIATION:** Anxiety disorders **DIFFERENTIAL DIAGNOSES:** Social phobia, obsessive-compulsive disorder, and depression			
Avoidant	▪ Timid ▪ Sensitive to rejection ▪ Socially withdrawn ▪ Feelings of inferiority	▪ Fears rejection by the doctor ▪ Avoids tests and treatment	A 35-year-old woman who works as a laboratory assistant lives with her elderly mother. She states that she was going out with a man but he left her because she was too shy. She reports that when coworkers ask her to join them for lunch, she wants to go but refuses because she is afraid that they will not like her.
Obsessive-compulsive	▪ Perfectionistic ▪ Orderly (makes lists) ▪ Stubborn ▪ Indecisive ▪ Ultimately inefficient	▪ Fears loss of control and may try to control the doctor during illness ▪ Follows the doctor's orders to the letter	A 33-year-old diabetic man reports that each night he makes up a written schedule for his behavior and for all of the food that he will eat for the next day. He tells the physician that his wife of 6 months recently moved out because he criticized her unwillingness to follow the same rigid schedule.
Dependent	▪ Poor self-confidence ▪ Allows others to make their decisions	▪ Has an excessive need to be cared for by others, resulting in	A 32-year-old female patient tells the doctor that her husband is very angry at her because she calls him at the office

PERSONALITY DISORDER	CHARACTERISTICS	INTERACTIONS WITH DOCTORS	PATIENT EXAMPLE
	and assume their responsibilities ■ May end up as an abused spouse	helplessness and the desire for attention from the physician during illness	many times a day to ask him to make trivial decisions for her. She also calls the doctor each morning to ask his advice.
Personality Disorder Not Otherwise Specified (NOS)			
Passive-aggressive	■ Procrastinates ■ Inefficient ■ Sullen ■ Outwardly compliant but inwardly defiant	■ Asks for help but then does not comply with the physician's advice	Two weeks after a 50-year-old overweight, hypertensive female patient agreed to start a diet program, she gains 4 pounds. She tells the doctor that she has not started dieting yet because her local grocery store did not have all of the recommended foods.

DSM-IV-TR, Diagnostic and Statistical Manual of Mental Disorders, Fourth Edition-Text Revision. Adapted from Fadem, B., & Simring, S. (2003). *High-yield psychiatry* (2nd ed.). Philadelphia: Lippincott Williams & Wilkins.

(i.e., manages) illness. For example, patients who have one of the Cluster A personality types are likely to respond to their illness by becoming even more withdrawn or suspicious. The physician may have to take more time establishing a trusting relationship with such patients. Patients with Cluster B personality types are more likely to become emotional and seductive when stressed by illness. For these patients, the doctor may have to set limits on inappropriate behavior and use closed-ended questions that limit the patient's responsiveness. Cluster C-type patients show increased anxiety and may be even more fearful than other patients about losing control and becoming dependent during illness. They may therefore respond to illness by becoming more controlling or angry (the obsessive-compulsive type) or more needy (the dependent type). For these patients, the doctor should not take the manifestations of these emotions personally, but should understand that they reflect the patients' underlying health concerns.

■ COMPLIANCE AND ADHERENCE

Compliance and adherence refer to the extent to which a patient follows the instructions of the physician. These instructions include taking medications on schedule, having a needed medical test or surgical procedure, and following directions for lifestyle changes, such as diet or exercise.

Factors affecting compliance

Although it may seem counterintuitive, compliance with medical advice is not related to patient intelligence, education, sex, religion, race, socioeconomic status, or marital status. It is, however, closely related to

TABLE 24-3	Factors Associated With Compliance With Medical Advice
FACTORS THAT INCREASE COMPLIANCE	**FACTORS THAT DECREASE COMPLIANCE**
Good physician-patient relationship (most important factor)	Perception of the physician as cold and unapproachable; anger at the physician
Feeling ill	Has few symptoms
Limitation of usual activities	Little disruption of activities
Written instructions for taking medication	Verbal instructions for taking medication
Acute illness	Chronic illness
Simple treatment schedule	Complex treatment schedule
Short time spent in the waiting room	Long time spent in the waiting room
Recommending one behavioral change at a time (e.g., this week, stop smoking)	Recommending multiple behavioral changes at the same time (e.g., stop smoking and start exercising and dieting)
Believing that the benefits of care outweigh its financial and time costs (the "Health Belief Model")	Believing that the financial and time costs of care outweigh its benefits
Peer support (particularly in adolescents with chronic illnesses)	Little peer support

Adapted from Fadem, S. (2001). *High-yield behavioral science* (2nd ed.). Baltimore: Lippincott Williams & Wilkins.

personality traits and defense mechanisms and even more closely with how well the patient likes the doctor.

Encouraging patient compliance

Patients who do not feel ill or who do not believe that they have a medical problem are less likely than patients with symptoms to comply with

TABLE 24-4	Review of Rules for the Doctor in the Doctor–Patient Relationship

Getting Information From Patients

- Sit at eye level with patients
- Do not put a table or desk between you and the patient
- Ask open-ended questions
- Avoid leading questions that suggest an answer
- Do not be judgmental
- Show support and empathy
- Speak less and let the patient speak more
- Clarify and summarize the information the patient has provided
- Anticipate a patient's unspoken questions and ask them
- Anticipate a patient's unspoken fears and address them

Giving Information To Patients

- Tell adult patients the truth about their diagnosis and prognosis
- Use vocabulary words the patient will understand
- Speak to adult patients directly, not through relatives or office staff
- Do not discuss issues concerning patients with anyone without the patients' permission
- Do not offer premature reassuring statements or platitudes
- Do not attempt to frighten patients into complying with medical recommendations
- Before beginning an examination or procedure, tell the patient what to expect
- Do not order a course of action; provide information and let the patient decide

Other Doctor–Patient Issues

- Do not blame the patient for failure to comply or for difficult behavior
- Respect the patient's autonomy
- Set limits on inappropriate behavior by the patient, e.g., threatening or seductive behavior
- Do not abandon the patient
- Do not refer the patient to another health professional for anything other than a medical reason
- Follow the patient's wishes or advance directives as closely as possible

medical advice. For example, if a patient who drinks alcohol excessively rationalizes this behavior to himself by believing that drinking is actually good for him, it is unlikely that he will follow suggestions to stop drinking. To get this patient to drink less alcohol, the physician must first address his willingness to stop drinking before recommending a treatment program.

In contrast, patients who are too anxious about the possibility of having an illness may also not follow doctors' recommendations. For example, when a patient whose parents both died of colon cancer refuses to have a colonoscopy because he "heard that it was uncomfortable," the doctor should identify the real reason for the patient's refusal. In this case, it is probably the realistic fear that cancer will be found. In such a patient, fear-provoking descriptions of untreated colon cancer are more likely to decrease rather than increase compliance with the recommended test. Factors associated with seeking help from a physician and then complying with medical advice are listed in Table 24-3. Table 24-4 provides a review of rules for the doctor's behavior in the doctor-patient relationship.

REVIEW QUESTIONS

1. A 50-year-old, dirty, disheveled patient who is being treated for psoriasis has had at least one complaint about the office or staff on every monthly visit. He frequently misses appointments without calling, and when he does come, he is often late. On this day, he complains that he had to wait too long, that it took forever for the nurse to find his records, and that the office is totally unorganized. The doctor's best response is to

   (A) not comment but proceed with the examination

   (B) acknowledge the patient's anger

   (C) refer the patient for psychiatric evaluation

   (D) ask the nurse to reschedule the patient's appointment for another day

   (E) tell the patient that there is no reason to be annoyed

   (F) tell the patient that you have never before had complaints about the office and staff

2. In telling the doctor about his daughter's death in a car accident when she was 18 years old, a 53-year-old man pauses in his narrative because he keeps breaking down crying. The doctor knows that the man is quite religious. The best thing for the doctor to say at this point is

   (A) "You have your religion to sustain you."

   (B) "I know you feel very sad now, but time is a great healer."

   (C) "Please take your time."

(D) "What a terrible loss."

(E) "Tell me more about your daughter."

3. A doctor would like to know whether a patient's back pain is related to exercise. Which of the following will produce the most comprehensive response from the patient?

(A) "Do you feel pain when you climb stairs?"

(B) "How often do you feel pain when you sit still?"

(C) "Tell me your thoughts about the relationship of your pain to exercise."

(D) "Is the pain more severe when you exercise early or later in the day?"

(E) "On a scale of one to ten, how much pain do you feel when you exercise?"

4. A 35-year-old single woman who has been smoking three packs of cigarettes a day for the last 15 years asks the doctor to help her stop smoking. The doctor asks the patient why she smokes so much. The patient responds, "All my life I have always felt very alone and empty inside; I smoke to fill myself up." The patient shows no evidence of a thought disorder but reveals that she often cuts her skin with a razor in order to "feel something" and has made three suicide attempts. This clinical picture is most consistent with which of the following personality types?

(A) Borderline

(B) Histrionic

(C) Avoidant

(D) Dependent

(E) Paranoid

(F) Passive-aggressive

(G) Schizoid

5. A well-educated, 50-year-old Latino female patient has a herniated disc. The disc causes her very little discomfort. The patient has a good relationship with her doctor, who, in an effort to avoid surgery, has recommended a complex series of exercises as well as medication to reduce the inflammation. This patient is most likely to comply with this treatment plan for which of the following reasons?

(A) The illness has few symptoms

(B) She likes the doctor

(C) The treatment schedule is complex

(D) She is well educated

(E) She is female

6. During a follow-up visit after a mastectomy, a 48-year-old married woman tells the surgeon that she feels "ugly" when she gets undressed in front of her husband at night. Most appropriately, the doctor should now say

   (A) "Do not be upset, you still look good."

   (B) "There are a number of new reconstructive procedures that can improve your appearance."

   (C) "You should be pleased that you have recovered well from the surgery."

   (D) "The most important thing is that we caught the disease in time."

   (E) "Tell me about how the surgery has affected your relationship with your husband."

7. When a 15-year-old girl comes to the doctor's office for an appointment, she asks the doctor to have her mother remain in the waiting room. What is the doctor's best cause of action?

   (A) Ask the girl if there is something she wants to say in private

   (B) Ask the mother to stay in the waiting room

   (C) Ask the mother if she has any questions about her daughter

   (D) Tell the mother that he will speak to her after he speaks to her daughter

   (E) Tell the girl that he cannot discuss private issues with her without her mother present

ANSWERS AND EXPLANATIONS

1-B. Before examining this patient, the physician should acknowledge his anger by saying, "You seem annoyed." The patient's anger at the doctor may be related to his own anxiety about having a serious illness and needing to go to a doctor. The doctor is responsible for dealing with illness-related emotional needs and problems of patients. There is no reason to refer this patient to another physician. Do not blame the patient, no matter how unpleasant, for anything, including coming late to appointments.

2-C. Allowing the patient to gather his thoughts by saying "please take your time" is the most appropriate statement by the doctor. Statements such as, "You have your religion to sustain you" or "I know you feel sad now, but time is a great healer" are efforts by the doctor to stop the patient from expressing sadness, in part because such expression makes her uncomfortable. Saying, "What a terrible loss" or "Tell me more about your daughter" may be appropriate after the patient has expressed his sadness and has had the opportunity to compose himself.

3-C. The most open-ended of these questions is, "Tell me your thoughts about the relationship of your pain to exercise." All of the other choices are more direct and closed-ended and will elicit less information from the patient.

4-A. This woman who has always felt empty and alone (not merely loneliness) but shows no evidence of a thought disorder shows a borderline personality type. Self-injurious behavior and suicide attempts are also characteristic of this personality type.

5-B. Patients are most likely to comply with medical advice because they like the doctor. Compliance is also associated with symptomatic illnesses and simple treatment schedules. There is no clear association between compliance and ethnicity, education, or gender.

6-E. The physician should not offer this patient falsely reassuring statements such as, "You still look good," You have recovered well," "The most important thing is that we caught the disease in time," or "You can have reconstructive surgery." Most appropriately, the doctor should find out what is causing this patient to feel unattractive, which is probably that the surgery has affected her relationship with her husband.

7-B. The doctor's best response is to ask the mother to stay in the waiting room. The patient obviously wants to speak to the doctor privately. Parents usually understand why confidentiality between adolescents and their doctors is necessary. The doctor does not have to ask the mother if she has any questions about her daughter or tell her that he will speak to her after the examination.

REFERENCES

American Psychiatric Association. (1994). *Diagnostic and statistical manual of mental disorders* (4th ed.). Washington, DC: American Psychiatric Association

Ambuel, B., Mazzone, M. F. (2001). Breaking bad news and discussing death. *Primary Care, 28,* 249.

Baile, W. F., Buckman, R., Lenzi, R., Glober, G., Beale, E. A., & Kudelka, A. P. (2000). SPIKES—A six-step protocol for delivering bad news: Application to the patient with cancer. *Oncologist, 5,* 302–311.

Levinson, W. Gorawara-Bhat, R., & Lamb, J. (2000). A study of patient clues and physician response in primary care and surgical settings. *JAMA, 284,* 1021–1027.

O'Brien, R. (1994). The doctor-patient relationship. *Ann N Y Acad Sci, 729,* 22.

Oldman, J. M. (1994). Personality disorders. Current perspectives. *JAMA, 272,* 1770.

Ong, L. M., de Haes, J. C., Hoos, A. M., & Lammas, F. B. (1995). Doctor-patient communication: A review of the literature. *Soc Sci Med, 20,* 903.

Rennie, D. & Dan, B. B. (1992). Models of the physician-patient relationship. *JAMA, 268,* 1410–1413.

Suchman, A. L., Markakis, K., Beckman, H. B., & Frankel, R. (1997). A model of empathic communication in the medical interview. *JAMA, 277,* 678.

Zinn, W. (1993). The empathic physician. *Arch Intern Med, 153,* 306–312.

25

Psychosomatic Medicine

E veryone knows or has heard of somebody who became ill after a stressful experience. The medical student who always seems to have a cold during exam week, or the elderly man who is diagnosed with a rapidly metastasizing cancer and dies 6 months after the death of his wife, are familiar themes. Although these examples and the folk wisdom of many cultures suggest that people under psychological stress are likely to become ill, it is only in the past few decades that medical research has provided compelling evidence of this psyche (mind) and soma (body) relationship.

Physicians must be aware of the close association between the mind and body in all aspects of medical practice. Not only are stressed people more likely to become medically ill, but medical illnesses or their treatments can themselves lead to or exacerbate psychological symptoms. Thus, the psychological symptoms displayed by a patient can sometimes be the first indication of a serious medical illness.

PSYCHOLOGICAL FACTORS THAT AFFECT MEDICAL CONDITIONS

The Diagnostic and Statistical Manual of Mental Disorders, Fourth Edition-Text Revision (DSM-IV-TR) has identified several psychological factors likely to affect the course or treatment of an individual's medical condition. These factors include psychiatric illnesses, such as depression, and poor health behaviors, such as smoking. They also include stress-related physiological responses and maladaptive personality traits and coping styles. Descriptions and clinical examples of these factors are given in Table 25-1.

Depression and medical illness

Depression affects both the body and the brain. It has been associated with a variety of physical changes, some of which have medical consequences (McEwen, 2000). For example, the risk in depressed patients of death after a myocardial infarction (MI) is higher than in nondepressed patients and is equivalent to that of patients with a history of previous MI or of left ventricular dysfunction (Frasure-Smith et al., 1993). Depressed patients are also more likely to develop diabetes, osteoporosis, and stroke (Krishnan et al., 2002).

Stress

In physics, the term **"stress"** refers to forces that are brought against an object in equilibrium. In psychiatry, stress refers to life events, or **stressors,** that have the force to alter the expected course of an individual's goals, employment, relationships, and health.

Stressful life events

It is obvious that events such as September 11 are extreme psychological stressors (Galea et al., 2002). However, even "ordinary" life events cause stress, some more than others. Several schemes have been devised to quantify such stress. According to research by Holmes and Rahe (1965), life events have positions in a hierarchy called the **Social Readjustment Rating Scale.** The position of an event in the hierarchy is determined by its power to cause a person to alter or readjust his or her life. For example, the event with the highest score, death of a spouse with 100 points, requires the most readjustment and thus represents the highest level of stress for an individual. Stressful life events also include positive occurrences, such as the birth of a wanted child (Table 25-2).

Holmes and Rahe suggested that the more life adjustments patients need to make, the higher their risk for medical and psychiatric illness. Eighty percent of patients who accumulated a score of 300 points or more in 1 year developed an illness in the following year. Because not all of the

TABLE 25-1 DSM-IV-TR Criteria for Psychological Factors Affecting the Course or Treatment of a Medical Condition

PSYCHOLOGICAL FACTOR	EXAMPLES	CLINICAL PORTRAIT
Mental disorder or psychological symptom (Axis I or Axis II disorder or symptom of the disorder)	■ Depression ■ Anxiety ■ Psychosis	A 43-year-old depressed patient who has had an MI states there is no point in living, and he stops taking his medication. One week later he develops severe chest pain and has another MI.
Maladaptive health behavior	■ Smoking ■ Sedentary lifestyle ■ Unhealthy diet ■ Excessive alcohol or drug use	A 48-year-old man who weighs 290 pounds and has atherosclerosis relates that whenever he gets upset or tense, he eats cookies and high-calorie snack food. He has recently gained another 20 pounds and reports shortness of breath and chest pain with even slight exertion.
Stress-related physiological response	■ Increased activity of the autonomic nervous system leading to increased heart rate and blood pressure ■ Increased release of ACTH leading to immune system depression	A 58-year-old patient who has had a previous MI develops severe chest pain and shortness of breath 1 week after she is laid off from the job that she has held for 15 years.
Personality trait	■ Obsessive-compulsive personality ■ Type A personality (time-pressured, competitive, sometimes also hostile) ■ Hostility is key component in increased risk for heart disease	An active, aggressive 38-year old car salesperson, hospitalized for an MI, becomes angry and belligerent when the doctor tells him that he may need to slow down. He signs out of the hospital against medical advice, returns to his job, and has another, more severe MI.

TABLE 25-1	DSM-IV-TR Criteria for Psychological Factors Affecting the Course or Treatment of a Medical Condition (Continued)

PSYCHOLOGICAL FACTOR	EXAMPLES	CLINICAL PORTRAIT
Coping style	■ Inability to express feelings ■ Regression (the return to developmentally earlier patterns of behavior; see Chapter 8)	A 65-year-old woman who has coronary artery disease refuses to leave the house for any reason unless her daughter accompanies her. When her daughter is on a business trip, she develops chest pain, does not seek treatment, and has a severe MI.

ACTH, adrenocorticotropic hormone; DSM-IV-TR, Diagnostic and Statistical Manual of Mental Disorders, Fourth Edition-Text Revision; MI, myocardial infarction.

TABLE 25-2	Magnitude of Stress Associated With Selected Life Events According to the Holmes and Rahe Social Readjustment Rating Scale

RELATIVE STRESSFULNESS	LIFE EVENT (POINT VALUE)
Very high	■ Death of a spouse (100) ■ Divorce (73) ■ Marital separation (65) ■ Death of a close family member (63)
High	■ Major personal loss of health due to illness or injury (53) ■ Marriage (50) ■ Job loss (47) ■ Retirement (45) ■ Major loss of health of a close family member (44) ■ Birth or adoption of a child (39)
Moderate	■ Assuming major debt (e.g., taking out a mortgage) (31) ■ Promotion or demotion at work (29) ■ Child leaving home (29)
Low	■ Changing residence (20) ■ Vacation (15) ■ Major holiday (12)

THE PATIENT A 65-year-old man is brought to the hospital after collapsing in a local restaurant. The patient is unable to move his right arm or leg and is having difficulty speaking. The history, obtained from his son, reveals that aside from mild hypertension, the patient's health had been good until the previous year. During that year both the patient's wife and his older brother died. After his wife's death, the patient retired from his job and moved to a different city. The move entailed taking out a mortgage on an apartment. During the move, the patient fell and fractured his hip and was hospitalized for 6 weeks. Neurologic examination and neuroimaging studies indicate that this patient has had a left-hemisphere stroke.

COMMENT According to the Holmes and Rahe scale, many of the social experiences this man had in the past year placed him at high risk for physical illness in the present year. These experiences include the death of two close family members—his wife (100 points) and brother (63 points)—as well as retirement (45 points), moving (20 points), and assuming a large debt (31 points). The fall and subsequent hospitalization (53 points) led to an accumulation of 312 points, well above the 300 point cutoff for risk of physical illness devised by Holmes and Rahe.

TREATMENT Supportive physiological measures should be given to the patient, along with treatment to prevent another stroke. Psychological counseling can help this patient deal with the stressors in his life as well as a serious new stressor, loss of his own physical health (53 points).

patients with high scores became ill, factors noted earlier, such as personality and coping styles, affect the relationship between life stress and illness.

Effects of stress on physiological function

In 1976, Hans Selye described the **general adaptation syndrome**—homeostatic mechanisms that the body uses in response to social stress. These mechanisms include neuroendocrine responses. An immediate effect of stress is to increase secretion of catecholamines such as epinephrine. This increase can exacerbate cardiovascular disorders such as congestive heart failure, cardiac arrhythmias, and hypertension; and pain disorders such as migraine headache. A later effect of stress is increased secretion of cortisol, which can lead to altered immune system activity and decreased ability to resist infection or cancer (see later text).

Stress and immune system function

Studies in the field of **psychoneuroimmunology (PNI)** have further characterized the relationship between stress and immune system function (Solomon, 2000; Wong, 2002). The major tenet of PNI is that external stress leads to stimulation of the hypothalamus, which in turn leads to the release of corticotropin-releasing factor (CRF). Release of CRF results in rapid release of adrenocorticotropic hormone (ACTH), which prompts the release of corticosteroids (e.g., cortisol) that modulate immune responses.

In PNI studies, measures of alterations in immune responses include decreased lymphocyte response to mitogens and antigens and impaired function of natural killer cells. It is of interest that medical students show decreased natural killer cell cytotoxicity and decreased cell-mediated immunity before and during examination periods (Vitaliano, 1988).

Use of stress reduction to treat physical illness

The idea that life stress can affect the course of physical illness implies that patients can improve the outcome of their illnesses if they successfully reduce their life stress. Although psychologically empowering, this belief also implies that the patient is responsible if her illness worsens. The latter perception can lead to disappointment, guilt, and depression if the stress-reduction strategy fails.

Evidence exists both for and against the notion that behavioral stress reduction strategies improve the outcome of illness. In an often-cited study, 86 women terminally ill with breast cancer who received standard cancer treatment and also participated in a supportive peer group lived longer than a group of women who received only standard treatment (Spiegel et al., 1981). However, in a more recent study of similar design using 300 women, there was no significant increase in median survival time for those in support groups (17.9 months) compared with those in control groups (17.6 months) (Goodwin et al., 2001).

■ MEDICAL CONDITIONS ASSOCIATED WITH PSYCHOLOGICAL SYMPTOMS

The social problems caused by medical illness often result in psychological difficulties. For example, a self-employed carpenter who is unable to work because of a bone infection becomes anxious and depressed because he cannot pay his bills. When these psychiatric symptoms lead to alcohol abuse and failure to take his medications, the patient's physical condition deteriorates, and his recovery is delayed.

Common psychological complaints in medically ill patients include depression, anxiety, and disorientation. Sometimes the latter is caused by delirium (see Chapter 14). Often, the treating physician can deal with a patient's psychological problems by talking with the patient and helping to organize and activate his or her social support systems. Specific psychotropic medications, such as antianxiety agents and antidepressants, also can help. For severe psychiatric problems, such as psychotic symptoms, a multidisciplinary approach, including a **consultation-liaison psychiatrist** who specializes in psychiatric symptoms in medical patients, may be needed.

Certain patient populations are more likely to be psychologically stressed than others. These populations include hospitalized patients, especially surgical patients, and those who are being treated in the intensive care unit (ICU) or coronary care unit (CCU). Patients with AIDS, patients on renal dialysis, and patients who have chronic pain are also at high risk for psychological stress and symptoms.

Surgical patients

Surgery is a stressful experience for anyone. However, some patients are at even greater psychological and medical risk for the effects of stress than others. These patients include those who believe that they will not survive surgery and patients who do not admit that they are worried before surgery. To reduce the risk for these patients, the doctor should encourage them to talk about their fears and address these fears as honestly as possible (see Chapter 24). Education beforehand about what to expect during and after the procedure in terms of mechanical support, pain relief, and other measures can also improve the outcome for surgical patients.

Patients undergoing renal dialysis

Patients on renal dialysis are at increased risk for psychological problems, such as depression. Among the reasons for this risk is the daunting recognition by these patients that they are dependent on other people and on machines for life itself. Psychological and medical risk for dialysis patients can be reduced through the establishment of good communication between the doctor and patient, as well as the use of in-home dialysis units. Such units are less likely to disrupt the patient's life than hospital-based treatment.

Patients in intensive care units or coronary care units

Because of the disorienting nature of the ICU or CCU environment and the life-threatening characteristics of their illnesses, patients treated in these units are at increased risk for psychiatric symptoms, particularly delirium, or **"ICU psychosis."** Several steps can be taken to decrease this risk. First, enhancing sensory and social input by encouraging the patient to talk and to have visitors and by providing orienting environmental cues, such as windows and clocks, can be helpful. The patient should also be able to maintain as much control as possible over his or her environment (e.g., adjusting the lighting level and self-administering pain medication).

Patients with AIDS

Individuals who are HIV-positive or have AIDS must deal with a particular combination of psychological stressors. Not only do they have a fatal illness, but they may also experience guilt over how they contracted the illness (e.g., sex with multiple partners, intravenous drug use) or the possibly of having infecting others. These patients must also deal with complex, painful, and often costly treatment regimens. In addition, if the patients are addicted to substances, they must undergo uncomfortable withdrawal from the drug. AIDS patients also often contend with fear of contagion from family, friends, and even medical personnel. Homosexual patients who are HIV-positive may be burdened further by the need to reveal their sexual orientation to others (i.e., to **"come out"**). Medical and psychological counseling, peer support groups, reassurance from the physician that the patient will not be abandoned, and psychoactive medication for specific symptoms can reduce medical and psychological risk for these patients.

■ PATIENTS WITH CHRONIC PAIN

Chronic pain, defined in the DSM-IV-TR as pain lasting at least 6 months, is commonly reported by patients. Chronic pain is associated primarily with physical factors but is often influenced by psychosocial factors. For example, the ability of a person to tolerate pain is decreased by depression, anxiety, and life stress in adulthood and by physical and sexual abuse in childhood.

Religious, cultural, and ethnic factors can also influence a patient's expression of pain as well as patient and support system responses to the pain. Certain cultures encourage the expression of pain, whereas others see value in remaining stoic (see Chapter 18).

Treating pain

Pain relief has physiological and psychological benefits. People who experience pain after a medical or surgical procedure have a higher risk of morbidity and a slower recovery from the procedure (Acute Pain Management Guideline Panel, 1992; Michaloliakou et al.,1996).

Relief of pain caused by physical illness is best achieved by analgesics (e.g., opioids) or nerve-blocking surgical procedures. Newer pain relief measures include implants that provide electrical stimulation of large-diameter afferent nerves, which may block the perception of pain (**the gate control theory** of pain control), as well as antidepressant and antiseizure medication (see later text).

Many patients with chronic pain are undermedicated because physicians fear that patients will become addicted to narcotics. This fear is generally unfounded. In a large study of more than 11,000 Medicare inpatients who received narcotics, only four cases of addiction occurred (Porter & Jick, 1980). Most patients with chronic pain easily discontinue the use of opioids as the pain remits and are probably at much higher risk for depression than they are for drug abuse.

Administration of pain medication

The schedule and route of administration of pain medication are important variables in the medication's effectiveness in reducing pain. For example, scheduled administration of the analgesic before the patient requests it (e.g., every 3 hours) may be more effective than medication administered when the patient requests it (on demand), because it separates the experience of pain from the receipt of medication.

Infants and children feel pain and remember pain as much as adults do and can receive anesthesia and analgesia safely. However, surveys in the 1970s and 1980s showed that they were less likely to receive analgesics than adults. One reason for this is that children may be more afraid of the receipt of pain medication (e.g., injection) than of the pain of the illness, injury, or surgical procedure itself. Therefore, the most useful ways of administering pain medications to children are orally (e.g., a fentanyl [Sublimaze] "lollipop") or transdermally (e.g., a skin cream to prevent pain from injections or spinal taps) (Berde & Sethna, 2002).

Placebo effects

A **placebo response** is defined as a subjective responsiveness to an inactive pharmacologic agent. Placebo responses to medications purported to relieve pain are common in medical practice. The mechanism by which cognitive cues, such as receipt of a pill or injection, can activate the placebo effect is not well understood. However, it apparently involves "real" changes in neural function, such as release of endogenous opioids (Sher, 1997; see Chapter 5). Neuroimaging studies (see Chapter 6) show that placebos activate brain regions containing high concentrations of opioid receptors (e.g., the brainstem and rostral anterior cingulate cortex) similarly to opioid analgesics (Petrovic et al., 2002). Despite these biologically useful actions of placebos, it is unethical to give a patient a placebo without first notifying him that he may be receiving either a placebo or an active medication (e.g., in a research study).

Other treatments for chronic pain

The neurotransmitters **serotonin** and **glutamate** are implicated in the experience of pain. Agents that alter levels of these neurotransmitters (e.g., antidepressants and antiseizure medications) are useful in pain management. Antidepressants, particularly tricyclics and venlafaxine (Effexor) (Ansari, 2000), are particularly useful for patients with arthritis, facial pain, headache, and irritable bowel syndrome. These drugs act in at least two ways to relieve pain. First, they can directly stimulate efferent inhibitory pain pathways. Second, they can decrease pain indirectly by improving the symptoms of depression, common in chronic pain patients. Glutamate is also implicated in chronic pain because **N-methyl-D-aspartate (NMDA) receptor modulators**, such as gabapentin (Neurontin), are effective in relieving pain, particularly when it results from injury to the central or peripheral nervous system (i.e., neuropathic pain) (Nicoldi et al., 1997).

Patients who have pain caused by physical illness also benefit from behavioral, cognitive, and other psychological therapies, such as biofeedback, hypnosis, psychotherapy, meditation, and relaxation training (see Chapter 17). Patients who participate in these therapies need less pain medication, become more active, and return more quickly to their pre-pain lifestyles.

■ OTHER PSYCHOSOMATIC RELATIONSHIPS

Medical conditions that present with psychological symptoms

Emotional symptoms such as depression (see Table 13-3), anxiety, psychosis, and personality changes can be signs of medical illness. For example, an elderly woman with no history of psychiatric illness who becomes unusually irritable and suspicious may be experiencing the first symptoms of Alzheimer's disease. Medical illnesses that present with psychiatric symptoms include not only neurologic problems such as dementia, but also toxic states, neoplasms (particularly pancreatic or other gastrointestinal cancers), rheumatologic illnesses, and connective tissue disorders (Table 25-3) (Case 25-2). Also, because most primary psychiatric disorders present early in life, a first episode of depression, anxiety, or especially psychosis in persons older than 50 years should occasion an aggressive medical workup before assuming that the disorder is primarily psychiatric.

Medication-induced psychological symptoms

Psychotropic medications are designed to relieve psychiatric symptoms; however, they can also produce these symptoms. For example, antipsychotics, antidepressants, and stimulants can produce agitation, anxiety, insomnia, and even psychotic symptoms. These and the antianxiety agents can also result in sedation, problems with concentration, and sexual dysfunction. Nonpsychotropic agents can also produce psychiatric symptoms in patients (Table 25-4).

CASE 25-2

THE PATIENT After a 1-week vacation to the Caribbean, a 25-year-old African-American woman with no history of psychiatric symptoms seems agitated and anxious. She tells her sister that a television newscaster is publicly discussing her behavior. She subsequently is admitted to the hospital with fever, fatigue, joint pain, and a butterfly-shaped rash across the bridge of her nose. Hematologic findings include mild anemia and presence of antinuclear antibodies (ANA).

COMMENT These signs, symptoms, and laboratory test results suggest that this patient has systemic lupus erythematosus (SLE), a connective tissue disorder. SLE is more common in African-American women of reproductive age. Personality changes and psychotic symptoms, such as the notion that people on television are referring to her (an idea of reference; see Table 12-3), are also symptoms of SLE. The sun exposure that this patient experienced on her vacation can exacerbate the symptoms of this disorder.

TREATMENT Immediate treatment includes antipsychotic agents to relieve her delusions and agitation. Long-term treatment of SLE includes antiinflammatory agents, such as corticosteroids and nonsteroidal antiinflammatory agents (NSAIDs), as well as education and support in coping with her chronic illness.

TABLE 25-3	Psychological Symptoms Associated With Medical Conditions

PSYCHOLOGICAL SYMPTOM	ASSOCIATED MEDICAL CONDITION
Anxiety	■ Anemias ■ Cardiac arrhythmias ■ Chronic infections with fever ■ Cushing's disease ■ Hyperthyroidism ■ Hypoglycemia or hyperglycemia ■ Pheochromocytoma ■ Pulmonary diseases ■ Severe blood loss
Depression	■ AIDS ■ Brain lesions, particularly in the left frontal lobe ■ Collagen-vascular diseases ■ Chronic pain (e.g., headache) ■ Hypoadrenalism (Addison's disease) ■ Hyperadrenalism (Cushing's disease) ■ Hypothyroidism ■ Hypoparathyroidism ■ Hyperparathyroidism ■ Huntington's disease ■ Immune system disorders ■ Infectious illnesses (e.g., influenza, mononucleosis) ■ Multiple sclerosis ■ Pancreatic and other gastrointestinal cancers ■ Parkinson's disease ■ Vitamin deficiencies
Personality changes	■ Brain infections, neoplasms, or trauma causing delirium ■ Dementia (e.g., Creutzfeldt-Jakob disease) ■ Huntington's disease ■ Temporal lobe epilepsy ■ Tertiary syphilis ■ Wilson's disease (explosive anger)
Mania or psychotic symptoms	■ AIDS ■ Acute intermittent porphyria ■ Cushing's disease ■ Huntington's disease ■ Multiple sclerosis ■ Neoplasms ■ Systemic lupus erythematosus

TABLE 25-4 Psychiatric Symptoms Induced by Nonpsychotropic Agents

CLASS OF AGENT	SPECIFIC AGENTS	SYMPTOM
Analgesic	Pentazocine, propoxyphene	Psychotic symptoms
Antiarrhythmics	Procainamide, quinidine	Confusion and occasionally delirium
Antiasthmatic	Albuterol, terbutaline, theophylline	Confusion, anxiety
Antibiotics	Antitubercular agents (e.g., iproniazid)	Psychotic symptoms (e.g., paranoia), memory loss
	Chloramphenicol, metronidazole	Confusion, depression, irritability
	Tetracycline	Depression
	Nitrofurantoin	Confusion, headache, sleepiness
Anticholinergics	Atropine, scopolamine, trihexyphenidyl, benztropine	Drowsiness, agitation; poor concentration in low doses; psychotic symptoms in high doses (atropine toxic psychosis); delirium
Anticonvulsants	Phenacemide and phenytoin	Mood symptoms, confusion, psychotic symptoms (less common)
Antihistamines	Diphenhydramine, hydroxyzine, phenylephrine, phenylpropanolamine	Sleepiness
	Phenylephrine, phenylpropanolamine	Psychotic symptoms, anxiety
Antihypertensives	Guanethidine, methyldopa, clonidine, some diuretics	Mild depression, fatigue, sexual dysfunction
	β-blockers (e.g., propranolol)	Depression, fatigue, psychotic symptoms (less common)
	Reserpine	Severe depression, confusion

TABLE 25-4 Psychiatric Symptoms Induced by Nonpsychotropic Agents
(Continued)

CLASS OF AGENT	SPECIFIC AGENTS	SYMPTOM
Antineoplastics	Fluorouracil	Confusion, disorientation, mood changes
Antiparkinson agents	L-dopa	Anxiety, psychosis, delirium, mania, depression
Cardiac glycosides	Digitalis	Mild depression, fatigue; delirium is associated with toxicity (particularly in the elderly)
Calcium channel blockers	Nifedipine, verapamil	Depression
Hypoglycemics	Insulin	Anxiety, confusion
Nonsteroidal anti-inflammatory drugs (NSAIDs)	Salicylates	Euphoria, depression, confusion (in very high doses)
	Indomethacin	Confusion, dizziness, psychotic symptoms, depression (less common)
	Phenylbutazone	Anxiety
Peptic ulcer drugs	Cimetidine	Depression, psychotic symptoms
Steroid hormones	Androgens	Aggressiveness, agitation
	Corticosteroids (use)	Hypomania, euphoria, depression, confusion, psychotic symptoms
	Corticosteroids (withdrawal)	Fatigue, headache, and vomiting imitating a brain tumor (i.e., "pseudotumor cerebri")
	Progestins	Depression, fatigue
	Thyroid hormones	Anxiety, psychotic symptoms

Adapted from Fadem, B., & Simring, S. (2003). *High-yield psychiatry* (2nd ed.). Philadelphia: Lippincott, Williams & Wilkins.

REVIEW QUESTIONS

1. A 35-year-old firefighter who was seriously burned while fighting a house fire 9 months ago takes an opioid-based medication daily to help control his pain. Which of the following is most likely to be true about this patient?

   (A) He is receiving too much pain medication

   (B) Psychological therapies will be of little benefit to him

   (C) His expression of pain is related exclusively to the extent of his pain

   (D) He is at high risk for depression

   (E) He is at high risk for addiction to opioids after the pain remits

2. A 62-year-old dermatologist with no history of psychiatric problems reports that he no longer engages in activities he formerly enjoyed. He states that his family would "probably be better off" without him, and he expresses guilt over the patients he was unable to help. He has problems sleeping, has a poor appetite, and has lost 12 pounds. The most appropriate next step in the management of this patient is

   (A) psychotherapy

   (B) evaluation for a gastrointestinal neoplasm

   (C) an antidepressant

   (D) evaluation of thyroid function

   (E) a hypnotic benzodiazepine

3. A 28-year-old woman with no psychiatric history develops rapid heart rate and acute anxiety, which have been present for the past 4 months. The patient has lost 8 pounds and reports having trouble sleeping. Physical examination reveals exophthalmus (bulging eyes) and a neck mass. The most appropriate next step in the management of this patient is

   (A) psychotherapy

   (B) evaluation for a gastrointestinal neoplasm

   (C) an antidepressant

   (D) evaluation of thyroid function

   (E) a hypnotic benzodiazepine

Questions 4–5

A 65-year-old male patient is scheduled for thoracic surgery. After the surgery, he will be in the intensive care unit (ICU) for about 12 hours and will require a mechanical ventilator.

4. During his stay in the ICU after surgery, this patient is most likely to experience which of the following psychiatric problems?

(A) Panic disorder

(B) Obsessive-compulsive disorder (OCD)

(C) Hypochondriasis

(D) Somatization disorder

(E) Delirium

5. To reduce this patient's likelihood of psychological problems in the ICU, the physician should

(A) limit visits from family

(B) reduce exposure to ambient light

(C) explain the need for mechanical ventilation prior to surgery

(D) discourage communication between patient and staff

(E) have the nurses control the patient's lighting level

ANSWERS AND EXPLANATIONS

1-D. This chronic pain patient is at high risk for depression but at relatively low risk for drug addiction. Pain patients tend to be undermedicated, and this patient is more likely receiving too little rather than too much pain medication. Psychological therapies can be of significant benefit to chronic pain patients. This patient's expression of pain is related not only to the extent of his pain, but to religious, cultural, and ethnic factors.

2-B. This patient, who had no previous history of psychiatric illness, now has symptoms of depression, including sleep problems, inappropriate guilt, suicidal ideation, and significant weight loss. Because of his age and because pancreatic cancer and other gastrointestinal cancers often present with depression, this patient should be evaluated for such conditions before his depression is treated. Psychotherapy, antidepressants, and benzodiazepines can treat the associated symptoms but do not address the underlying illness.

3-D. This patient has symptoms of an overactive thyroid, including a neck mass (enlarged thyroid gland), exophthalmus, rapid heart rate and weight loss. People with thyroid hyperactivity may also present with anxiety and insomnia, symptoms that should remit with appropriate treatment. As in question 2, psychotherapy, antidepressants, and benzodiazepines do not address the underlying illness.

4-E, 5-C. Because of the disorienting nature of the ICU, delirium is commonly seen in patients. Panic disorder, OCD, hypochondriasis, and somatization disorder are no more common in ICU patients than in the general population. To reduce this patient's likelihood of psychological problems in the ICU, the physician should explain the need for and function of the mechanical ventilator and any other mechanical support that he will need. The physician should also encourage visits from family and communication between patient and staff. The patient should be encouraged to control aspects of his environment (e.g., lighting level). Outside stimuli such as light should be increased rather than decreased (e.g., placing the patient's bed near a window).

REFERENCES

Acute Pain Management Guideline Panel. (1992). *Acute pain management: Operative or medical procedures and trauma: Clinical practice guideline.* Rockville, MD: Agency for Health Care Policy and Research, Public Health Service, U. S. Dept. of Health and Human Services.

Ansari, A. (2000). The efficacy of newer antidepressants in the treatment of chronic pain: A review of current literature. *Harvard Rev Psychiatry, 7,* 257–277.

Berde, C. B., & Sethna, N. F. (2002). Analgesics for the treatment of pain in children. *N Engl J Med, 347,* 1094–1103.

Frasure-Smith, N., Lesperance, F., & Talajic, M. (1993). Depression following myocardial infarction: Impact on 6-month survival. *JAMA, 270,* 1819–1825.

Galea, S., Ahern, J., Resnick, H., Kilpatrick, D., Bucuvalas, M., Gold, J., & Vlahov, D. (2002). Psychological sequelae of the September 11 terrorist attacks in NYC. *N Engl J Med, 346,* 982–987.

Goldstein, M. G., & Niaura, R. (1992). Psychological factors affecting physical condition: Cardiovascular disease literature review. Part I. *Psychosomatics, 33,* 134–145.

Goodwin, P. J., Leszcz, M., Ennis, M., Koopmans, J., Vincent, L., Guther, H., et al. (2001). The effect of group psychosocial support on survival in metastatic breast cancer. *N Engl J Med, 345,* 1719–1726.

Holmes, T. H., & Rahe, R. H. (1967). The social readjustment rating scale. *J Psychosomatic Res, 11,* 213–218.

Kiecolt-Glaser, J. K., & Glaser, R. (1986). Psychological influences on immunity. *Psychosomatics, 27,* 621–624.

Krishnan, K. R., Delong, M., Kraemer, H., Carney, R., Spiegel, D., Gordon, C., et al. (2002). Comorbidity of depression with other medical diseases in the elderly. *Biol Psychiatry, 52,* 559–588.

McEwen, B. S. (2000). The neurobiology of stress: from serendipity to clinical relevance. *Brain Res, 886,* 172–189.

Michaloliakou, C., Chung, F., & Sharma, S. (1996). Preoperative multimodal analgesia facilitates recovery after ambulatory laparoscopic cholecystectomy. *Anesth Analg, 82,* 44–51.

Niaura, R., & Goldstein, M. G. (1992). Psychological factors affecting physical condition: Cardiovascular disease literature review. Part II. *Psychosomatics, 33,* 146–155.

Nicoldi, M. (1997). An NMDA modulator, gabapentin (Neurontin), clearly facilitates resolution of chronic migraine. *Pharmacol Res, 35,* (Suppl.), 64.

Petrovic, P., Kalso, E., Petersson, K. M., & Ingvar, M. (2002). Placebo and opioid analgesia, imaging a shared neuronal network. *Science, 295,* 1737–1740.

Schleifer, S. J., Keller, S. E., Camerino, M., Thornton, J. C., & Stein, M. (1983). Suppression of lymphocyte stimulation following bereavement. *JAMA, 250,* 374–377.

Selye, H. (1976). *The stress of life.* New York: McGraw-Hill.

Spiegel, D., Bloom J. R., & Yalom, I. D. (1981). Group support for patients with metastatic cancer: A randomized prospective outcome study. *Arch Gen Psychiatry, 38,* 527–533.

Shekelle, R. B., Gale, M., Ostfeld, A. M., & Paul, O. (1983). Hostility, risk of coronary heart disease and mortality. *Psychosomat Med, 45,* 109.

Solomon, G. F. (2000). Psychoneuroimmunology. In M. G. Gelder, J. J. Lopez-Ibor, & N. Andreasen (Eds.), *New Oxford textbook of psychiatry.* London: Oxford University Press.

Stein, M., Schleifer, S. J., & Keller, S. E. (1987). Brain, behavior and immune process. In R. Michels, & J. O. Cavenar, (Eds.), *Psychiatry.* Philadelphia: Lippincott.

Vitaliano, P. P., Maiuro, R. D., Russo, J., Mitchell, E. S., Carr, J. E., & Van Citters, R. L. (1988). A biopsychosocial model of medical student distress. *J Behav Med, 11,* 311–331.

Wong, C. M. (2002). Post-traumatic stress disorder: Advances in psychoneuroimmunology. *Psychiatr Clin North Am, 25,* 369–383.

Ethical and **26**
Legal Issues
in Medicine

A ccording to the Code of Medical Ethics of the American Medical Association, **ethical conduct** for physicians is a standard based on moral principles or practices and matters of social policy involving moral issues. In contrast, **legal conduct** is behavior that conforms to written law and to the regulations that interpret and set standards for such law. Unethical conduct and illegal conduct involve behavior that does not conform to these standards.

Legal and ethical principles are often closely associated, although ethical standards characteristically exceed legal obligations. For example, if a physician refuses to treat a patient who is HIV-positive because she is afraid of infection, her behavior is legal but unethical. Although there is no legal duty for a doctor to treat a patient and thus no civil cause of action in a court of law, this doctor could face professional discipline by her peers in the form of censure or other action by her local or state medical society or board.

Certain behavior by physicians may not be illegal or unethical but may still be inappropriate. For example, accepting expensive gifts from patients or treating close family members, while inappropriate, do not necessarily constitute unethical behavior.

■ PROFESSIONAL BEHAVIOR

Doctors are expected to observe the law and to show appropriate and professional (i.e., ethical) behavior when interacting with patients. The professional behavior of a doctor may come into question if he or she treats patients while not functioning normally, crosses boundaries in the doctor-patient relationship, or does not follow the standards of care of the community.

Impaired physicians

It is always unethical and in some circumstances illegal for physicians or physicians-in-training to practice medicine when their judgment or abilities are impaired. Causes of impairment include drug or alcohol abuse, physical or mental illness, and impairment in functioning associated with old age. If a physician is impaired, he must immediately and voluntarily remove himself from contact with patients.

If an impaired doctor continues to have contact with patients, colleagues with knowledge of the impairment have the responsibility to prevent that doctor from practicing medicine and to obtain help for the doctor. Colleagues also need to ensure that the impaired doctor does not see patients prior to getting help, and that he or she does, in fact, seek and receive appropriate treatment.

How and where to report impaired colleagues varies by the venue it occurs in and by the nature of the threat. If the impairment or unethical conduct by the physician or physician-in training threatens the welfare of hospitalized patients, it should be reported to the authorities overseeing the clinical situation (e.g., the hospital's chief of the medical staff). An impaired medical student should be reported to the dean of the medical school or the dean of students, and an impaired resident should be reported to his or her residency training director.

If the behavior by the impaired colleague violates state licensing laws, it should also be reported to the state licensing board or to the impaired physicians program, usually part of the state medical society. If the unethical conduct violates criminal statutes, it must be reported to law enforcement agencies.

Medical malpractice

Medical malpractice occurs when a patient is harmed because of a physician's actions or inactions. Medical malpractice is a **tort,** or civil wrong, not a crime. Therefore, a finding for the plaintiff (the patient) results in a financial award or **damages** to the patient from the defendant physician or his insurance carrier. Such a finding does not typically result in a jail term or loss of license for the physician.

For a malpractice claim to be substantiated, the **four "D"s** of malpractice must be present—dereliction, duty, damages, and directly. First, there must be negligence, or **dereliction,** where the doctor deviated from the normal standards of care for that community. There must also be an established physician-patient relationship (i.e., a **duty**). Finally, the patient must be injured (**damaged**), and the injury must be caused **directly** by the doctor's negligence, not by another factor.

Because the invasive nature of their intervention may potentially cause physical injury to patients, physicians in high-risk specialties such as those in surgery, obstetrics, and emergency medicine are the specialists most likely to be sued for malpractice. Specialists who use few if any invasive procedures, such as psychiatrists and family practitioners, are much less likely to be sued.

If a doctor makes an error while treating a patient, the risk of a malpractice suit can be reduced by prompt, full disclosure. For example, if a patient has an allergic reaction to medication because the prescribing physician did not check the patient's history for allergies, the doctor should disclose this mistake to the patient and apologize. If a physician has knowledge that another doctor made such an error, the physician should encourage the other doctor to disclose it. An effective way to ensure such disclosure is for the physician to arrange a joint meeting between herself, the treating doctor, and the patient or related persons (Wu, 1997).

When a jury finds for the plaintiff in a malpractice case, the patient can be awarded compensatory damages only or both compensatory and punitive damages. **Compensatory damages** are funds given to reimburse the patient for medical bills or lost salary and to compensate the patient for pain and suffering. **Punitive (or exemplary) damages** are designed to punish the physician and set an example for the medical community. These are awarded only in cases of wanton carelessness or gross negligence. For example, if a surgeon impaired by alcohol cuts a vital nerve leaving a patient permanently paralyzed, punitive damages may be awarded in addition to compensatory damages. Although compensatory damages are covered by most medical malpractice insurance carriers, the physician himself is responsible if punitive damages are awarded to a patient.

In recent years, the number of malpractice suits has increased, for several reasons. First, there is a general increase in lawsuits and in the size of pay outs to successful plaintiffs in malpractice actions (Smarr, 2003). Second, a breakdown has occurred in the traditional physician-patient relationship, in part because the growth of managed care and similar systems has reduced the amount of time a doctor can spend with an individual patient. In addition, technological advances in medicine have reduced the amount of personal contact that patients have with their doctors. This increase in lawsuits and awards has caused malpractice carriers to exit from the market and the cost of malpractice insurance to rise, making it difficult for physicians, particularly those in high-risk specialties, to obtain affordable insurance. In some states, high insurance premiums have forced some physicians to give up the practice of medicine (Mello et al., 2003) and have compelled groups of others to press for caps on malpractice awards using formal protests and work stoppages (Margolin & Schuppe, 2003).

Professional boundaries

No matter what behavior a patient shows toward the doctor, it is the doctor's responsibility to maintain a professional separation or boundary between herself and the patient. For this reason, a physician should not treat himself, family members, or close friends. However, such treatment is not ethically or legally proscribed.

Sometimes an ill patient will behave in sexually inappropriate ways toward a physician (see Chapter 24). Although seductive-acting patients may genuinely be attracted to the doctor, more commonly their behavior is caused by unconscious transference reactions or use of inappropriate defense mechanisms to deal with feelings of vulnerability, dependence, and fear associated with their illness (see Chapter 8).

Doctors can also be attracted to their patients. However, because of the inherent inequality of the doctor-patient relationship, romantic or sexual relationships with current or even former patients are inappropriate and are prohibited by the ethical standards of most specialty boards. Patients who claim that they had a sexual relationship with a physician can file an ethics complaint, a medical malpractice complaint, or both.

Doctors should also avoid socializing outside of the medical setting with any patient who might misinterpret such contact. In a similar way, accepting valuable gifts from patients is not appropriate, although it may be appropriate to accept a small token of appreciation from a patient, such as eggs produced by home-raised chickens.

If for any reason a doctor wishes to or must terminate a relationship with a patient (e.g., because the doctor is retiring), she must give notice to the patient or to family members in sufficient time to allow the patient and family to obtain the services of another doctor.

Good Samaritan laws

Physicians are not legally required to treat patients in emergencies, but those who do are shielded from the liability of malpractice suits by statutes known as **Good Samaritan laws.** To be shielded by these laws, the Samaritan doctor's action in the emergency must meet certain criteria. First, the procedure that the doctor employs must be standard and generally accepted by the medical profession. The actions taken by the physician also must be within his or her competence and training, and the doctor cannot be paid for the emergency services. Finally, the doctor usually must stay with the patient until other physicians, not paramedical personnel, take over the patient's care.

■ LEGAL COMPETENCE

To be **legally competent** to make health care decisions, a patient must understand the risks, benefits, and likely outcomes of such decisions. All adults (persons 18 years of age and older) are assumed to be legally competent to make health care decisions for themselves except if they are actively psychotic, suicidal or in a coma. Minors (persons younger than 18 years of age) usually are not considered legally competent.

Emancipated minors

Emancipated minors are under 18 years of age but are considered competent adults and thus can make decisions concerning their own medical care. To be considered emancipated, a minor usually must fulfill at least one of the following requirements. He or she must be: 1) self-supporting; 2) in the military; or 3) married. Minors are also considered emancipated if they have children whom they care for, although in most states, simply being pregnant does not automatically confer emancipation.

Questions of competence

A person can meet the legal standard for competence to accept or refuse medical treatment even if she is mentally ill or retarded or is incompetent in other areas of her life. For example, a person who has schizophrenia may be competent to make health care decisions but not be competent to manage her own finances.

If doubt exists, a judge must decide whether an individual is or is not competent. Physicians are often consulted by judges for information about whether patients have the capacity to make health care decisions, but physicians cannot decide whether someone is legally competent.

Involuntary hospitalization

In psychiatric emergencies, patients who will not or cannot agree to be hospitalized can be hospitalized against their will or without consent with the certification of one or two physicians for up to a few months (depending on state law) before a court hearing. For involuntary hospitalization, a patient usually must be dangerous to self or others or unable to provide self-care (not merely self-neglect). Even if a psychiatric patient voluntarily chooses to be hospitalized, he may be required to wait for up to a few days (depending on state laws) before he is permitted to sign out against medical advice.

Patients who are confined to mental health facilities, whether voluntarily or involuntarily, retain most of their civil rights, including the right to receive or refuse treatment (e.g., medication, electroconvulsive therapy,

TABLE 26-1	The Mental Health Bill of Rights (May Vary in Detail From State to State)

PATIENTS WHO ARE HELD IN A MENTAL HEALTH FACILITY INVOLUNTARILY HAVE THE
■ Right to receive appropriate treatment
■ Right to refuse treatment
■ Right to privacy
■ Right to manage one's own finances, unless declared legally incompetent
■ Right to receive visitors
■ Right to communicate with the outside world
■ Right to be paid for work done in the facility

and surgical procedures). However, if the patient is suicidal, he or she may not be considered competent to refuse treatment. In addition, medication may be administered against such patients' wishes to prevent danger to themselves or to others. The **Mental Health Bill of Rights** for confined patients can be found in Table 26-1.

Criminal law

A crime requires both an **evil intent** (mens rea) and an **evil deed** (actus reus). For example, if a post-partum woman murders her infant because she explains that "Satan told me to kill the child," she has committed an evil deed but did not have evil intent. A judge or jury may determine that by virtue of her mental state, the woman lacked the requisite state of mind to have committed a crime.

Every adult is presumed competent to stand trial (even persons with mental retardation or mental illness). An adult is determined unfit to stand trial (legally incompetent) if she does not understand the charges against her or is not able to cooperate with counsel in the preparation of her defense.

A person who is found legally insane must have a mental illness, and as a result of this illness must meet one of the **statutory criteria** (Table 26-2) under state or federal law. Most states and federal jurisdictions have a different and more liberal set of standards under which an individual with mental illness can qualify for **diminished capacity,** which may modify the punishment.

■ INFORMED CONSENT

Except for life-threatening emergencies in which the patient is unconscious or otherwise incapable of consenting or in which risk-disclosure is so psychologically threatening that it is medically contraindicated, physicians must obtain consent from competent, adult patients before proceeding with any medical or surgical treatment. However, before patients can consent, they must be informed of and understand several things (see later text). This

TABLE 26-2	Statutory Criteria for Legal Insanity	
TEST	DEFINITION	COMMENTS
M'Naghten	Determines whether the person understands the nature and quality of his actions and, if so, whether he knows that the actions were wrong	▪ The strictest test ▪ Is the standard criterion in most jurisdictions
The American Law Institute (ALI) Model Penal Code	Determines whether the person appreciates the wrongfulness of his behavior (cognitive prong) Alternatively, determines whether the person is able to conform his conduct to the requirements of the law (volitional prong)	After the John Hinckley case (attempted assassination of President Reagan), most jurisdictions with the ALI test dropped the volitional prong
Durham	Evaluates whether the person's criminal behavior is the "product" of a mental illness	▪ The most lenient test ▪ Has been abandoned in almost all jurisdictions

Adapted from Fadem, B., & Simring, S. (2003). *High-yield psychiatry* (2nd ed.). Philadelphia: Lippincott Williams & Wilkins.

combination of information provided by the physician and acquiescence by the patient is called **informed consent.** Although a signature may not be required for minor medical procedures, patients usually sign a document of consent for major medical procedures or for surgery. Other hospital personnel, such as nurses, usually cannot obtain informed consent.

Components of informed consent

Before patients can give consent to be treated by a doctor, they must be informed

- ▪ of and understand the health implications of their diagnosis
- ▪ of the health risks and benefits of the treatment or procedure
- ▪ of the alternatives to the treatment or procedure
- ▪ of the likely outcome if they do not consent to the treatment or procedure
- ▪ that they can withdraw consent at any time before or during the treatment or procedure

Refusal to consent

Competent patients have the right to refuse to consent to a needed test or procedure for religious or other reasons, even if their health will suffer or death will result from such refusal.

However, before accepting the patient's refusal, the doctor should try to understand the reason behind it. If the refusal is the result of depression, fear, pain, or intolerance of the treatment, the physician should treat the depression or attempt to make the treatment more effective and acceptable to the patient (Chapter 25). If these steps have been taken and the patient still refuses intervention, the physician must follow the patient's wishes.

Like other competent patients, pregnant women have the right to refuse diagnostic, medical, or surgical intervention necessary to protect the health or life of the fetus (e.g., cesarean section), even if the fetus will die or be seriously injured without the intervention (see Case 26-1).

Other issues concerning consent

Although patients have the right to appropriate medical interventions, they cannot choose inappropriate interventions. For example, if a patient wants a diagnostic test or procedure that he clearly does not need and has no reasonable chance of benefitting him, the physician is not ethically bound to do it, even if it is noninvasive and paid for by the patient's health insurance company. If the patient insists, the doctor should determine the reason for the patient's request and address that issue with the patient.

If a patient is in a teaching hospital, he or she has the right to refuse to be interviewed, tested, or examined by resident doctors or medical stu-

---

CASE 26-1

THE PATIENT A clearly competent, pregnant, 25-year-old woman tells her obstetrician that over the past year she has repeatedly abused intravenous drugs and has had at least 10 sexual partners. The doctor explains to the patient that, because she may have been exposed to HIV through sexual contact or infected needles, the fetus she is carrying also is at high risk for infection. The doctor then suggests that the woman be tested for HIV so that, if the test is positive, she can be treated with an antiviral agent that can significantly reduce the danger of HIV transmission to the unborn child (see Table 19–6). The woman states that her boyfriend has said he will leave her if she is infected with the virus and she refuses to be tested for HIV.

COMMENT Although the doctor should discuss how the infection can affect the child and urge the patient to be tested, he cannot compel this pregnant woman to have an HIV test. Even if this patient agreed to be tested and was positive for HIV, she cannot be compelled to be treated. Like other competent patients, this patient has the right to refuse medical tests or treatment even if the fetus will die or be seriously injured as a result.

INTERVENTION The most appropriate action for the doctor to take in this case is to note in the patient's chart that she has refused to be tested and to continue providing appropriate prenatal care. Once the child is born, however, the mother cannot refuse to have it tested, and if necessary treated, for HIV (see later text).

---

dents. It is not appropriate for the resident or student to judge or challenge such refusal, which is also the right of incarcerated patients.

Patients must give consent before entering a research study. However, such consent cannot be construed as carte blanche. For example, if a patient's condition worsens in a research study because of lack of treatment or placebo treatment (as in the Tuskegee Institute study, see Chapter 20) or exposure to experimental treatment, the patient's participation in the study must end and the patient must be given the standard treatment for his or her condition.

Unexpected findings

As noted, patients must be informed in order to give consent before any medical or surgical procedure can be performed. In some instances, however, an unexpected finding necessitates a medical or surgical procedure or a diagnostic test for which the patient has not given consent.

If the unexpected finding does not constitute an emergency (e.g., an unsuspected probable ovarian malignancy is found during a laparotomy and needs to be biopsied or removed), the patient must give informed consent before the additional procedure or procedures can be performed. In this example, the anesthetized patient must be allowed to wake up so that the doctor can discuss the findings with her. If the unexpected finding requires emergency action (e.g., a "hot" appendix is found serendipitously during a laparotomy), the doctor can perform the procedure on an emergency basis without consent from the patient.

Organ donation and transplant

Most people who need organ transplant surgery will never have it because there are not enough organs available for all of the people who need them (Sheehy et al., 2003). One reason for this organ shortage is that relatively few people make their organs available for transplant when they die. To donate one's organs after death, a person must sign an organ donor card or inform relatives or other surrogates of his or her wish to donate. Parents, legal guardians, or their surrogates can donate the organs of a child who is legally dead. At the very least, the relatives must avow that they know of no reason why the organs cannot be donated. In the absence of such documentation or information, organs usually cannot be harvested from a person who is legally dead.

Consenting living adults and, with parental consent, living minors can be sources of organs or tissues for certain types of transplant. The restrictions on using a living minor as a donor include the following:

■ The minor should be the only possible source of the organ or tissue
■ The donation cannot result in serious risks of immediate or long-term complications or harm to the minor
■ The donation or transplant should provide "clear benefit" to the recipient, who should be a close family member

- The procedure must be standard (not experimental) and have a reasonable chance of success

The field of organ donation and transplant is rapidly changing. Legal and ethical questions involving live donor and artificial organ transplant are currently being addressed in the courts and in professional societies. Table 26-3 includes questions addressing current issues surrounding organ donation and transplant.

■ TREATMENT OF MINORS

Under ordinary circumstances, parents or legal guardians (hereinafter "parents") must give consent for surgical or medical treatment of a minor. Exceptions to this rule include emergency situations, certain issues involving reproduction and drug abuse in teenagers, and occasions when parents refuse medically necessary testing or treatment.

Exceptions to parental consent requirements

In an emergency situation, such as a life-threatening illness or accident, when a delay in treatment can potentially harm a minor child, treatment can proceed even if the parents cannot be located to give consent.

Parents cannot refuse to consent to an established (but not an experimental) medical procedure when to do so would endanger the minor child. If parents refuse to consent and there is time to do so, a court order to do the procedure can be obtained from a judge, within hours if necessary. If there is no time to obtain a court order, the doctor can proceed with the treatment without obtaining a court order or consent from the parents. For example, if for religious or other reasons parents refuse to consent to a needed blood transfusion for a child and there is no alternative appropriate treatment, the doctor can give the child the transfusion without parental consent.

Genetic testing of children

Children at risk for genetic disorders can pose ethical questions for physicians. For example, can parents forego genetic testing for a minor who is at risk for a serious genetic illness? The age of onset of the illness and the availability of the treatment are important factors in this decision. For example, if the illness has a pediatric onset and treatment is available, genetic testing should be offered or even required. However, if the genetic disorder has a pediatric onset and no treatment is available, parents should have the discretion as to whether to test the child. When a child is at risk for a genetic condition with an adult onset and there are no preventive therapies or treatments available for it, (e.g., Huntington's disease) genetic testing usually should not be done. In the last case, the parents should nevertheless be informed of available tests and be given the opportunity to discuss the issue with the physician (Table 26–4).

TABLE 26-3	Ethical and Legal Issues Involving Organ Donation and Transplant

CLINICAL SCENARIO	ANSWERS
A mentally retarded adult (or minor child) would like to donate skin to a sibling who was seriously burned in a house fire. The donation has a good chance of success and the donor's skin is likely to regenerate without scarring. Can he or she donate?	■ Yes, he can donate as long as he will not be harmed by the donation. ■ Yes, he can donate as long as his parents or legal guardian do not object. ■ Yes, he can donate if there is no other appropriate source for the donation.
A 14-year-old-boy, who is a perfect match, refuses to donate his bone marrow to his critically ill sister. Without the transplant, the sister will die. With the transplant, she has a good chance of surviving. The parents want him to donate the bone marrow. Can the boy be compelled to donate? Could he be compelled to donate if he were an adult (age 18 or over)?	■ Yes, he can be compelled to donate if he is the only appropriate source of bone marrow for his sister. ■ Yes, he can be compelled to donate if he will not be harmed seriously by the donation. ■ No, he could not be compelled to donate if he were an adult.
A 16-year-old boy whose parents were killed in an accident would like to donate the organs of his 8-year-old brother who was in the accident and has been declared legally dead. Can the boy donate his brother's organs?	■ Yes, he can donate his brother's organs if the 16 year old has knowledge that or believes that his parents would have wanted to donate the younger child's organs.
A surgeon would like to substitute a kidney earmarked for transplant into a 50-year-old patient for a kidney slated to be used for her current 30-year-old patient. The younger patient's designated donated kidney is found to be unsuitable for transplant. Can the doctor make the substitution?	■ No, the doctor cannot make the substitution because the organ is promised to the older patient and it would be unethical to use it for the younger patient.
The parents of an anencephalic neonate on life support wish to donate the child's organs and tissue. Can the parents make this donation? Can the physician maintain the child on ventilator support to sustain organ viability until a determination of brain death is made?	■ Yes, it is appropriate for the parents to make this donation because, in contrast to most other brain-damaged persons, this child has no potential for future consciousness. ■ Yes, the physician can maintain ventilator support but can only re-move the organs and tissue after the determination of death is made.

TABLE 26-4	Ethics of Genetic Testing for Children: Should Genetic Testing Be Done on a Child at Risk for a Genetic Disorder?	
ONSET OF THE DISORDER	PREVENTIVE THERAPY OR TREATMENT AVAILABLE	CONDUCT GENETIC TESTING
Childhood	Yes	Yes
Childhood	No	Parental discretion
Adulthood	No	No

Seriously ill newborns

When a child is born with a serious medical condition, the parents and the physician may have to decide whether to initiate or continue life-sustaining treatment. In the often-cited case of "Baby Doe," the parents of a newborn with Down's syndrome and a life-threatening tracheoesophageal fistula refused corrective surgery, which led to death of the infant and a revamping of legal and ethical standards concerning decision-making for disabled newborns.

The two major questions that are now typically used in such decisions are: 1) What is best for the child? and 2) What will be the child's quality of life? The latter must be evaluated from the child's, not its parents', perspective. For example, if the child will have more pain and suffering than joy or is neurologically unable to experience joy, it is ethical not to initiate or to stop life-sustaining treatment. In contrast, if the child will have mental retardation (e.g., Down's syndrome) but will be able to experience pleasure, and if his life-threatening physical problems can be corrected surgically, the surgery must be done, even if the parents object. Thus, today, Baby Doe would be saved. If the outcome for a child cannot be predicted with any certainty, as in cases of very premature infants, such treatment should be initiated or continued until such a prediction can be made.

■ CONFIDENTIALITY

The ethical standards of the profession require that physicians maintain the confidentiality of their patients. Without patients' permission, doctors cannot reveal information about them even to close relatives or to their medical insurance carriers. For example, if a doctor determines that the fetus a woman is carrying is not her husband's child, the doctor cannot reveal this information to her questioning husband. Similarly, doctors cannot reveal information about a patient to the patient's employer, even if the doctor is being paid by that employer.

Confidentiality of teenagers

Even though people under the age of 18 years are minors, it is ethical for doctors to keep certain information about them confidential from their parents. For example, doctor-patient confidentiality usually can be maintained when treating a minor for drug or alcohol dependence or for mental illness. Also, with the exception of abortion, which in most states requires parental consent or notification, doctor-patient confidentiality can be maintained in situations involving reproductive issues such as sexually transmitted diseases (Table 26-5).

In any situation in which a doctor must breach the confidentiality of a minor to protect him or her, the doctor should inform the minor in advance that confidentiality will be broken.

Appropriate breaches of confidentiality

In some situations, physicians are not required to maintain the confidentiality of competent patients. These situations include the following:

- The patient is suspected of child or elder abuse
- The patient is at significant risk of suicide
- The patient poses a serious threat to another person

When a patient threatens others, the physician must first ascertain the credibility of the threat or danger. If the threat or danger is credible, the doctor must notify the appropriate law enforcement officials or social service agency. In two landmark cases, the California Supreme Court ruled that a physician must also warn (**Tarasoff vs. the Regents of University of California I**) and protect (**Tarasoff vs. the Regents of University of California II**) the intended victim.

■ REPORTABLE ILLNESSES

Most states require physicians to report certain illnesses to their state health departments. These disorders are called **reportable illnesses.** Af-

TABLE 26-5	Situations in Which Parental Consent Usually Is Not Required for the Treatment of Minors

1. Emergencies in which the child could be harmed by delaying intervention
2. Treatment of drug and alcohol dependence or abuse
3. Treatment of sexually transmitted disease
4. Prescription of contraceptives
5. Pregnancy testing
6. Medical care during pregnancy
7. Medical care during and after delivery
8. Treatment for mental illness

ter receiving this information, state health departments report these data to the federal **Centers for Disease Control and Prevention (CDC)** for statistical purposes.

The requirements for reporting specific illnesses vary from state to state. In all states, varicella, hepatitis, measles, mumps, rubella, salmonellosis, shigellosis, and tuberculosis are reportable. Sexually transmitted diseases, which are reportable in all states, include syphilis, gonorrhea, chlamydia, and AIDS. HIV-positive status is not reportable in all states, and genital herpes is not reportable in most states.

HIV-infected physicians

When a doctor has an infectious disease that could potentially be transmitted to and prove harmful to a patient, the doctor should not engage in behavior that would significantly increase the chance of such transmission. The issue of infected doctors treating patients has become even more significant since the AIDS epidemic began.

Although a Florida dentist apparently transmitted AIDS to some of his patients, no physician-to-patient transmission of HIV has ever been confirmed in the United States. Thus, as long as an HIV-infected physician follows appropriate and accepted procedures for infection control, he is unlikely to pose a risk to his patients. Because of this, the doctor himself or colleagues of the doctor with knowledge of his HIV status usually are not required to inform either patients or the medical establishment about the doctor's HIV-positive status.

HIV-infected patients

As discussed at the beginning of this chapter, it is unethical for a doctor to refuse to treat HIV-positive patients because of issues such as fear of infection. Doctors also are expected to maintain the confidentiality of their HIV-positive patients, in life and in death (e.g., on autopsy reports).

Exceptions to this rule exist. Doctors do not have to maintain the confidentiality of their HIV-positive patients who habitually put other persons in danger of infection by engaging in high-risk behavior. For example, if an HIV-positive patient tells a doctor that he is having unprotected sex with a partner who does not know about his infection, the doctor must see that the patient informs the partner. To do this, the doctor must first try to persuade the patient to tell the partner.

- **If the patient agrees,** the doctor should set up an appointment to see the patient and partner together to ensure that the patient discloses to the partner and to provide the opportunity for the doctor to answer any questions that the partner may have.
- **If the patient refuses** to tell the partner, the doctor must notify public health authorities. If they do not act on this information, in some jurisdictions, the physician must inform the endangered partner.

ADVANCE DIRECTIVES

Advance directives are instructions given by patients in anticipation of the need for a medical decision. A durable power of attorney and a living will are examples of advance directives.

Durable power of attorney and living will

Durable power of attorney is a legal document in which a competent person designates another person (e.g., spouse or friend) as her legal representative (i.e., **health care proxy**) to make decisions about her health care when she can no longer do so.

A **living will** is a document in which a competent person gives directions for his future health care if he becomes incompetent to make decisions when he needs care. If there is no advance directive, the doctor must follow standard procedures, including all measures needed to save the life of the patient.

Health care facilities that receive Medicare payments (most hospitals and nursing homes) are required to ask patients whether they have advance directives and, if necessary, have personnel available to help patients prepare such documents. Such facilities must also inform patients of their right to refuse treatment or resuscitation.

Surrogates

If an incompetent patient has no advance directive, health care providers or family members who knew the patient (such persons are considered surrogates) must determine what the patient would have done if she were competent (**the substituted judgment standard**). If no information is available about the patient's wishes, the decision must be made based on what a reasonable person would wish for himself or herself after weighing each course of action (**the best interest standard**). The personal wishes of surrogates are irrelevant to the medical decision.

When a health care proxy or surrogate has been making decisions for an incompetent patient and the patient regains function (competence) even briefly or intermittently, the patient regains the right during those periods to make decisions about her health care.

DEATH AND EUTHANASIA

Physicians are required to certify the cause of death (e.g., natural, suicide, accident) and sign the death certificate. If a patient wishes to donate his or her organs at death, legal death must be determined by at least one doctor other than the patient's doctor.

Legal standard of death

In the United States, when a person's heart is beating, the legal standard of death is irreversible cessation of all functions of the entire brain, including

THE PATIENT A legally competent 65-year-old man signs a document that states that he does not want any measures taken to prolong his life should he sustain severe brain damage. Five months later, he has a stroke. He goes into a coma and requires life support. Extensive evaluation reveals that he will never recover consciousness. Although they know the patient's wishes, the patient's wife and his adult children urge the physician to keep the man alive.

COMMENT Under these circumstances, the patient's wishes are clear; he does not want any measures taken to prolong his life.

INTERVENTION The physician should carry out the patient's prior request and not provide life support. This decision is based on the patient's prior instructions as put forth in his living will. The wife's or adult children's wishes are not relevant to this decision.

---

the brainstem ("**brain death**"). This standard differs by state but commonly includes **absence of** the following:

- Response to external events or painful stimuli (comatose state)
- Spontaneous respiration (necessitating controlled ventilation)
- Cephalic reflexes (e.g., pupillary, corneal, pharyngeal, cough, swallow)
- Electrical potentials of cerebral origin over 2 μv from symmetrically placed electrodes more than 10 cm apart
- Cerebral blood flow for more than 30 minutes

If the patient is dead according to the legal standard, the physician is authorized to remove life support. A court order or relative's permission for such removal is not necessary.

Euthanasia

According to the code of ethics of the American Medical Association and medical specialty organizations, **euthanasia** (i.e., mercy killing or physician-assisted suicide) is a criminal act and is never appropriate.

When Dr. Jack Kevorkian challenged the law in Michigan regarding physician-assisted suicide by actually administering a lethal injection to a patient himself, he was convicted of murder. Although not strictly legal in any state, physician-assisted suicide is not generally an indictable offense as long as, and unlike Dr. Kevorkian, the physician does not actually perform the killing (e.g., the patient injects himself). Although it is illegal and unethical to administer medication with the purpose of shortening a patient's life, it is an accepted part of medical practice to provide medically needed analgesia to a terminally ill patient even if it coincidentally may shorten the patient's life (the so-called **double effect**) (Quill, 2003). In addition, under most circumstances, food, water, and medical care as well as life support can be withheld from a terminally ill patient who has no reasonable prospect of recovery but is not legally dead.

There is no ethical distinction between withholding and withdrawing life-sustaining treatment. Thus, if a competent patient requests that he not be put on a ventilator or if he requests cessation of artificial life support, it is both legal and ethical for a physician to comply with this request. Such action by the physician is not considered euthanasia.

REVIEW QUESTIONS

1. A 40-year-old woman undergoes surgery to repair a herniated disc. After the surgery, she has partial paralysis of one leg and sues the surgeon for malpractice. The lawsuit will be successful if the patient can prove that
   (A) the patient will lose a significant amount of time from work because of the paralysis
   (B) the paralysis is permanent
   (C) the physician was not board-certified in neurosurgery
   (D) the patient's sexual function is negatively affected by the paralysis
   (E) the physician did not follow the usual standards of professional care

2. A competent, pregnant, 33-year-old patient at term begins to have contractions and comes to the hospital for a vaginal delivery. Her physician discovers that the patient has an active genital herpes infection and suggests a cesarean section. He explains to the patient that without the surgery, the fetus is at high risk for infection and death. The patient refuses the surgery. The most appropriate action for her physician to take at this time is to
   (A) ask a judge to issue a court order to do the surgery
   (B) tell the patient that she can be criminally prosecuted if the child dies
   (C) get permission from the patient's husband to do the surgery
   (D) deliver the child vaginally
   (E) refer the patient to another doctor

3. A 13-year-old girl who was injured while riding her bicycle is brought to the emergency department by her neighbor. She has internal injuries that require immediate surgery. Her parents cannot be located. The most appropriate action for the physician to take at this time is to
   (A) obtain consent for the surgery from the neighbor
   (B) obtain consent for the surgery from the chief operating officer of the hospital

(C) do the surgery without obtaining consent

(D) keep the patient comfortable until the parents can be located

(E) obtain consent from the child herself

Questions 4–5

A married 16-year-old female has been in the intensive care unit in a coma for 2 weeks after sustaining brain damage in a car accident. She has had a flat line electroencephalogram (EEG) for 24 hours, shows no pupillary or corneal reflexes, and requires ventilator support. Despite repeated consultations with her religious advisor, the patient's father, with whom the young couple lives, insists that the physician not withdraw life support. The patient's mother who lives in another state says that her daughter would want life support only if she could live a normal life.

4. The most appropriate action for the doctor to take at this time is to

(A) get a court order to withdraw life support

(B) withdraw life support

(C) get the hospital ethics committee to authorize withdrawal of life support

(D) get the patient's husband to authorize withdrawal of life support

(E) get the patient's father to authorize withdrawal of life support

5. If life support is discontinued, it is justified because

(A) the physician declared the patient brain dead

(B) the mother had expressed her daughter's wishes

(C) the hospital ethics committee decided to stop life support

(D) the best interest standard was applied

(E) the mother did not live with the patient

ANSWERS AND EXPLANATIONS

1-E. The lawsuit will be successful if the patient can prove that the physician did not follow the usual standards of professional care. An unfavorable outcome alone (e.g., paralysis of the leg as an unavoidable complication of the surgical procedure) or negative effects on functioning because of the injury do not constitute malpractice. Licensed physicians are legally allowed to perform any medical or surgical procedure; they do not have to be boarded in a specialty.

2-D. The most appropriate action for the physician to take is to deliver the child vaginally. Competent pregnant women, like all competent adults, can refuse medical treatment, even if the fetus will die as a result. Neither the patient's husband (even if he is the father) nor the court has the right to alter this decision. Frightening the patient by telling her that she can be criminally prosecuted if the child dies or referring her to another doctor is not appropriate in this case.

3-C. Only the parent can give consent for surgical or medical treatment of a minor. In an emergency such as this, if the parent or guardian cannot be located, treatment may proceed without consent. The neighbor or chief operating officer has no legal standing to make health care decisions for this child. Waiting to act until the parents are reached could be harmful to the child.

4-B, 5-A. After explaining the situation to family members, the most appropriate action for the doctor to take in this unfortunate circumstance is to withdraw life support. If the physician has declared the patient dead, she is legally dead, and discontinuation of life support is justified. Because the patient is already dead, the best interest standard or wishes of the deceased, the relatives of the deceased, or the hospital ethics committee do not apply.

REFERENCES

American Medical Association. (2002–2003). *Code of medical ethics: Current opinions.* Chicago: AMA Press.

American Medical Association. (2002). *Code of medical ethics.* Chicago: AMA Press.

Gabbard, G. O., Nadelson, C. (1995). Professional boundaries in the physician-patient relationship. *JAMA, 273,* 1445–1449.

Gutheil, T. G., Gabbard, G. O. (1993). The concept of boundaries in clinical practice: Theoretical and risk-management dimensions. *Am J Psychiatry, 150,* 188.

Margolin, J., & Schuppe, J. (2003, July 7). Malpractice bill stuck in deadlock. *The Star Ledger.*

Mello, M. M., Studdert, D. M., & Brennan, T. A. (2003). The new medical malpractice crisis. *N Engl J Med, 348,* 2281–2284.

Quill, T. E. (2001). *Caring for patients at the end of life: Facing an uncertain future together.* London: Oxford University Press.

Sheehy, E., et al. (2003). Estimating the number of potential organ donors in the United States. *NEJM, 349:* 667–674.

Smarr, L. E. (2003). Statement of the Physician Insurers Association of America before a joint hearing of the Unites States Senate Judiciary Committee and Health, Education, Labor and Pensions Committee, February 11, 2003.

Wu, A. W., Cavanaugh, T. A., McPhee, S. J., Lo, B., Micco, G. P. (1997). To tell the truth: ethical and practical issues in disclosing medical mistakes to patients. *J Gen Intern Med, 12,* 787–788.

Systems of Health Care Delivery **27**

T he United States has the most advanced medical technology and the most highly trained physicians in the world. However, when compared with people in many other developed countries, Americans have shorter life expectancies (Table 27-1) and a greater probability of dying in childhood and in adulthood (Table 27-2). The explanation for this counterintuitive concurrence lies to some extent in the structure of the American health care system.

The United States is one of the few industrialized countries that does not have publicly mandated and funded health care insurance coverage for all citizens. The elderly, the chronically disabled, and the indigent have government-funded health care insurance through Medicare and Medicaid (see later text). Other Americans, however, must either obtain health insurance through their employers or pay out-of-pocket for their health care. This situation in part explains why Americans average fewer visits to physicians per year than people in other developed countries, often relying instead on over-the-counter medications and home treatments.

Throughout this book, the relationship between behavior and illness has been discussed. This chapter addresses the challenges facing ill Americans in obtaining the world's finest health care and, significantly, in paying for that care.

TABLE 27-1	Life Expectancy (in Years) at Birth in Selected Member States (in Alphabetical Order) of the World Health Organization		
	LIFE EXPECTANCY (YEARS)		
Member State	**Both Sexes**	**Males**	**Females**
Australia	80.0	77.4	82.5
Canada	79.3	76.5	81.9
France	79.3	75.6	82.9
Germany	78.2	75.1	81.1
Italy	79.3	76.2	82.2
Japan	81.4	77.9	84.7
Spain	78.9	75.3	82.6
Sweden	80.0	77.7	82.3
United Kingdom	77.5	75.1	79.9
United States	77.0	74.3	79.5

Adapted from Annex Table 1. The World Health Organization. (2002). *Basic indicators for all member states.* The World Health Report.

■ DEMOGRAPHICS OF HEALTH

Socioeconomic status, gender, and age are important variables in health and in obtaining health care.

Socioeconomic status and health

Socioeconomic status, a construct determined primarily by occupation, education, and income, correlates directly with health status. People in lower socioeconomic groups typically have poorer mental and physical health and decreased life expectancies than those in higher socioeconomic groups.

In the United States, approximately 85% of people in low socioeconomic groups are African American or Latino. Thus, these ethnic groups are at higher risk than the white population for several medical conditions (see Chapter 20) and for dying young (see Chapter 4). Among white Americans, those with lower incomes are at higher risk for illness.

Patients with higher incomes are more likely to seek treatment in a timely fashion, whereas low-income patients are more likely to delay seeking treatment. Because of this delay, by the time a poor person is seen, he

TABLE 27-2 Probability of Dying in Two Age Groups in Selected Member States (in Alphabetical Order) in the World Health Organization

| | PROBABILITY OF DYING (PER 1,000 PEOPLE) | | | |
| | UNDER AGE 5 YEARS | | BETWEEN AGES 15 AND 59 YEARS | |
MEMBER STATE	Males	Females	Males	Females
Australia	7	5	94	54
Canada	6	5	98	59
France	5	4	134	60
Germany	5	4	121	61
Italy	6	5	100	51
Japan	5	4	97	47
Spain	5	4	124	48
Sweden	4	3	84	54
United Kingdom	7	6	109	69
United States	9	7	144	83

Adapted from Annex Table 1. The World Health Organization. (2002). *Basic indicators for all member states.* The World Health Report.

or she is often severely ill, making treatment more difficult and expensive. High-income patients are also more likely to visit private doctors' offices than are low-income patients, who tend to go to hospital emergency rooms (ER). Although hospital ER visits are more expensive than private doctors' office visits, doctors in private practice can refuse to see patients who cannot pay them. In contrast, most hospital ERs are responsible for stabilizing every patient who presents for treatment, even those unable to pay.

In addition to the added difficulty that the poor face in obtaining health care, poorer diet and habits, such as smoking and alcohol abuse, are seen more commonly in low socioeconomic groups and contribute to increased risk for physical and emotional illness.

Gender and health

The sex difference in life expectancy (see Table 27-1) starts early; males are more likely than females to die in the first 5 years of life and in young and middle adulthood (see Table 27-2). There also are sex differences in the risk of having certain illnesses in adulthood. For example, women are at higher risk than men for developing autoimmune disorders (Table 27-3).

Men are more likely to have heart disease than women. However, when women, particularly those under age 55 years, have their first heart attack, they are less likely than men to undergo diagnostic and therapeutic procedures and more likely than men to die (Vaccarino et al., 1999). This sex difference in death rate after heart attack has been attributed to sex differences in reactions to medications, presentation of symptoms, and other physiological factors. However, it has also been attributed to missed or delayed diagnoses of heart problems in women resulting from the societal stereotype that only men have heart disease (Wong, 2001).

Smoking rates in American women, lower than in men in past years, now equal or exceed those of men. Thus, unsurprisingly, as in men, the most common cause of cancer death in American women is lung cancer. Table 27-4 lists incidence rates and death rates for different types of cancer in women and men.

No matter what the illness, gender differences exist in the frequency of seeking medical care. With the same symptom severity, women seek medical treatment more often than men.

TABLE 27-3	Female/Male Ratios of Common Autoimmune Disorders
DISORDER	**FEMALE:MALE RATIO**
Hashimoto thyroiditis	10:1
Primary biliary cirrhosis	9:1
Chronic active hepatitis	8:1
Graves' hyperthyroidism	7:1
Systemic lupus erythematosus	6:1[a]
Scleroderma	3:1
Rheumatoid arthritis	2.5:1
Idiopathic thrombocytopenia purpura	2:1[a]
Multiple sclerosis	2:1
Autoimmune hemolytic anemia	2:1

[a]Ratio is age specific.
Adapted from Institute of Medicine. (2001). *Exploring the biological contributions to human health: Does sex matter?* Washington, DC: National Academy Press, p. 150.

	CASES	DEATHS
SEX	**TOTAL = 1,284,900**	**TOTAL = 555,500**
Female	■ Breast (31%)	■ Lung and bronchus (25%)
Total cases = 647,400	■ Lung and bronchus (12%)	■ Breast (15%)
Total deaths = 267,300	■ Colorectal (12%)	■ Colorectal (11%)
	■ Uterus (6%)	■ Pancreas (6%)
	■ Non-Hodgkin's	■ Ovary (5%)
	lymphoma (4%)	■ Non-Hodgkin's
	■ Melanoma (4%)	lymphoma (4%)
	■ Ovary (4%)	■ Leukemia (4%)
	■ Others (about 27%)	■ Others (about 30%)
Male	■ Prostate (30%)	■ Lung and bronchus (31%)
Total cases = 637,500	■ Lung and bronchus (14%)	■ Prostate (11%)
Total deaths = 288,200	■ Colorectal (11%)	■ Colorectal (10%)
	■ Urinary bladder (7%)	■ Pancreas (5%)
	■ Melanoma (5%)	■ Non-Hodgkin's
	■ Non-Hodgkin's	lymphoma (5%)
	lymphoma (4%)	■ Leukemia (4%)
	■ Kidney (3%)	■ Esophagus (3%)
	■ Others (about 26%)	■ Others (about 31%)

TABLE 27-4   Cancer Cases and Deaths By Sex and Site[a]

[a]These are approximate percentages. Basal and squamous cell skin cancers and in situ carcinoma except urinary bladder are excluded.
Adapted from American Cancer Society. (2001). *Surveillance research;* and from Howe, H. L., Wingo, P. A., Thun, M. J., Ries, L. A., Rosenberg, H. M., Feigal, E. G., & Edwards, B. K. (2001). Annual report to the nation on the status of cancer (1973 through 1998), featuring cancers with recent increasing trends. *J Natl Cancer Inst, 93,* 824–842.

Age and health

Children are more likely than young and middle-aged adults to require medical treatment. However, of all age groups, the elderly are at highest risk for physical and mental illness. Although they comprise only 12% of the population, the elderly currently incur more than 30% of all health care costs. Because of the increasing number of elderly Americans (see Chapter 4), that percentage is expected to rise to 50% by the year 2020. The leading causes of death by age group are listed in Table 27-5.

■ HEALTH CARE DELIVERY SYSTEMS

Hospitals

The United States has close to 6,000 hospitals and almost 1,000,000 hospital beds. Hospital facilities fall into four basic groups: **community hospitals, federal government hospitals, non-federal psychiatric hospitals,** and **non-federal long-term care hospitals** (Table 27-6). Currently, at least

TABLE 27-5	Leading Causes of Death by Age Group (Across Sex and Ethnic Group)
AGE GROUP	CAUSES OF DEATH IN DECREASING ORDER OF FREQUENCY (APPROXIMATE NUMBER)
Infants (<1 year of age)	Congenital anomalies (7,100) SIDS (4,700) Respiratory distress syndrome (1,800)
Children (1–4 years of age)	Accidents (2,600) Congenital anomalies (800) Cancer (primarily leukemia and CNS malignancies) (500)
Children (5–14 years of age)	Accidents (3,500) Cancer (primarily leukemia and CNS malignancies) (1,100) Homicide and legal intervention (700)
Adolescents and young adults (15–24 years of age)	Accidents (most in motor vehicles) (14,000) Homicide and legal intervention (8,400) Suicide (4,800)
Adults (25–44 years of age)	Accidents (27,300) AIDS (27,200) Cancer (21,900)
Adults (45–64 years of age)	Cancer (133,100) Heart disease (105,000) Stroke (14,700)
Elderly (65 years of age)	Heart disease (620,000 and over) Cancer (lung, breast, prostate, and colorectal, in decreasing order) (317,500) Stroke (131,500)

CNS, central nervous system; SIDS, sudden infant death syndrome.

one third of hospital beds, especially in city hospitals, are unoccupied. This current surplus of beds is caused in part by restrictions on length of hospital stays imposed by health insurance entities. In 2001, the average hospital stay was 5.7 days, down from 6.1 days in 1997 (American Hospital Association, 2003).

Nursing homes and other health care facilities

The United States currently has approximately 25,000 nursing homes, with a capacity of more than 1.5 million beds. These institutions provide inpatient long-term care, particularly for the elderly, but also for the chronically disabled.

TABLE 27-6 Hospitals Meeting American Hospital Association Criteria for a Hospital Facility

TYPE	NUMBER	COMMENT
Community hospitals ■ Non-government not-for-profit ■ Investor-owned (for-profit) ■ State and local government	 2,998 754 1,156	Category includes all non-federal and short-term general and other special hospitals (e.g., obstetrics and gynecology, rehabilitation, orthopedic) and academic medical centers or other teaching hospitals accessible to the general public
Federal government hospitals	243	Veterans Administration and military hospitals that are federally owned and reserved for individuals who have served (veterans) or are currently serving in the military
Non-federal psychiatric hospitals (often owned and operated by state governments)	491	For chronically mentally ill patients Decreasing number of hospitals resulting primarily from increasing use and effectiveness of psychoactive medications, leading to deinstitutionalization
Non-federal long-term care hospitals	140	For chronically physically ill patients

Adapted from American Hospital Association. (2003). Hospital statistics. Chicago: American Hospital Association.

Because of the aging of the American population (see Chapter 4), the number of nursing homes and beds is increasing. Despite this and because of the high expense of nursing home care (which is not funded by Medicare; see later text), only about 5% of the elderly use such care. Most elderly Americans spend the last years of their lives in their own residences; a smaller number spend their last years being cared for by family members.

Nursing homes are classified by the level of care that they provide, which also determines their costs. **Residential care facilities** provide limited care, such as meals, housekeeping, and personal care, and they typically cost about $35,000 per year. **Skilled care facilities** provide professional nursing care and can cost more than $75,000 per year.

Rehabilitation centers, halfway houses, and **visiting nurse's associations** provide less expensive alternatives to hospital and nursing home care for elderly and disabled people. Rehabilitation centers and halfway houses provide short-term care to help hospitalized patients reenter society. Visiting nurse associations provide nursing care in the patient's own home, as well as physical and occupational therapy and social work services. For the chronically disabled and those older than age 65 years, these alternative care facilities are funded by Medicare (see later text).

Hospice care

Hospice is a health care facility that provides inpatient and outpatient supportive care to terminally ill patients. Terminal illness in this context refers to patients who are expected to live less than 6 months. Diagnostic tests or treatments aimed at cure are not part of hospice care.

The hospice concept, which originated in England, offers patients death with dignity in their own homes, with family present and with as little pain as possible. To do this, hospice provides care by physicians, nurses, social workers, and volunteers who give peer and family support, grief counseling, and administration of pain medication to patients as needed. For people over age 65 years, hospice care is paid for under Medicare.

Physicians

Currently, there are 126 medical schools and 16 colleges of osteopathic medicine in the United States, graduating annually more than 15,000 **medical doctors (MDs)** and 1,800 **doctors of osteopathy (DOs)**. Both MDs and DOs are correctly called physicians.

Training and practice are essentially the same for DOs and MDs; however, osteopathic medicine stresses the interrelatedness of body systems and the use of musculoskeletal manipulation in the diagnosis and treatment of physical illness.

There are currently more than 700,000 physicians in the United States. Approximately 25% of these are foreign medical school graduates. Demographically, the ratio of physicians to patients is higher in the northeastern states and in California than in the southern and mountain states; many rural regions have no physicians at all.

Primary care physicians, including family practitioners, internists, and pediatricians, provide initial care to patients. They currently account for at least one third of all physicians and are expected to make up one half of all physicians within the next few years.

Overall, physicians have an average annual income of about $200,000 annually. Pediatricians and family practitioners typically earn less than this average figure, and surgical specialists typically earn more (Table 27-7).

■ COSTS OF HEALTH CARE

Health care expenditures in the United States make up more than 15% of the total economy, a higher percentage than in any other industrialized

TABLE 27-7 Average Annual Income For Some Medical Specialties in 1997

SPECIALTY	AVERAGE ANNUAL INCOME
Pediatrics	$137,100
Family practice	$138,300
Internal medicine	$143,900
Dermatology	$166,500
Gastroenterology	$198,700
Orthopedic surgery	$273,500
Neurosurgery	$317,700
Cardiovascular surgery	$363,300

Adapted with permission from Kilmore, P.T. (1998, April 22). The Hay Group. *The New York Times*.

society. These costs have been increasing steadily, and they showed the fastest rise in 10 years in 2001. The major reason for this increase is the increased use of and costs for services, medical goods, and advances in medical technology needed to care for the increasing elderly population.

Hospitalization is the most expensive component of health care in the United States. Physician costs are the next most expensive, followed in decreasing order by nursing home care, medications, and personal medical equipment. The percentage of funds spent in each area of health care has changed over the last 20 years. For example, between 1982 and 2000, hospital spending decreased by about 10% while prescription drug costs almost doubled (Fig. 27-1). Currently, the cost of prescription drugs exceeds those of nursing homes and home health care combined (Pear, 2003).

■ PAYMENT FOR HEALTH CARE

Sources of payment for health care include the federal government and state governments through Medicare and Medicaid, as well as private health insurance companies. Approximately 15% of Americans have no health insurance and must pay for the costs of health care themselves. The health insurance plans of others may not pay all medical costs, leaving those individuals **"underinsured"** and therefore responsible for the remainder of the charges.

No matter how an individual is insured, the privacy of health information (e.g., insurance claims, referral authorization requests) is protected

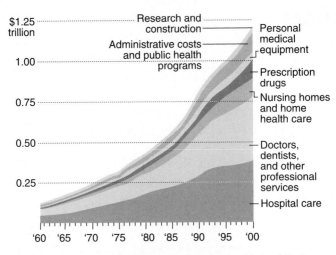

FIGURE 27-1. Annual health care spending in the United States, 1960–2000. Figures have been adjusted for inflation in 1996 dollars.

(Source: U. S. Department of Health and Human Services, and Pear, R. (2002, January 8). Propelled by drug and hospital costs, health spending surged in 2000. The New York Times.)

by **The Standards for Privacy of Individually Identifiable Health Information ("Privacy Rule")**. This rule sets national standards for insurance plans and companies as well as health care providers to protect the privacy of individually identifiable health information held or transmitted in any form (e.g., paper, oral or electronic). This rule also implements the requirements **of the Health Insurance Portability and Accountability Act of 1996 (HIPAA)** (Department of Health and Human Services, 2003).

Federal and state-funded insurance coverage

The largest percentages of personal health care expenses are paid by the federal and state governments through **Medicare** and **Medicaid.** These programs provide medical insurance to certain groups of people; namely, the elderly, the chronically disabled, and the indigent. Eligibility requirements and coverage provided by these programs are outlined in Table 27-8.

    Diagnosis-related groups (DRGs) are a method of cost control used by Medicare to pay hospital bills. With this system, the amount paid to the provider by Medicare is based on an estimate of the cost of care for each illness, rather than the actual charges incurred.

Private health insurers

Individuals who wish to be covered by health insurance but are not eligible for Medicare or Medicaid must obtain private health insurance. This insurance can be either purchased by the individual or obtained through a group plan paid for by the individual's employer (often with a copay-

TABLE 27-8 Medicare and Medicaid

SOURCE OF FUNDING	ELIGIBILITY	COVERAGE
Medicare		
Federal government (through the Social Security system)	■ People eligible for Social Security benefits (e.g., those 65 years of age regardless of income) ■ People of any age with chronic disabilities or debilitating illnesses ■ Covers at least 34 million people	■ Part A: Inpatient hospital costs, home health care, nursing home care for a limited time (about 3 months) after hospitalization, hospice care ■ Part B: Dialysis, physical therapy, laboratory tests, outpatient hospital care, physician bills, ambulance service, medical equipment ■ Part B is optional and has a 20% copayment and a $100 deductible ■ Neither Part A nor B covers all outpatient prescription drug costs or long-term nursing home care
Medicaid (MediCal in California)		
Both federal and state governments (the state contribution is determined by average per capita income of the state)	■ Indigent (very low income) people ■ One-third of all monies are allocated for nursing home care for indigent people ■ Covers at least 25 million people ■ No copayment or deductible	■ Inpatient and outpatient hospital costs ■ Physician services ■ Home health care, hospice care ■ Laboratory tests, dialysis ■ Ambulance service, medical equipment ■ Prescription drugs ■ Long-term nursing home care ■ Dental care, prescription eyeglasses, hearing aids

ment from the insured). Many insurance plans also have a **deductible,** which is the amount the patient must pay out-of-pocket before the insurance company begins to cover expenses, and a **copayment** or percentage, typically 20% of the total bill that the patient must pay.

Blue Cross/Blue Shield (BC/BS) is a nonprofit, private insurance carrier regulated by insurance agencies in each state. Blue Cross pays for hospital costs and Blue Shield pays for physician fees and diagnostic tests.

THE PATIENT A 70-year-old woman who retired from her long-term teaching job 2 years ago is hospitalized with a fractured hip. The patient, who is covered by Medicare Parts A and B, as well as a Blue-Cross/Blue-Shield (BC/BS) plan to cover deductibles and copayments not covered by Medicare, has $100,000 in savings. She was brought to the hospital by ambulance, stayed in the hospital for 5 days, and required physical therapy and a "walker" for help with mobility for the next 6 weeks. After 6 months at home, it is determined that this patient is unable to care for herself and requires care in a nursing home, probably for the rest of her life.

COMMENT Because she is over 65 years old and eligible for Social Security benefits, this patient can expect that Medicare Part A will cover her inpatient hospital costs. Part B covers ambulance services, physician fees, medical equipment (the "walker"), and therapy and BC/BS will pay the uncovered portion of these costs. The patient herself is responsible for long-term nursing home costs because neither Medicare nor BC/BS will cover these costs.

INTERVENTION After the patient's $100,000 is exhausted to pay for the nursing home (probably within 3 years at $35,000-$75,000 per year), she will be indigent and therefore eligible for Medicaid. Medicaid will pay for her nursing home care and will supplement Medicare to pay for all other health care for the rest of her life.

Blue Cross/Blue Shield covers up to half of the working population in the United States, and almost half of its subscribers are enrolled in some type of managed care plan (see later text). In addition to BC/BS, individuals can take out a health insurance policy with one of at least 1,000 other private insurance carriers, such as Aetna and Prudential.

Because most people get health insurance through their employers, if they lose their job, they lose their insurance coverage. Sometimes unemployed persons can continue to belong to their former employer's group plan (group plans are typically less expensive than individual plans) for a limited time via the **Consolidated Omnibus Budget Reconciliation Act (COBRA)** health benefits provision. However, the cost of such health insurance is high and, for the now unemployed individual, often prohibitive.

Insurance carriers typically offer a **traditional fee-for-service indemnity plan,** in which individuals choose physicians and pay them for each visit or procedure, and at least one type of **managed care plan** (see later text). Traditional plans commonly place no restrictions on provider or referral choice, but they have higher premiums than managed care plans that have restrictions.

Managed care plans

Managed care is a system, developed to a great extent over the past 15 years, in which all aspects of an individual's health care are coordinated by providers. Managed care plans include **health maintenance organizations (HMOs)**, **preferred provider organizations (PPOs)**, and **point of service (POS) plans** (Table 27-9).

The major purpose of managed care is to control costs both for the patient and for the provider. To do this, managed care plans typically restrict the treatments they will pay for. These restrictions can lead to differences in treatment between managed care and fee-for-service patients. For example, some studies show that procedures such as angiography may be used less frequently among patients enrolled in managed care plans than among those with fee-for-service coverage (Guadagnoli et al., 2001). In part because of such restrictions, managed care is less popular with the public and with physicians than with the insurance companies and government entities from which it evolved (Robinson, 2001).

If a doctor believes that a treatment not covered by a managed care company will materially benefit his or her patient, the doctor should advocate for coverage of such care with the company. Attempts by some managed care plans to restrict the relay of information about uncovered treatment options by the doctor to the patient, (i.e., **"gag clauses"**) are ethically unacceptable (American Medical Association, 2003).

■ PREVENTION OF ILLNESS

Because fewer patient visits and early treatment ultimately result in lower costs, the philosophy of managed care stresses prevention of illness rather than acute treatment. Types of prevention include primary, secondary, and tertiary prevention.

CASE 27-2

THE PATIENT   A 48-year-old woman with metastatic ovarian cancer has been treated with several chemotherapeutic agents but is now unresponsive to them. The patient's physician believes that a bone marrow transplant (BMT) has a good chance of prolonging the patient's life but knows that the patient's HMO will refuse to pay for the transplant. When the doctor contacts the case manager at the HMO, she instructs him not to discuss the BMT option with the patient because it is not covered by the plan, and she suggests that the doctor recommend instead a chemotherapy regimen that is covered by the plan.

COMMENT   A physician has an ethical responsibility to inform a patient of all treatment alternatives and options that he or she feels are appropriate (e.g., BMT in this case) even if they are not covered by the patient's managed care plan.

INTERVENTION   The doctor should contact the case manager or supervisor at the HMO and advocate for coverage of the bone marrow transplant. If the company still refuses, the doctor should pursue alternative strategies that will allow the patient to have the treatment.

TABLE 27-9	Managed Care Plans and Percentage of Employees Enrolled in Each Type		
TYPE OF PLAN (% ENROLLED)	**DEFINITION**	**COMMENTS**	
Health Maintenance Organization (HMO) (33% for both staff and Independence Practice Association [IPA] models)[a]	■ Physicians and other health care personnel are paid a salary to provide medical services to a group of people who are enrolled voluntarily and who pay an annual premium ■ HMOs can operate their own hospitals and clinics ■ Services include hospitalization, physician services, preventive medical services, and often dental, eye, and podiatric care	■ These plans are the most restrictive for the patient in terms of choice of doctor ■ Patient is assigned a "gatekeeper" (a primary care doctor from within the network who decides if and when a patient needs to see a specialist)	
HMO IPA model	■ Physicians in private practice are hired by an HMO to provide services to HMO patients ■ About 65% of HMOs have IPA components	■ Private-practice physicians receive a fee, or capitation, for each HMO patient they see	
Preferred Provider Organization (PPO) (31%)	■ A third-party payer (e.g., a union trust fund, insurance company, or corporation) contracts with physicians in private practice and hospitals to provide medical care to its subscribers ■ Participants choose physicians from a listing of member practitioners (the network) ■ Physicians in the network receive capitation for each patient they see	■ These plans guarantee doctors in private practice a certain volume of patients ■ By paying a larger share of the cost, patients can choose a doctor who is not in the network ■ There is no "gatekeeper" physician	

TABLE 27-9 Managed Care Plans and Percentage of Employees
Enrolled in Each Type (Continued)

TYPE OF PLAN (% ENROLLED)	DEFINITION	COMMENTS
Point-of-Service (POS) Plan (17%)	▪ Variant of a PPO in which a third-party payer contracts with physicians in private practice to provide medical care to its subscribers ▪ Physicians in the network receive capitation for each patient they see	▪ As with a PPO, patients can choose a doctor who is not in the network by paying an extra fee ▪ As with an HMO, there is a "gatekeeper" physician

[a]Percentages from Kilborn, P. T. (1997, August 17). Workers getting greater freedom in health plans. *The New York Times.*

Primary prevention

Primary prevention is aimed at reducing the incidence (new cases) of a disorder by reducing its associated risk factors. For example, providing smallpox immunization for health care workers is a primary prevention strategy that will prevent the disease from occurring in this group. Improved obstetrical care to avoid premature birth and its associated problems is primary prevention strategy aimed at decreasing the incidence of prematurity.

Secondary prevention

Secondary prevention is aimed at reducing the severity of a disorder. For example, mammography is a secondary prevention strategy. It does not prevent breast cancer from occurring, but because it permits early identification and treatment of the disease, it ultimately reduces the personal and medical costs of treatment. Early identification of phenylketonuria (PKU) in infants to prevent mental retardation is another secondary prevention strategy. Identification of a child with PKU leads to diet modifications that will prevent the negative sequelae of this metabolic abnormality.

Tertiary prevention

Tertiary prevention is a strategy aimed at improving the outcome of an existing disorder. For example, an educational program for mentally ill adults aimed at helping them enter the work force does not prevent the condition nor reduce its severity. However, this tertiary strategy can ultimately improve the outcome for a patient with mental illness as well as reduce the cost to society of caring for that person.

REVIEW QUESTIONS

1. A 34-year-old man who has been disabled for more than 2 years is now eligible for Social Security disability income and for Medicare Part A. He opts to pay an extra fee to obtain Medicare Part B because he can expect that it will cover

   (A) hospital care

   (B) home health care

   (C) hospice care

   (D) long-term nursing home care

   (E) physical therapy

2. Which of the following patients can be expected to use the most Medicare services and funds during his or her lifetime?

   (A) Asian-American man

   (B) Asian-American woman

   (C) White man

   (D) White woman

   (E) Native-American man

3. A 40-year-old married doctor with two children must choose a health insurance plan from several options provided by the hospital where he works. In which of the following plans will he have the most choice in choosing a doctor?

   (A) A health maintenance organization (HMO)

   (B) A preferred provider organization (PPO)

   (C) A point-of-service (POS) plan

   (D) A fee-for-service plan

4. An attending physician who has recently started working in a hospital emergency department sees five patients during his first hour on the service. Which of these middle-aged patients is likely to be the most ill when first seen by the resident?

   (A) An unemployed man who lives in a homeless shelter

   (B) A woman who works as a mailroom clerk

   (C) A male physician

   (D) A successful actress

   (E) A male accountant

5. Which of the following are the three leading causes of death in the United States in people aged 45 to 64 years of age in order of magnitude (higher to lower)?

   (A) AIDS, heart disease, cancer

(B) Cancer, heart disease, stroke

(C) Cancer, heart disease, AIDS

(D) Heart disease, cancer, AIDS

(E) Heart disease, cancer, stroke

ANSWERS AND EXPLANATIONS

1-E. Medicare Part A covers inpatient hospital costs, home health care, nursing home care for a limited time (about 3 months) after hospitalization, and hospice care. Part B covers physical therapy, dialysis, laboratory tests, outpatient hospital care, physician bills, ambulance service, and medical equipment. Neither Part A nor Part B Medicare currently covers long-term nursing home care.

2-B. Medicare pays for health care services for persons 65 years of age and older and others (see question 1) who are eligible to receive Social Security benefits. Because statistically she is likely to have a longer life than a white or Native-American man or woman, or an Asian-American man (see Table 4-1), an Asian-American woman is likely to use the most Medicare services during her lifetime.

3-D. Patients have the most choice in choosing a doctor in a traditional fee-for-service indemnity plan. This type of plan has no restrictions on provider choice or referrals. Health maintenance organizations (HMOs), preferred provider organizations (PPOs), and point-of-service (POS) plans have restrictions on doctor choice. HMOs are the most restrictive of managed care plans for the patient in terms of choice of doctor. Rather than choosing a doctor from the network as in the PPOs and POS plans, the patient is usually assigned a doctor in HMOs.

4-A. A man from a low socioeconomic group, such as this homeless man, is likely to be most ill when the resident first sees him. Compared with high-income patients and female patients, low-income patients and male patients are more likely to delay seeking treatment. Delay in seeking treatment commonly results in more severe illness.

5-B. In order of magnitude, cancer, heart disease, and stroke are the leading causes of death in middle-aged people (ages 45 to 64 years). In the elderly population and all age groups, the leading causes of death are heart disease, cancer, and stroke, in that order.

REFERENCES

American Hospital Association. (2003). *Hospital statistics.* Chicago: American Hospital Association.

American Medical Association. (2003). *Code of medical ethics.* American Medical Association. Current Opinions.

Department of Health and Human Services (HHS). (2003). *Summary of the HIPAA privacy rule.* Washington, DC: HHS publication.

Flegal, K. M., Carroll, M. D., Ogden, C. L., & Johnson, C. L. (2002). Prevalence and trends in obesity among US adults, 1999–2000. *JAMA, 288,* 1723–1727.

Guadagnoli, E., Landrum, M. B., Peterson, E. A., Gahart, M. T., Ryan, T. J., & NcNeil, B. J. (2001). Appropriateness of coronary angiography after myocardial infarction among Medicare beneficiaries: managed care vs. fee for service. *N Engl J Med, 343,* 1460–1466.

Howe, H. L., Wingo, P. A., Thun, M. J., Ries, L. A., Rosenberg, H. M., Feigal, E. G., & Edwards, B. K. (2001). Annual report to the nation on the status of cancer (1973 through 1998), featuring cancers with recent increasing trends. *J Natl Cancer Inst, 93,* 824–842

Institute of Medicine. (2001). *Exploring the biological contributions to human health: Does sex matter?* Washington, DC: National Academy Press.

Kilborn, P. T. (1997, August 17). Workers getting greater freedom in health plans. *The New York Times.*

Kilborn, P. T. (1998, April 22). Doctor's pay regains ground despite the effects of HMOs. *The New York Times.*

Leary, W. E. (1999, January 21). Study urged on cancer and races: Health panel cites higher rates in poor. *The New York Times.*

National Center for Health Statistics. (1999). *Health, United States, 1999, with health and aging chartbook.* (Publication No. PHS-99-1232). Hyattsville, MD: National Center for Health Statistics.

National Center for Health Statistics. (2000). *Health, United States, 2000, with health and aging chartbook.* (Publication No. PHS-2000-1232). Hyattsville, MD: National Center for Health Statistics.

Ogden, C. L., Flegal, K. M., Carroll, M. D., & Johnson, C. L. (2002). Prevalence and trends in overweight among US children and adolescents, 1999–2000. *JAMA, 288,* 1728–1732.

Pear, R. (2002, January 8). Propelled by drug and hospital costs, health spending surged in 2000. *The New York Times.*

Pear, R. (2003, January 7). Spending on health care increased sharply in 2001. *The New York Times.*

Robinson, J. C. (2001). The end of managed care. *JAMA, 285,* 2622–2628.

Vaccarino, V., Parsons, L., Every, N. R., Barron, H. V., & Krumholz, H. M. (1999). Sex-based differences in early mortality after myocardial infarction. *N Engl J Med, 341,* 217–225.

Wong, Y., Rodwell, A., Dawkins, S., Livesey, A., & Simpson, I. A. (2001). Sex differences in investigation results and treatment in subjects referred for investigation of chest pain. *Heart, 85,* 149–152.

Appendix: Medical Epidemiology and Biostatistics

Medical epidemiology is the study of the factors affecting the occurrence and distribution of diseases in human populations. The basic measures in epidemiology are rates (e.g., incidence rates and prevalence rates) and measures of risk (e.g., relative risk, attributable risk, and odds risk ratio). Biostatistics summarize and evaluate data obtained from epidemiologic and other studies.

■ INCIDENCE AND PREVALENCE

Incidence rate is a ratio of the number of new (incident) cases of a disorder or event to the number of potential new cases (people at risk). Prevalence rate is a ratio of the number of present cases of a disorder or event to the number of potential cases.

Calculating incidence and prevalence rates

To calculate **incidence rate,** the number of individuals who develop an illness in a given period (commonly 1 year) is divided by the total number of individuals at risk for the illness during that period. For example, the number of intravenous (IV) drug abusers newly diagnosed as HIV-positive in 2004 is divided by the number of IV drug abusers in the population during 2004, to yield the incidence rate for HIV infection among IV drug abusers in 2004.

To calculate **prevalence rate,** the number of individuals in the population who have an illness (e.g., are HIV-positive) is divided by the total population at risk for the illness. Specific prevalence measures include point prevalence and period prevalence.

- **Point prevalence** is the number of individuals who have an illness at a specific point in time (e.g., the number of people who are HIV-positive on August 31, 2004) divided by the total population who could potentially have the illness on that date.
- **Period prevalence** is the number of individuals who have an illness during a specific time period (e.g., the number of people who are HIV-positive in 2004) divided by the total population who could have the illness midyear in 2004.

Association between incidence and prevalence

Prevalence is equal to the incidence rate multiplied by the average duration of the disease process. Therefore, if the disease lasts a long time, prevalence is greater than incidence. For example, because HIV-positive status typically lasts a lifetime, its prevalence is much higher than its incidence. In contrast, the prevalence of influenza, an acute illness, is approximately equal to its incidence.

Health interventions that prevent a disease from occurring in the first place (i.e., primary prevention [see Chapter 27]) result in reduced incidence of illness. Ultimately, the prevalence of that illness will be reduced as well. For example, both development of a vaccine for HIV and reduction in behavioral risk factors, such as increased use of condoms, will reduce the number of new cases (incidence) of HIV and ultimately its prevalence in the population.

There are at least two ways that people with a specific illness can leave the population of prevalent cases. They can either recover or die. For example, the prevalence of HIV in the population will decrease if either a cure for the illness is found or the death rate from HIV increases. Table A-1 summarizes factors affecting incidence and prevalence of an illness such as HIV.

Quantifying risk in population studies

Relative risk, attributable risk, and the odds (or odds risk) ratio are measures used to quantify risk in population studies. Relative risk and attributable risk are calculated for cohort studies, whereas the odds ratio is calculated for case-control studies (Table A-2).

Relative risk compares the incidence rate of a disorder among individuals exposed to a risk factor (e.g., smoking) with the incidence rate of the disorder in nonexposed individuals. **Attributable risk** is useful for determining what would happen in a study population if the risk factor

Effects of Events on Incidence and Prevalence of HIV Infection

WHAT IF?	EFFECT ON INCIDENCE	EFFECT ON PREVALENCE
A vaccine to prevent HIV is developed	Decreased	Decreased
Government campaigns result in increased use of condoms in the population	Decreased	Decreased
A new antiviral agent cures HIV	None	Decreased
A new antiviral agent does not cure HIV but does increase the life expectancies of patients with the illness	None	Increased

TABLE A-2 **Relative Risk, Attributable Risk, and Odds Ratio**

TYPE OF ANALYSIS	USED TO ANALYZE	EXAMPLE
Relative risk	Cohort studies	If the incidence rate of lung cancer among smokers in Newark, NJ in 2004 is 20:1000 and the incidence rate of lung cancer among nonsmokers in Newark in 2004 is 2:1000, the relative risk is 20:2, or 10. That is, the risk of lung cancer is 10 times higher for smokers than for nonsmokers.
Attributable risk	Cohort studies	Given the data above, the risk of lung cancer attributable to smoking (the attributable risk) is 20:1000 minus 2:1000, or 18:1000. That is, 18:1000 cases of lung cancer can be attributed to smoking.
Odds ratio	Case-control studies	Of 200 patients treated in a hospital, 50 have lung cancer; of these patients, 45 are smokers; of the remaining 150 patients, 60 are smokers; the odds ratio for smoking and the risk of lung cancer is:

	Smokers	Nonsmokers
People with lung cancer	A = 45	B = 5
People without lung cancer	C = 60	D = 90

$$\frac{(A)\,(D)}{(B)\,(C)} = \frac{(45)\,(90)}{(5)\,(60)} = 13.5 = \text{Odds ratio}$$

If you have lung cancer, you are 13.5 times more likely to have smoked than if you do not have lung cancer, i.e., the risk of lung cancer is 13.5 times higher for smokers than for nonsmokers in this population.

were removed (e.g., determining how common lung cancer would be in a study if people did not smoke). To calculate attributable risk, the incidence rate of the illness in nonexposed individuals is subtracted from the incidence rate of the illness in those who have been exposed to a risk factor. Because incidence data are not available in a case-control study, the **odds ratio** or **odds risk ratio** can be used as an estimate of relative risk.

■ BIAS, RELIABILITY, AND VALIDITY

Goals of medical research include 1) identifying significant relationships between risk factors and illness; and 2) evaluating the effectiveness of new treatments. For practical reasons, not all members of a population can be studied. Therefore, such identification and evaluation must be done by utilizing subgroups of individuals that ideally represent the entire population. The evaluation instruments used for such assessment must be bias-free, reliable, and valid.

Bias in research studies

A biased test or study is one constructed so that one outcome is more likely to occur than another. The results of such tests or studies thus do not convey the truth. Ways that research studies can be biased include selection, recall, and sampling bias.

Selection bias can occur if subjects are permitted to choose whether to go into a drug or a placebo group rather than being assigned to one randomly. For example, in a study on the effectiveness of estrogen replacement therapy (ERT) on menopausal symptoms, menopausal women who have many hot flashes are more likely to choose the ERT group rather than the placebo group because they want relief. Thus, women with more symptoms end up in the ERT group, making it more difficult to show a positive effect of ERT. Selection bias can also occur if, rather than making random assignments, the investigator purposely chooses which patients go into the drug group and which patients go into the placebo group. For example, a physician investigator, believing that a new drug for relief of menopausal symptoms being tested in clinical trials will be effective, will put all of her most serious cases into the new drug group. Thus, women with more symptoms end up in the new drug group, making it more difficult to show a positive effect of the new drug.

In **recall bias,** knowledge of the presence of a disorder alters the way the subject remembers his or her history. For example, if because their children are affected, mothers of children with cleft palate overestimate how much medication they took during pregnancy, the overestimation can make it appear (erroneously) that certain medications are related to cleft palate deformities.

In **sampling bias,** subjects who volunteer to be in a study may not represent the population being studied. Factors unrelated to the subject of the study may have led them to volunteer but could also distinguish the subjects from the rest of the population. Because of these factors, the results of the study may not be applicable to the entire population. For example, college students who volunteer for an experiment on the physiological bases of sexual response are likely to be more sexually active than students who do not volunteer. Because the students who volunteered may not be representative of the entire population of college students, the results of the experiment may not be true for that whole population (i.e., may not be generalizable).

Reducing bias in research studies

Several strategies can be used to reduce bias in research studies. These include use of blind studies, crossover studies, and randomized studies.

The expectations of patients can influence the effectiveness of treatment. **Blind studies** attempt to reduce this influence. In a **single-blind study,** the subject does not know what treatment he or she is receiving. In a **double-blind study,** neither the subject nor the clinician-evaluator knows what treatment the subject is receiving.

In a blind drug study, a patient may receive a **placebo** (an inactive substance) (see also Chapter 5) rather than the active drug. People receiving the placebo are the control group, those receiving the active drug are the experimental group. In a **crossover study,** subjects are randomly assigned to one of two groups, group 1 or group 2. Subjects in group 1 first receive the drug and subjects in group 2 first receive the placebo. Later in the study, the groups switch or crossover—those in group 1 now receive the placebo, and those in Group 2 receive the drug. Because subjects in both groups receive both the drug and the placebo, each subject acts as his or her own control.

To ensure that the proportion of sicker people to healthier people is the same in the treatment and control groups, a **randomized study** is used, in which patients are randomly assigned to a group. The number of patients in each group does not have to be equal.

Reliability and validity of research studies

Reliability refers to the reproducibility of results.

- **Interrater reliability** measures whether the results of the test are similar when the test is administered by a different rater or examiner.
- **Test–retest reliability** measures whether the results of the test are similar when the person is tested repeatedly.

Validity measures whether the test assesses what it was designed to assess (e.g., does a new IQ test really measure IQ or does it instead measure educational level?) (see Chapter 10).

■ SENSITIVITY, SPECIFICITY, AND PREDICTIVE VALUES

Sensitivity and specificity are components of validity and measure the ability of a test to identify people who have a disorder (sensitivity) and people who do not have a disorder (specificity). Predictive values can determine the likelihood that a person with a positive test has the disorder (positive predictive value) and the likelihood that a person with a negative test does not have the disorder (negative predictive value) (Example A-1, Fig. 1-A).

Sensitivity

Sensitivity measures how well a test identifies truly ill people.

- **True positives (TP)** occur when a test correctly identifies ill people as ill.
- **False negatives (FN)** occur when a test incorrectly identifies ill people as well.
- Sensitivity is calculated using only people who are in fact ill (TP and FN) by dividing the number of TP by the sum of the number of TP and FN.

EXAMPLE A-1   Sensitivity, Specificity, Predictive Value, and Prevalence

---

A new blood test to detect the presence of prostate cancer was given to 1000 patients. Although 200 of the patients actually had prostate cancer, the test was positive in only 160 patients (true +); the other 40 ill patients had negative tests (false −) and thus were not identified by this new test. Of the 800 patients who did not have prostate cancer, the test was negative in 720 patients (true −) and positive in 80 patients (false +).

Use this information to calculate the sensitivity, specificity, positive predictive value, and negative predictive value of this new blood test and the prevalence of prostate cancer in this population.

	Patients with prostate cancer	Patients without prostate cancer	Total patients
Positive test	160 (true +)	80 (false +)	240 (those with + test)
Negative test	40 (false −)	720 (true −)	760 (those with − test)
Total patients	200	800	1000

$$\text{Sensitivity} = \frac{160 \text{ (true +)}}{160 \text{ (true +)} + 40 \text{ (false −)}} = \frac{160}{200} = 80.0\%$$

$$\text{Specificity} = \frac{720 \text{ (true −)}}{720 \text{ (true −)} + 80 \text{ (false +)}} = \frac{720}{800} = 90.0\%$$

$$\text{Positive predictive value} = \frac{160 \text{ (true +)}}{160 \text{ (true +)} + 80 \text{ (false +)}} = \frac{160}{240} = 66.67\%$$

$$\text{Negative predictive value} = \frac{720 \text{ (true −)}}{720 \text{ (true −)} + 40 \text{ (false −)}} = \frac{720}{760} = 94.7\%$$

$$\text{Prevalence} = \frac{200 \text{ (total of those with prostate cancer)}}{1000 \text{ (total patients)}} = 20.0\%$$

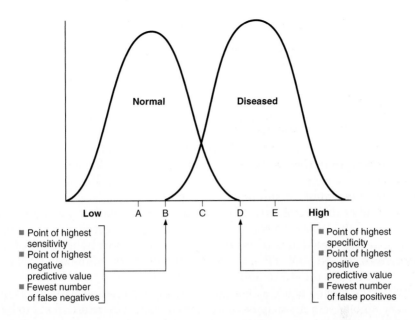

FIGURE A-1. Graphic representation of screening test scores (from low to high) of a population of normal people and diseased people. A, B, C, D and E represent possible diagnostic cutoff points.

- Tests with high sensitivity can rule out disease and are most useful in cases where a false-negative diagnosis can lead to severe consequences (e.g., not identifying serious, treatable, or transmissible disorders).
- A test with high sensitivity typically is used first to ensure identification of all possible cases.

Specificity

Specificity measures how well a test identifies truly well people.

- **True negatives (TN)** occur when a test has correctly identified well people as well.
- **False positives (FP)** occur when a test has incorrectly identified well people as ill.
- Specificity is calculated using only people who are in fact well (TN and FP) by dividing the number of TN by the sum of the number of TN and FP.
- Tests with high specificity can rule in disease and are most useful in cases where a false-positive diagnosis can lead to dangerous, painful, or unnecessary treatment.
- A test with high specificity is typically used later in the diagnostic process to eliminate the false-positive results and to avoid unnecessary interventions.

Predictive value

The **predictive value** of a test is a measure of the percentage of test results that match the actual diagnosis. Predictive values (but not sensitivity or specificity) vary according to the prevalence of the disorder in the population.

- **Positive predictive value (PPV)** is the probability that someone with a positive test actually has the illness. It is calculated by dividing the number of TP by the sum of the number of TP and FP.
- **Negative predictive value (NPV)** is the probability that a person with a negative test is actually well. It is calculated by dividing the number of TN by the sum of the number of TN and FN.
- The higher the **prevalence** of a disorder in a population, the higher the PPV and the lower the NPV of a test used to detect it (e.g., in Example A-1, if the prevalence of prostate cancer increased by a factor of 10, there would be 1600 TP and 400 FN; however, the number of TN and FP would remain at 720 and 80, respectively).
- When the prevalence of a disorder is low in a population, even tests with very high specificity may have low PPV because there are likely to be a high number of false-positives relative to true positives (e.g., in Example A-1, if the prevalence of prostate cancer decreased by a factor of 10, there would only be 16 TP, but the number of FP would remain at 80).

■ CLINICAL PROBABILITY AND ATTACK RATE

Clinical probability is the number of times an event actually occurs divided by the number of times the event can occur (Example A-2).

   Attack rate is a type of incidence rate used to describe disease outbreaks. It is calculated by dividing the number of people who become ill during a study period by the number of people at risk during the study period. For example, if 20 of 40 people who drank apple juice and 10 of 50 people who drank orange juice become ill after a picnic, the attack rate is 50% for apple juice and 20% for orange juice.

■ RESEARCH METHODS

The purpose of research is to identify relationships between factors. These factors, which include events, characteristics, and outcomes, are called variables. Types of research studies include cohort, case control, and cross sectional (Table A-3).

Variables

A variable is a quantity that can change under different experimental situations; variables can be independent or dependent. An **independent variable** is a predictive factor that affects an outcome (e.g., the amount of fat in the diet). A **dependent variable** is the outcome that reflects the ef-

After 3 years of clinical trials of a new medication to treat erectile dysfunction, it is determined that 20% of patients taking the new medication develop hypertension. If two patients (patients A and B) take the drug, calculate the following probabilities.

1. The probability that both patient A and patient B will develop hypertension:
This is calculated by multiplying the probability of A developing hypertension by the probability of B developing hypertension (the multiplication rule for independent events)
The probability of A developing hypertension = 0.20.
The probability of B developing hypertension = 0.20.
The probability of both A and B developing hypertension = 0.20 × 0.20 = 0.04.

2. The probability that at least one of the two patients (either A or B or both A and B) will develop hypertension:
This is calculated by adding the probability of A developing hypertension to the probability of B developing hypertension and then subtracting the probability of both A and B developing hypertension (see 1. above) (the addition rule).
= 0.20 + 0.20 − 0.04 = 0.36.

3. The probability that neither patient A nor patient B will develop hypertension:
This is calculated by multiplying the probability of patient A being normotensive by the probability of patient B being normotensive: probability of both being normotensive = 1 − probability of A being hypertensive × 1 − probability of B being hypertensive = 0.80 × 0.80 = 0.64.

fects of changing the independent variable (e.g., body weight under different dietary fat regimens).

Cohort studies

Cohort studies begin with the identification of specific populations (cohorts) who are free of the illness under investigation at the beginning of the study. After assessment of exposure to a risk factor (a variable linked to the cause of an illness [e.g., smoking]), incidence rates of illness between exposed and nonexposed members (controls) of a cohort are compared. For example, healthy adults are followed from early adulthood through middle age to compare the health of those who smoke versus those who do not smoke. Cohort studies can be **prospective** (taking place in the present time) or **historical** (some activities have taken place in the past) (Table A-3).

A **clinical treatment trial** is a special type of cohort study in which some members of a cohort with a specific illness are given one treatment and other members of the cohort are given another treatment or a placebo. The results of the two treatments are then compared. For example, the difference in survival rates between men with lung cancer who receive a new drug and men with lung cancer who receive a standard drug are compared.

TABLE A-3	Research Study Design	
TYPE OF STUDY	**POPULATION AT THE INITIATION OF THE STUDY**	**EXAMPLE**
Prospective (concurrent) cohort study	Subjects who are free of illness	A study is designed to determine whether students who start to smoke at age 16 years will have more respiratory complaints by their twenty-first birthdays than students who do not start to smoke.
Historical (nonconcurrent) cohort study	Subjects who are free of illness	A study is designed to determine whether chemical exposure 30 years ago is associated with an increased incidence of lung cancer in 2000 men who worked in a paint manufacturing plant.
Case-control study	Subjects who have an illness (i.e., cases) and subjects who do not have the illness (i.e., controls)	A study is designed to determine whether more women with lung cancer (cases) report a history of smoking during teenage years than women without lung cancer (controls).
Cross-sectional study	Subjects studied at a specific point in time (may or may not have the illness)	A study is designed to determine whether smokers have more colds than nonsmokers according to a random telephone sample

Case-control studies

Case-control studies begin with the identification of subjects who have a specific disorder (cases) and subjects who do not have that disorder (controls). Information on the prior exposure of cases and controls to risk factors is then obtained. For example, the smoking histories of people with and without lung cancer are compared (see Table A-3).

Cross-sectional studies

Cross-sectional studies begin when information is collected from a group of individuals who provide a "snapshot" in time of disease activity. Such studies can provide information on the relationship between risk factors and health status of a group of individuals at one specific point in time (Table A-3). They can also be used to calculate the prevalence of a disease in a population.

▪ ELEMENTS OF STATISTICAL ANALYSES

Descriptive statistics summarize the data obtained from research studies. **Inferential statistics** provide a way to generalize results to an entire population by observing a sample of that population.

Measures of central tendency: mean, median, and mode

The **mean** is the average and is obtained by adding a group of numbers and then dividing by the quantity of numbers in the group. The **median,** or the 50th percentile value, is the middle value in a sequentially ordered group of numbers (i.e., the value that divides the data set into two equal groups). The **mode** is the value that appears most often in a group of numbers.

Measures of dispersion

Standard deviation (s) is the average distance of observations from their mean. Standard deviation is calculated by squaring each variation (or deviation from the mean in a group of scores), then adding the squared deviations. This sum is then divided by the number of scores in the group minus one, and the square root of the result is determined. A **standard normal value, or z score,** is the difference between an individual score and the population mean in units of standard deviation. **Standard error** is the standard deviation divided by the square root of the number of scores in a sample. A **confidence interval** specifies the limits between which a given percentage of the population would be expected to fall (Table A-4).

Normal distribution

A normal distribution, also referred to as a **Gaussian** or **bell-shaped** distribution, is a theoretic distribution of scores in which the mean, median, and mode are equal. In a normal distribution, approximately 68% of the population scores fall within one standard deviation of the mean; approximately 95% of scores fall within two standard deviations of the mean; and 99.7% of scores fall within three standard deviations of the mean (Fig. A-2). The highest point in the distribution of scores is the modal peak.

Estimating the mean: confidence intervals or limits

The mean of a sample is only an estimate. Therefore, the confidence interval specifies the limits between which a given percentage (e.g., 95% is conventionally used in medical research) of the population would be expected to fall. Confidence limits generally are equal to the mean of the

TABLE A-4	Formulas for Standard Deviation, Standard Error, z Score, and Confidence Interval	
MEASURE	**COMMENT**	**FORMULA**
Standard deviation (S)	Average distance of observations from their mean	$S = \sqrt{\dfrac{\Sigma\,(X-\bar{X})^2}{n-1}}$
Standard error (SE)	Estimate of the quality of the sample	$SE = \dfrac{S}{\sqrt{n}}$
z score (z)	Difference between one score in the distribution and the population mean in units of standard deviation	$z = \dfrac{(X-\bar{X})}{S}$
Confidence interval (CI)	Specifies the high and low limits of the interval in which the true mean lies	$CI = \bar{X} \pm z\,(SE)$
$\bar{X}$ = mean	n = number of samples	

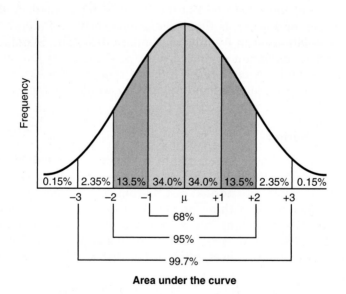

Area under the curve

FIGURE A-2. The normal (Gaussian distribution. The number of standard deviations (S) (−3 to +3) from the mean is shown on the x axis. The percentage of the population that falls under the curve within each S is shown.

(From Fadem, B. (2003). High-yield behavioral science. 2nd ed. Baltimore: Lippincott Williams & Wilkins, p. 114.)

sample ($\bar{X}$) plus or minus the z score multiplied by the standard error. For the 95% confidence interval, a z score of 2 is used; the 99% confidence interval uses a z score of 2.5; and the 99.7% confidence interval uses a z score of 3.

For example, if 25 men selected at random had a mean body weight of 180 pounds with a standard deviation of 10, the 95% confidence interval for this sample would be:

$$180 \pm 2 \left(\frac{10}{\sqrt{25}} \right) = 180 \pm 4, \text{ or } 176 \text{ to } 180 \text{ pounds.}$$

The 99.7% confidence interval for this sample would be:

$$180 \pm 3 \left(\frac{10}{\sqrt{25}} \right) = 180 \pm 6, \text{ or } 174 \text{ to } 186 \text{ pounds.}$$

Precision and accuracy

Precision is the degree to which the mean is resistant to random variation. The higher the confidence desired (99.7% versus 95%), the wider the limits of the interval and the less precise the estimate of the mean. **Accuracy** refers to the likelihood of bias. An inaccurate result means that the estimate of the mean is biased. For example, a patient takes his blood pressure at home and obtains readings of 130/80, 140/90, 136/88, 142/90, and 134/86. However, his doctor consistently obtains readings of 120/80. Therefore, the patient's estimate of his mean blood pressure is neither precise (readings vary greatly from each other) nor accurate (the mean the patient obtained is different from his true blood pressure obtained by the doctor).

Skewed distributions

In a skewed distribution, the modal peak shifts to one side (Fig. A-3). If the distribution is positively skewed (skewed to the right), the tail is toward the right and the modal peak is toward the left (i.e., scores cluster toward the low end). If the distribution is negatively skewed (skewed to the left), the tail is toward the left and the modal peak is toward the right (i.e., scores cluster toward the high end). A bimodal distribution has two modal peaks (e.g., two distinct populations).

■ HYPOTHESIS TESTING

A **hypothesis** is a statement based on inference, existing literature, or preliminary studies that suggests a difference between two groups. The possibility that this difference occurred by chance is tested using statistical procedures.

The null hypothesis

The **null hypothesis,** which postulates that no difference exists between two or more groups, can be either **rejected** or **not rejected** after statistical

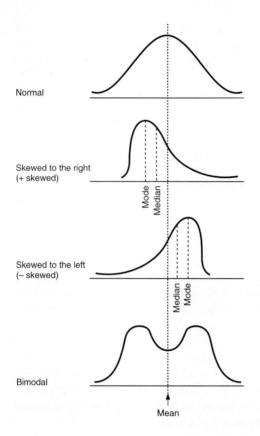

FIGURE A-3. Frequency distributions.

(From Fadem, B. (2003). High-yield behavioral science. 2nd ed. Baltimore: Lippincott Williams & Wilkins, p. 115.)

analysis. For example, in a study of a new antihypertensive, the null hypothesis assumes that the mean blood pressure in the group that receives the new drug is not significantly different from the mean blood pressure of the group that gets the placebo. A **type I (a) error** occurs when the null hypothesis is rejected even though it is true (e.g., the new drug really does not lower blood pressure). A **type II (b) error** occurs when the null hypothesis is not rejected although it is false (e.g., the new drug really does lower blood pressure) but there may not have been enough power to detect this difference (Example A-3).

Statistical probability

The **P (probability) value** is the chance of a type I error occurring. α is a preset level of significance usually set at 0.05 **($P < 0.05$)** by convention. **Power** (1 minus β) is the ability to detect a difference between groups if it is truly there. The larger the sample size, the more power a researcher has to detect this difference. If a P value is equal to or less than 0.05, it is unlikely that a type I error has been made (i.e., a type I error is made 5 or fewer times out of 100). A P value equal to or less than 0.05 (e.g., $P \leq 0.01$) is generally considered to be statistically significant.

A group of 20 patients who have similar systolic blood pressures at the beginning of a study (Time 1) is divided into two groups of 10 patients each. One group is given daily doses of an experimental drug meant to lower blood pressure (experimental group); the other group is given daily doses of a placebo (control group). Blood pressure is measured 2 weeks later (Time 2).

The **null hypothesis** assumes that there are no significant differences in blood pressure between the two groups at Time 2.

Do not reject the null hypothesis:	if, at Time 2, patients in the experimental group show systolic blood pressures similar to those in the placebo group
Reject the null hypothesis:	if, at Time 2, patients in the experimental group have significantly lower blood pressures ($P < 0.05$) than those in the placebo group

■ STATISTICAL TESTS

Statistical tests are used to analyze data from medical studies. The results of statistical tests indicate whether to reject or not reject the null hypothesis. Statistical tests can be parametric or nonparametric.

Parametric tests use population parameters (e.g., mean scores) and are usually used to identify the presence of statistically significant differences between groups when the distribution of scores in a population is normal and when the sample size is large. Commonly used parametric statistical tests include **t-tests, analysis of variance (ANOVA),** and **linear correlation** (Example A-4).

Linear correlation refers to the degree of relationship between two continuous variables and can be assessed using linear correlation coefficients (*r*) that range between plus 1 and minus 1. If the two variables move in the same direction, *r* is positive (e.g., as height increases, body weight increases, or as calorie intake decreases, body weight decreases). If the two variables move in opposite directions, *r* is negative (e.g., as time spent exercising increases, body weight decreases) (Fig. A-4).

If the distribution of scores in a population is not normal or if the sample size is small, nonparametric statistical tests are used to evaluate the presence of statistically significant differences between groups. Commonly used nonparametric statistical tests include **Wilcoxon's** (rank sum and signed-rank), **Mann-Whitney,** or **Kruschal-Wallis** tests. To analyze categorical data or compare proportions, the **chi-square** (Example A-3) or **Fisher's Exact** tests (used when sample size is small) are used.

A consumer group would like to evaluate the success of three different commercial weight loss programs. To do this, male and female subjects are assigned to one of three programs (group A, group B, and group C). The mean weight of the subjects is not significantly different among the three groups at the start of the study (Time 1). Each group follows a different diet regimen. At Time 1 and at the end of the 6-week study (Time 2), the subjects are weighed and their blood pressure measurements are obtained. Examples of how statistical tests can be used to analyze the results of this study are given below.

t-test: Difference between the means of two samples
Independent (nonpaired) test: Tests the mean difference in body weights of subjects in group A and subjects in group B at Time 1 (i.e., two groups of subjects are sampled on one occasion).
Dependent (paired) test: Tests the mean difference in body weights of people in group A at Time 1 and Time 2 (i.e., the same people are sampled on two occasions).

Analysis of variance: Differences between the means of more than two samples.
One-way analysis: Tests the mean differences in body weights in subjects in group A, group B, and group C at Time 2 (i.e., one variable: group).
Two-way analysis: Tests the mean differences in body weights of men and women and in body weights of group A, group B, and group C at Time 2 (i.e., two variables: sex and group).

Correlation: The mutual relation between two continuous variables
Tests the relation between blood pressure and body weight in all subjects at Time 2. Correlation coefficients (r) are negative (0 to -1) if the variables move in opposite directions and positive (0 to $+1$) if the variables move in the same direction (see Fig. A-4).

Chi-square test: Differences between frequencies in a sample and
Fisher's exact probability: Differences between frequencies in a small sample.
Test the difference among the percentage of subjects with body weight of 140 lbs or less in groups A, B, and C at Time 2.

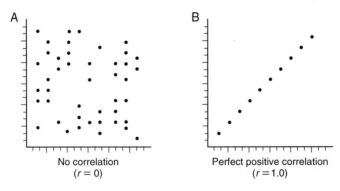

A — No correlation ($r = 0$)

B — Perfect positive correlation ($r = 1.0$)

FIGURE A-4.   Scatter plots demonstrating linear correlations.

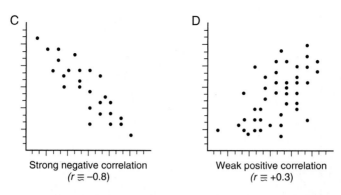

C

Strong negative correlation
(r ≅ −0.8)

D

Weak positive correlation
(r ≅ +0.3)

FIGURE A-4 *Continued.* Scatter plots demonstrating linear correlations.

REVIEW QUESTIONS

1. In the United States, disease X has the same incidence rate in white and African-American people but the prevalence rate of disease X is lower in African-American than in white individuals. The most likely explanation for this difference in prevalence rate is that when compared to white people, African-American people have

   (A) more resistance to disease X

   (B) past immunity to disease X

   (C) increased access to health care

   (D) increased likelihood of recovering from disease X

   (E) increased likelihood of dying from disease X

2. A highly contagious, life-threatening disease has just been identified in the population, and a screening test is being developed to identify it early in its course. To decrease the number of deaths from the disease, the cutoff point for the test should be set at the point of highest

   (A) sensitivity

   (B) specificity

   (C) positive predictive value

   (D) negative predictive value

   (E) accuracy

Questions 3 and 4

Research by Schroeder and Kranse (*N Engl J Med* [2003], 349, 393–395) suggests that the cutoff value for prostate-specific antigen (PSA) used to identify patients likely to have prostate cancer should be lowered from 4 ng/mL to 3 ng/mL (Fig. A-5).

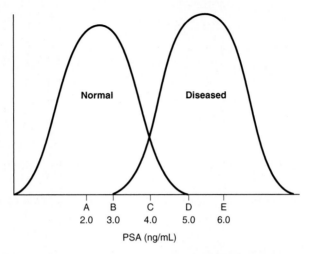

FIGURE A-5. Prostate-specific antigen (PSA) scores in a population of men.

3. With respect to the test, this change would
   (A) increase negative predictive value
   (B) decrease sensitivity
   (C) increase false negative rate
   (D) increase positive predictive value
   (E) increase specificity

4. With this change in the cutoff point, the incidence and prevalence of prostate cancer would

	Incidence	Prevalence
(A)	Increase	Increase
(B)	Decrease	Decrease
(C)	Increase	Not change
(D)	Not change	Not change
(E)	Increase	Decrease

Questions 5 and 6

A new test to detect prostate cancer in men aged >50 years has a sensitivity of 90% and a specificity of 75%. Autopsy studies suggest that the disease has a prevalence of 30% and a lifetime incidence of 10% for men in this age group.

5. The positive predictive value of this screening test is best estimated as
   (A) 12.5%
   (B) 30%
   (C) 60%

(D) 70%

(E) 85%

6. If this test is given only to men aged over 80 years in which the prevalence of prostate cancer is 70% and the incidence is 55%, the positive predictive value and sensitivity of this screening test will

Positive predictive value	Sensitivity
(A) Increase	Increase
(B) Decrease	Decrease
(C) Increase	Not change
(D) Not change	Not change
(E) Increase	Decrease

7. Two separate, randomized, double-blind trials were done to see whether administration of aspirin after a cerebrovascular accident (CVA) decreases risk for another CVA. Both trials showed that aspirin reduced the risk by 10%. This reduction was significant in one trial ($P < 0.05$); in the other, it was not significant. The best explanation for this difference between the results of the two trials is that

(A) the efficacy of aspirin was different between the two trials

(B) randomization did not evenly distribute the risk factors in the two trials

(C) the sample sizes in the two trials were different

(D) there was a placebo effect in one trial but not in the other

(E) the researchers were "blind" in one trial but not in the other

8. A case-control study is done to determine if elderly demented patients are more likely to be injured at home than elderly patients who are not demented. An odds ratio of 3 is obtained from the data. This figure means that, when compared with nondemented elderly patients, demented elderly patients

(A) should be institutionalized

(B) have one-third the risk of injury

(C) have the same risk of injury

(D) should be kept at home

(E) have three times the risk of injury

ANSWERS AND EXPLANATIONS

1-E. The prevalence rate of a disorder decreases either when patients recover or when they die. Compared with white patients, African-American patients tend to have decreased access to health care (see Chapters 20 and 27). They are therefore less likely to receive early treatment for disease X and thus more likely to die. Decreased prevalence in black patients is thus more likely to be caused by early death than by recovery from disease X. Resistance to an illness or past immunity to an illness affects the incidence rate, which is equal in both groups in this example.

2-A. Because the disease is life threatening and contagious, all diseased people must be identified quickly. To do this, the cutoff point for the screening test should be set at the point of highest sensitivity (i.e., the point at which there are the fewest number of false negatives). At this point, most of the diseased people will be identified, even though some truly well people are likely to mistakenly be identified as diseased (false positives).

3-A, 4-D. This reference interval change can be expected to both decrease the number of false negatives (truly ill people who test negative) and increase the number of false positives (truly well people who test positive). Such alterations will increase sensitivity (TP/TP + FN) and negative predictive value (TN/TN + FN) and will decrease specificity (TN/TN + FP) and positive predictive value (TP/TP + FP) of the test. A change in the cutoff value of the test would not affect the incidence or prevalence of prostate cancer in the population.

5-C. Using the following calculations, the positive predictive value (TP/TP + FP) of this test is 270/270 + 175 = 60%.

	DISEASE PRESENT	DISEASE ABSENT	TOTAL
Positive test	270 (TP)	175 (FP)	445
Negative test	30 (FN)	525 (TN)	555
Total	300	700	1000

6-C. Using the following calculations, if the prevalence of prostate cancer increases, positive predictive value increases. Sensitivity does not change because it is a characteristic of the test, not the population.

	DISEASE PRESENT	DISEASE ABSENT	TOTAL
Positive test	630 (TP)	75 (FP)	705
Negative test	70 (FN)	225 (TN)	295
Total	700	300	1000

If the prevalence of the disease increases, both TP and FN will increase to the same extent and sensitivity will not change. However, with increased prevalence the ratio of sick to healthy patients will increase; therefore, PPV will increase. Also, because with increased prevalence, the ratio of sick (FN) to healthy patients (TN) the negative test result group increases, NPV decreases.

7-C. The best explanation for this difference between the trials is that the sample sizes in the two trials were different. The larger the sample size, the higher the power, and the less likely a type I error will be made. This decreased likelihood is reflected in a lower p value and thus a higher likelihood of significance for studies with a large sample size. Problems with randomization, efficacy, blinding, or placebo effects would have differentially affected the risk observed in the two trials.

8-E. An odds ratio of 3 means that when compared to nondemented elderly persons, demented elderly persons have three times the risk of injury. This number does not indicate whether certain people should be institutionalized or remain at home.

INDEX

Page numbers in *italics* denote figures; those followed by "t" denote tables; and those followed by "q" or "a" denote questions or answers.

Fighting, definition, 351
Filipino Americans, 321
Fixed interval reinforcement, 139, 141t
Fixed ratio reinforcement, 139, 141t
Flooding, 170
Flumazenil (Mazicon, Romazicon), 302
Fluorouracil, 424t
Fluoxetine (Prozac, Sarafem), 292t
  manic episode precipitated by, 209q,
    210a
Fluphenazine (Prolixin), 285t, 287
Flurazepam (Dalmane), 301t
Fluvoxamine (Luvox), 293t
Folie à deux, 193
Folk medicine, beliefs and practices, 319t,
    320, 325q, 326a
Folstein Mini-Mental State Examination,
    98, 99t, 101q, 102a
Formal operations, 28
Fosamax (alendronate sodium), 47
Foster families/homes, 10
Fracture, in child and elder abuse, 358t
Fragile X syndrome, 31–32
Free association, 167t
Free-floating anxiety, 153t, 224
Freud, Sigmund
  theories of the mind, 121–123, 122t,
    130q–131q, 132a
  theory of development, 7
Frontal lobe, neuropsychiatric anatomy,
    68t, 69–70
Frontal release signs, 70
Frotteurism, 345t
Fugue, dissociative, 276, 277t
Functional magnetic resonance imaging, in
    psychiatric diagnosis, 95, 97t

Gabapentin (Neurontin), 421
"Gag clause," 463
Galantamine (Reminyl), 304, 304t
Galvanic skin response, in psychiatric diag-
    nosis, 94
Gambling, pathological, 355
Gamma aminobutyric acid (GABA), 80
  and aging, 54t
  and sedative abuse, 376
  and violence, 353
Gamma-glutamyltransferase, 388a
Gastric bypass, 257
Gastrointestinal cancer
  depression and, 423t, 426q, 427a
  gender and, 455t
Gaussian distribution, 479, 480
Gender
  and Alzheimer's disease, 271t
  and depression, 208q–209q, 210a

and health, 452t–455t, 453–454
and hemispheric specialization, 72–73,
    73
and homicide rate, 352, 353t
and life expectancy, 53
and obesity, 254, 255t–256t
and suicide risk, 215, 216
Gender identity, 331t
  development, 13
Gender identity disorder (GID), 180t, 332,
    346q, 347a
Gender role, 331t
General adaptation syndrome, 417
Generalization, stimulus, 137
Generalized anxiety disorder (GAD), 225t,
    227, 233t
Generativity, in middle adulthood, 46
Genetic factors
  in Alzheimer's disease, 271t
  and suicide risk, 217
Genetic influences, 63–67
  neuropsychiatric disorders, 66–67
  psychiatric disorders, 64–66, 65t
  research studies, 64
  substance abuse disorders, 67
Genetic testing, of children, 440, 442t
Genital differentiation, 329–330
Genitalia, ambiguous, 330–331
Geodon (ziprasidone), 289t
Geriatrics, 51
Gerontology, 51
Giftedness, 157
Glasgow Coma Scale, 73, 98, 100, 100t
Global assessment of functioning (GAF)
    scale, 181
Globus hystericus, in conversion disorder,
    244
Globus pallidus, neuropsychiatric anatomy,
    72
Glutamate, 80
  in Alzheimer's disease, 271t
  in chronic pain, 421
  in schizophrenia, 186–187
  and substance abuse, 373
Glutamic-oxaloacetic transaminase, 388a
Glycine, 80
Gonadal hormones
  and emotion, 336
  psychoactive effects, 303
  and sexual development, 330–332
  and sexuality, 334, 336
Good Samaritan laws, 434–435
Graves' hyperthyroidism, 454t
"Grid abdomen," in factitious disorder, 246
Grief reactions, in dying and death, 56–58,
    58t, 59q, 60a

Legal insanity, 436, 437t
Legal issues. *See* Ethical and legal issues
Leukemia, 455t
Levitra (vardenafil), for sexual dysfunction, 341
Levothyroxine (Levothroid, Synthroid), psychoactive effects, 303
Lewy body dementia, 273
Lexapro (escitalopram), 292t
Librium (chlordiazepoxide), 301t
Life events, stressful, and medical illness, 414, 416t, 417–418
Life expectancy, *53,* 53–54, 452t
Life support, withdrawal, 447q, 449a
Limbic lobe/system, neuropsychiatric anatomy, 68t, 70, *71*
Linear correlation, 485
Liothyronine (Cytomel), psychoactive effects, 303
Lithium, 296–297, 298t
    adverse effects, 297
    for bipolar disorder, 205
    laboratory tests, 92, 297, 300t
    mode of action, 284t
Living will, 445
Lobotomy, prefrontal, 69
Locus ceruleus, 77, *78,* 82q, 83a, 271t
Logical thought, acquisition, 24
Long-term care hospital, 457t
Longevity, *53,* 53–54
Loose associations, in psychosis, 185t
Lorazepam (Ativan), 301t
    for anxiety disorders, 232
Loss
    aging and, 52
    stages, 56
Love, in early adulthood, 45
Ludiomil (maprotiline), 291t
Lung cancer, gender and, 454, 455t
Luria-Nebraska Neuropsychological Battery, 98
Luvox (fluvoxamine), 293t
Lymphoma, non-Hodgkin's, 455t
Lysergic acid diethylamide (LSD), abuse, 374t, 376t, 385

Magical thinking, in psychosis, 184t
Magnetic resonance imaging, in psychiatric diagnosis, 95, *95,* 97t
Mahler, Margaret, theory of development, 7
Mal de pelea, 355
Malingering, 247, 248q, 250a
Malpractice, 432–434, 447q, 448a
Managed care plans, 462–463, 464t–465t
Mania
    differential diagnosis, 206

medical conditions associated with, 423t
neurotransmitter activity associated with, 76t
Manic episode, in bipolar disorder, 189t, 202, 203t, 209q, 210a
Maprotiline (Ludiomil), 291t
Marijuana
    abuse, 92t, 374t, 376t, 384–385
    and sexuality, 338, 340
Marital/couples therapy, 173
Marital status, and suicide risk, 215–216
Marriage, demographics and current trends, 42
Masked depression, 198, 201, 209q, 210a
Masochism, sexual, 345t
Masturbation, 28
Maternal-infant separation, 9–10
Mazicon (flumazenil), 302
Mean
    calculation, 479
    estimation, 479–481
Measures
    of central tendency, 479
    of dispersion, 479, 480t
Medial cortex, neuropsychiatric anatomy, 68t, 70
Median, 479
Medical College Admission Test (MCAT), 158
Medical doctor (MD), 458. *See also* Physician(s)
Medical illness. *See* Illness
Medicare/Medicaid, 460, 461t, 466q, 467a
Mediterranean origin, 323
Melanoma, 455t
Melanosis coli, laxative-induced, 258
Melatonin, and sleep, 110
Mellaril (thioridazine), 285t, 286
Memory
    false recovered, 277
    loss. *See* Amnesia
    in mental status examination, 150t
Menarche, 26
Menopause, 46–47, 47q, 48a
Menstruation, first, 26
Mental age (MA), 155, 162q, 163a
Mental disorders, caused by general medical condition not otherwise classified, 180t
Mental health, and suicide risk, 217
Mental Health Bill of Rights, 436t
Mental health facility, involuntary confinement, 435–436, 436t
Mental illness
    criminal law related to, 436, 437t
    substance abuse and, 373

Narcolepsy, 112t, 116–117
Narcotics. *See* Opioid(s)
Nardil (phenelzine), 293t
Native Americans
    ethnocultural issues, 322–323
    infant mortality, 4t
Natural environment phobia, 229t
Nefazodone (Serzone), 294t
Negative
    false, 474
    true, 475
Negative predictive value (NPV), 476,
        485q–486q, 488a
Negative reinforcement, 138, 143q, 144a
Negative symptoms, in schizophrenia, 182
Negative transference, 130
Neglect, signs, 358t
Negligence, in medical malpractice, 433
Neologisms, in psychosis, 185t
Neoplasms, psychological symptoms asso-
        ciated with, 423t
Neuroanatomy
    in Alzheimer's disease, 82q, 83a, 270,
        271t, *272*
    behavioral. *See* Behavioral neuroanatomy
Neurobiological associations, in anxiety
        disorders, 226
Neurofibrillary tangles, 271t
Neuroimaging studies, *95–96,* 95–97, 97t
Neuroleptic malignant syndrome, from an-
        tipsychotic agents, 288t
Neurologic changes
    in aging, 54–55, 54t
    in depression, 81q, 83a
    in schizophrenia, 81q, 82a–83a
Neurological evaluation
    electroencephalography, 97–98
    imaging studies, *95–96,* 95–97, 97t
    neuropsychological tests, *98–99,* 98–100,
        99t–100t
Neurological signs, soft, in intermittent ex-
        plosive disorder, 354
Neuronal loss, in Alzheimer's disease, 271t
Neuronal plasticity, 75
Neurontin (gabapentin), 421
Neuropeptides, 80
Neurophysiology, in Alzheimer's disease,
        271t
Neuropsychiatric anatomy, 67–74, 68t–69t,
        71, 73. See also Behavioral
        neuroanatomy
Neuropsychiatric disorders
    genetic influences, 66–67
    neurotransmitter activity associated with,
        76t

Neuropsychological tests, in psychiatric
        diagnosis, *98–99,* 98–100,
        99t–100t
Neurotransmitter(s), 74–80
    abnormalities
        in aging brain, 54–55, 54t
        in Alzheimer's disease, 271t
        in anxiety disorders, 226
        in depression, 209q, 210a
        in depression, 81q–82q, 83a
        neuropsychiatric conditions and, 76t
        in schizophrenia, 186–187
    amino acid, 80
    biogenic amine, 75–80, *77–79*
    neuropeptide, 80
    regulation, 75
    and sexuality, 338, 340t
    and violence, 353
New York Hospital, Zion vs., 105
Newborns, disabled, health care decisions
        for, 442
Nicotine addiction, 92t, 374t, 376t, 382
Nifedipine, 425t
Nightmare disorder, 114t
Nighttime awakenings, in elderly persons,
        118q, 119a
Nigrostriatal tract, 76, *77*
Nitrofurantoin, 424t
NMDA (*N*-methyl-D-aspartate), 80, 271t
NMDA receptor modulators, 421
Nocturnal myoclonus, 113t
Non-Hodgkin's lymphoma, 455t
Nondominant hemisphere, 72
Nonsteroidal antiinflammatory drugs
        (NSAIDs), psychological symp-
        toms induced by, 425t
Norepinephrine, 77, *78*
    and aging, 54t
    in Alzheimer's disease, 271t
    hyperactivity, in schizophrenia, 186
    psychopathology associated with, 93t
    and sexuality, 338, 340t
    and sleep, 111
Norepinephrine reuptake inhibitors, sero-
        tonin and, selective, 293t, 296
"Normal" behavior, concept of, 1–2
Normal distribution, 479, *480*
Norpramin (desipramine), 291t, 295
Nortriptyline (Aventyl, Pamelor), 291t
Nuclear family, 42
Nucleus basalis of Meynert, 82q, 83a
Null hypothesis, 481–482, Example A4
Nursing home, 52, 455–457
Nuviva (vardenafil), for sexual dysfunction,
        341

Obesity
  characteristics, 253–256, *254*
  in children, 263q–264q, 265a
  etiology, 256–257
  gender and, 254, 255t–256t
  health problems associated with, 256
  treatment, 257–258, 264q, 265a
Object permanence, 8, *9*
Obsessive-compulsive personality disorder,
    225t, 235q, 236a, 403t
Obstructive sleep apnea, 115
Occipital lobe, neuropsychiatric anatomy,
    69t
Occupation, and suicide risk, 216
Odds ratio, 471t, 472, 487q, 488a
Olanzapine (Zyprexa), 289t, 299t
"Old-old," 51
Older adults. *See* Elderly persons
Open-ended questions, 408q, 410a
  in clinical interview, 393
Operant conditioning, 137–140, 141t
  extinction in, 138
    resistance to, 140
  punishment in, 138
  reinforcement in
    negative, 138
    positive, 137–138
    schedules, 138–140, 141t, 142q, 144a
  shaping in, 140
Opioid(s)
  abuse, 380–382
    effects of use, 374t
    laboratory findings, 92t, 386t
    treatment, 375t, 381–382
    and violence, 354
    withdrawal reactions, 374t, 387q, 388a
  endogenous, 80
Oppositional defiant disorder, 32–33
Orap (pimozide), 285t
Orbitofrontal cortex, neuropsychiatric
    anatomy, 68t, 70
Organ donation and transplant, ethical and
    legal issues, 439–440, 441t–442t
Orgasm phase, of sexual response cycle,
    335t, 346q–347q, 348a
Orgasmic disorder, 339t, 346q, 347a
Orientation, in mental status examination,
    150t
Orientation times three, in cognitive disor-
    ders, 267
Orlistat (Xenical), for obesity, 257
Osteopathic physician, 458. *See also*
    Physician(s)
Osteoporosis, estrogen-replacement therapy
    and, 47q, 48a–49a

Ovarian cancer, 455t
Overgeneralization, 170
Overweight children, 254, 263q–264q, 265a
Oxazepam (Serax), 301t
Oxycarbamazepine (Trileptal), 298t,
    299–300

P (probability) value, 482
Pain, chronic
  depression and, 426q, 427a
  placebo effects, 421
  psychological symptoms associated with,
    423t
  treatment, 420–421
Pain disorder, 242t, 244
Pain medications, administration, 420–421
Pallidum, neuropsychiatric anatomy, 72
Palmar grasp reflex, 11
Pamelor (nortriptyline), 291t
Pancreatic cancer, 90t, 423t, 455t
Panic attack, 228, 235q, 236a
Panic disorder, 225t, 228, 233t
  with agoraphobia, 228, 233t
  sodium lactate test, 101q, 102a
  treatment, 235q, 236a
Papez circuit, neuropsychiatric anatomy,
    68t, 70, *71*
Parallel play, 11–12
Paralysis, sleep, in narcolepsy, 116
Paranoid personality disorder, 400t
Paranoid schizophrenia, 188t
Paraphilias, 344–345, 345t
Parapraxes, as proof of unconscious mind,
    122, 122t
Parasomnias, 111, 114t
Parasympathetic nervous system, 74
Parental consent, exceptions, 440, 443,
    443t, 447q, 449a
Parietal lobe, neuropsychiatric anatomy,
    69t
Parkinson's disease, psychological symp-
    toms associated with, 423t
Parnate (tranylcypromine), 293t
Paroxetine (Paxil), 292t
Partner abuse, 362–363, 363t, 364, 368q,
    369a
Passive-aggressive personality disorder,
    404t
Pathological gambling, 355
Patient(s)
  abandonment, 398
  compliance, 405–407, 405t
  desire for inappropriate treatment, 438
  giving information to, 395–398, 397t
  interviewing, *392,* 392–395

professional behavior, 432–435
role of
in child and elder abuse, 364,
367q–368q, 368a–369a
in death and dying, 59q–60q, 61a
in domestic abuse, 364, 368q, 369a
in dying and death, 58–59
in patient decision making, 398
in rape counseling, 365–366, 366t
sleep deprivation, 105–106
suicide risk, 220a, 220q
Piaget, Jean, theory of development, 7
Pickwickian syndrome, 115–116, 256
Pimozide (Orap), 285t
Placebo, in research studies, 473
Placebo effects, 80
in chronic pain treatment, 421
Plasticity, neuronal, 75
Plateau phase, of sexual response cycle,
335t
Play
cooperative, 12
parallel, 11–12
in school age child, 25
Playing doctor, 14
Point-of-Service (POS) plan, 465t
Population studies, risk quantification in,
470, 471t, 472
Porphyria, acute intermittent, 91t, 423t
Positive
false, 475
true, 474
Positive predictive value (PPV), 476,
485q–486q, 487q, 488a
Positive reinforcement, 137–138
Positive symptoms, in schizophrenia, 182
Positive transference, 130
Positron emission tomography (P, 102a
Positron emission tomography (PET)
for localization of brain activation, 101q,
102a
in psychiatric diagnosis, 95, 96
Post-traumatic stress disorder, 225t,
230–231, 234t, 235q–236q, 236a
versus dissociative disorders, 275
Postpartum blues, 4
Postpartum reactions, 4–5
Power, in statistics, 482
Power of attorney, durable, 445
Precision, in statistics, 481
Preconscious mind, in Freudian theory,
122
Predictive value, test, 475, 476, Example
A1
Preferred Provider Organization (PPO),
464t

Prefrontal cortex, 69
Prefrontal lobe syndrome, 70
Prefrontal lobotomy, 69
Pregnancy, during adolescence, 29, 29–30
Premature birth, 3–4
Premature ejaculation, 339t
Premenstrual dysphoric disorder (PMDD),
336
Premenstrual syndrome (PMS), 336
Prenatal life, 2, 3
Preschool child, 14–16
attachment in, 14
characteristics, 15t
separation in, 14
social interaction in, 14
Presentation, in mental status examination,
150t
Prevalence, 485q, 487a
of HIV infection, factors affecting, 470,
471t
and incidence, association between, 470
period, 470
point, 470
Prevalence rate, 470
Prevention of illness, 463, 465
Primary biliary cirrhosis, 454t
Primary care physician, 458. See also
Physician(s)
Primary gain, in somatoform disorders,
240, 242
Primary prevention, 465
Primary process thinking, in Freudian the-
ory, 122
"Privacy Rule," 459–460
Private health insurance, 460–462
Probability
clinical, 476, Example A2
statistical, 482
Proband, 64
Procainamide, 424t
Prodromal symptoms, in schizophrenia, 183
Professional behavior, 432–435
Professional boundaries, 434
Projection, as defense mechanism, 126,
128t
Propoxyphene, 424t
Propranolol (Inderal), 304
Prospective cohort studies, 477, 479t
Prostate cancer, 455t
Provigil (modanafil), 296
Prozac (fluoxetine), 292t
Pseudodementia
versus cognitive disorders, 268, 269t
in elderly person, 55, 278q, 279a
Pseudoparkinsonism, from antipsychotic
agents, 288t

Slow-wave sleep, *107,* 108
Smile, social, 8
Smoking, 36q, 37a–38a, 374t, 376t, 382
Social anxiety disorder, 228, 233t
Social challenges, in mental retarded children, 32
Social characteristics
  of infants, 12t
  of preschool children, 15t
  of toddlers, 13t
Social considerations, in homosexuality, 333–334
Social determinants, of violence, 352
Social development, 6
Social interaction
  in preschool children, 14
  in toddlers, 11–12
Social phobia, 225t, 228, 233t, 236q, 237a
Social Readjustment Rating Scale, 414, 416t, 417
Social smile, 8
Social status, and suicide risk, 215–216
Socioeconomic status, and health, 452–453, 466q, 467a
Sodium lactate, in diagnosis of panic disorder, 94, 101q, 102a
Sodomy, 364
Soft neurological signs, in intermittent explosive disorder, 354
Sole custody, 44
Somatization, as defense mechanism, 125–126, 129t
Somatization disorder, 241t, 242
Somatoform disorders, 180t, 240–245
  differential diagnosis, 244–245
  DSM-IV-TR classification, 240, 241t–242t
  etiology, 240, 242
  primary gain in, 240, 242
  secondary gain in, 242
  treatment, 245, 246t
  undifferentiated, 240
Somatostatin, 271t
Sonata (zaleplon), 302t, 303
Southeast Asian Americans, 319t
Specificity, test, 475, *475,* 485q–486q, 488a, Example A1
Speech, in mental status examination, 151t
Spinal cord injury, and sexuality, 343
Split custody, 44
Splitting, as defense mechanism, 126, 129t
Spontaneous recovery, in classical conditioning, 137
Squeeze technique, for sexual dysfunction, 341
Stagnation, in middle adulthood, 46
Standard deviation *(S),* 479, 480t

Standard error *(SE),* 479, 480t
Standard normal value (z score), 479, 480t
Standards for Privacy of Individually Identifiable Health Information, 459–460
Stanford Achievement Test, 158
Stanford-Binet Intelligence Scale, 148t
State-funded health insurance, 460, 461t
Statistical analyses, 479–481, *480,* 480t
Statistical probability, 482
Statistical tests, 483, 483t, 485
Statutory criteria, for legal insanity, 436, 437t
Statutory rape, 365
Stelazine (trifluoperazine), 285t
Steroid hormones, psychological symptoms induced by, 425t
Stimulant(s)
  abuse, 382–383
    effects of use, 374t
    laboratory findings, 92t, 386t
    treatment, 375t–376t, 383
    withdrawal reactions, 374t, 387q, 388a
  for attention-deficit/hyperactivity disorder, 34, 37q, 38a
  for depression, 296, 297t
Stimulus generalization, 137
Stranger anxiety, 8, 19q, 20a–21a
Strattera (atomoxetine), 296
Stress
  and immune system function, 417–418
  management, 174, 418
  and medical illness, 414, 416t, 417–418
  physiological effects, 417
  psychological, medical conditions associated with, 418–420
Stress disorders
  acute, 230–231
  characteristics, 230–231
  differential diagnosis, 231
  occurrence, 231
  post-traumatic, 225t, 230–231, 234t, 235q–236q, 236a
  prognosis, 231
Stress-related physiological response, 415t
Striatum, neuropsychiatric anatomy, 72
Structural theory, of mind, 122–123
Sublimation, as defense mechanism, 124, 127t, 131q, 132a
Substance abuse, 371–386, 386q–387q, 388a
  biology, 372–373
  classification, 373
  clinical features, 385, 385t
  DSM-IV definitions, 372t
  effects of use, 374t
  genetic influences, 67

Ventricles, enlarged, in Alzheimer's disease, 271t
Verbal ability
  development, 6, 158t
  of infants, 12t
  of preschool children, 15t
  of toddlers, 13t
Verbal response, in Glasgow Coma Scale, 100t
Viagra (sildenafil citrate), for sexual dysfunction, 341
Vietnamese Americans, 321
Vineland Social Maturity Scale, 157, 158t, 162q–163q, 163a
Violence
  in abused children, 362
  biological determinants, 352–354, 353t
  domestic, 362–363, 363t, 364
  social determinants, 352
Virilizing adrenal hyperplasia, congenital, 331
Visiting nurse association, 458
Vitamin deficiency, 423t
Voyeurism, 345t

Wechsler Adult Intelligence Scale-Revised (WAIS-R), 156–157, 156t
Wechsler Intelligence Scale for Children-Revised (WISC-R), 157
Wechsler Preschool and Primary Scale of Intelligence (WPPSI), 157

Weight loss, for obesity, 257–258, 264q, 265a
Wellbutrin (bupropion), 294t
White Americans
  family types, 43t
  infant mortality, 4t
  obesity data, 255t
White-coat hypertension, 143q, 144a
Wide-Range Achievement Test (WRAT), 158
Will, living, 445
Wilson's disease, 91t, 423t
Withdrawal reactions
  in alcohol abuse, 374t, 377–378
  clonidine for, 82q, 83a
  definition, 372t
  in substance abuse, 373, 374t, 387q, 388a
Wolffian duct system, 330
Word salad, in psychosis, 185t
Work, in early adulthood, 45

Xanax (alprazolam), 301t
  for anxiety disorders, 231–232
Xenical (orlistat), for obesity, 257

Z score, 479, 480t
Zaleplon (Sonata), 302t, 303
Zion vs. New York Hospital, 105
Ziprasidone (Geodon), 289t
Zoloft (sertraline), 293t
Zolpidem (Ambien), 302t, 303
Zung Self-Rating Depression Scale, 149, 152
Zyprexa (olanzapine), 289t, 299t